Manual of Bone Densitometry Measurements

Springer
London
Berlin
Heidelberg
New York
Barcelona
Hong Kong
Milan
Paris
Singapore
Tokyo

J.N. Fordham (Ed.)

Manual of Bone Densitometry Measurements

An Aid to the Interpretation of Bone Densitometry Measurements in a Clinical Setting

With 49 Figures

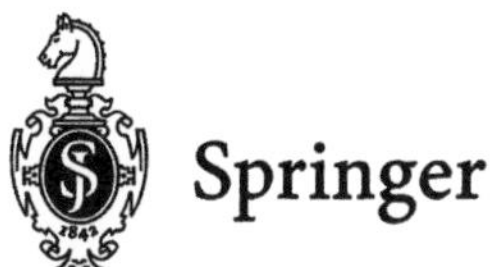

Springer

John N. Fordham, MD, FRCP, BSc
Consultant Rheumatologist, South Cleveland Hospital,
Marton Road, Middlesbrough, Cleveland TS4 3BW, UK

Cover illustrations: Front cover: Ch. 8, Figures 3 and 4 (fractures of the proximal femur and distal radius). Back cover inset: Tees Transporter Bridge in sunlight, epitomising its trabecular structure.

ISBN-13: 978-1-4471-1196-2   e-ISBN-13: 978-1-4471-0759-0
DOI: 10.1007/978-1-4471-0759-0

British Library Cataloguing in Publication Data
Manual of bone densitometry measurements: an aid to the
    interpretation of bone densitometry measurements in a
    clinical setting
    1. Bone densitometry – Measurement
    I. Fordham, John
    616.7′1′075
ISBN-13: 978-1-4471-1196-2

Library of Congress Cataloging-in-Publication Data
Manual of bone densitometry measurements: an aid to
the interpretation of bone densitometry measurements
in a clinical setting/John Fordham (ed.)
    p. cm.
    Includes bibliographical references and index.
    ISBN-13: 978-1-4471-1196-2 (acid-free paper)
    1. Bone densitometry – Handbooks, manuals, etc.
2. Osteoporosis – Diagnosis – Handbooks, manuals, etc.
3. Bones – Diseases – Diagnosis – Handbooks, manuals, etc.
I. Fordham, John, 1947–
RC931.O73 M355 2000
616.7′1075–dc21   00–026565

® Springer-Verlag London Limited 2000
Softcover reprint of the hardcover 1st edition 2000

Typeset by EXPO Holdings, Malaysia
Printed and bound at the Cromwell Press, Trowbridge, Wiltshire
28/3830-543210 Printed on acid-free paper SPIN 10682024

Preface

The importance of osteoporosis in the United Kingdom as a cause of death and disability is now well recognised. There are in excess of 200,000 osteoporotic-related fractures in the UK per annum associated with an estimated cost of £942,000,000. Following hip fracture it is known that about 50% of patients are unable to live independently and about 20% of such patients die within the first 6 months. These figures, compelling as they are, reflect poorly on current medical practices which manifestly have failed to identify patients with low bone density at risk of fracture. The hope is that the technical advances which have enabled bone mineral density, and other allied indices, to be measured with high precision and accuracy offers the chance of identifying patients at risk of fracture and guiding the clinician to make treatment decisions which may reduce the patients' risk of fracture.

In the UK, services for identifying patients at risk of fracture are still in their infancy and are not uniformly available throughout the country. This situation is, however, likely to improve particularly following the publication of the Royal College of Physicians report "Osteoporosis – clinical guidelines for prevention and treatment" and the recognition in "Our Healthier Nation" that osteoporosis prevention should be included as a target to achieve a reduction of 20% in accidents by 2010. It is also hoped that the National Osteoporosis Society's initiative of a Service Framework for Osteoporosis for implementation by primary care groups, local health groups and primary care trusts will provide the impetus for a more uniform and consistent use of bone densitometry to identify patients at risk and to guide appropriate interventions.

It is clear, however, that in secondary care there is a similar need for increased awareness of osteoporosis especially in those specialities directly involved in dealing with the consequences of fractures. The relevance of bone densitometry in different clinical settings will obviously vary. However, on a pragmatic level, the WHO definition of osteoporosis and osteopenia are based on DXA measurements and therefore the widespread application of these criteria does offer the prospect of some uniformity of approach to patient management.

At the patient-clinician level it is important not to over-interpret the measurements but rather to use these as a guide to management in the clinical context taking into account other concurrent risk factors. There are a large number of unanswered questions including the use of allied techniques, notably ultrasound, compilation of reference ranges, and use of axial or peripheral sites, all of which ensure a continuing and lively debate. In the meantime, services for patients will continue to develop. It is against this backcloth that this manual has been prepared. The contributors come from different backgrounds and present different perspectives on the use of bone densitometry. It is hoped that the manual will provide a useful, practical aid to those setting up and running osteoporosis services with an emphasis on a pragmatic approach.

Ultimately the clinical usefulness of bone densitometry measurements in osteoporosis services will only be reflected by a decline in the incidence of fractures with reduction in the associated suffering and costs.

Acknowledgements

I would like to acknowledge my debt to Mrs Penny Shields and Miss Angela Coverdale for secretarial support. Also the help and guidance from Nick Mowat and Nick Wilson. I would also like to record the help given by Dr Stuart Wood and Dr Mike Kirby in the early stages of this Manual. Lastly Melanie Fordham for her constant support and encouragement during all stages of production of this work.

Contents

List of Contributors   ix

1. **Bone Mineral Density Measurement in the Management
   of Osteoporosis: A Public Health Perspective**
   R. Madhok and T. Allison   1

2. **Measurement of Bone Density: Current Techniques**
   J.G. Truscott 17

3. **Methodological and Reporting Considerations**
   D.S. Simpson and J.G. Truscott 37

4. **Definitions and Interpretation of Bone Mineral Density
   in a Clinical Context**
   R. Eastell 55

5. **The Use of Bone Density Measurements in Male and
   Secondary Osteoporosis**
   R.M. Francis 67

6. **The Use of Bone Mineral Density Measurements in the
   Context of Osteoporosis Services**
   J.N. Fordham 89

7. **Developing Clinical Practice Guidelines (CPGs) for Bone
   Mineral Density Measurement and Osteoporosis
   Management**
   R.A. Hughes 121

8. **Use of Bone Mineral Density Measurement in
   Orthopaedic Practice**
   S.M. Hay 147

9. **Use of Bone Mineral Density Measurement in Primary
   Care**
   P. Brown 171

10. **Bone Densitometry in the Elderly**
    T. Masud and P.D. Miller 199

Index 221

List of Contributors

Dr T. Allison
Consultant in Public Health
    Medicine
East Riding Health Authority
East Yorkshire HU10 6DT
UK

Dr P. Brown
General Practitioner
138 Overland Road
Mumbles
Swansea SA3 4EU
UK

Professor R. Eastell
Consultant Physician
Clinical Sciences Centre
Northern General Hospital
Herries Road
Sheffield S5 7AU
UK

Dr J.N. Fordham
Consultant Rheumatologist
South Cleveland Hospital
Marton Road
Middlesbrough
Cleveland TS4 3BW
UK

Dr R.M. Francis
Consultant Physician
Musculoskeletal Unit
Freeman Hospital
High Heaton
Newcastle Upon Tyne NE7 7DN
UK

Mr S.M. Hay
Consultant Orthopaedic Surgeon
The Robert Jones and Agnes
    Hunt Orthopaedic Hospital
Oswestry
Shropshire SY10 7AG
UK

Professor R. Madhok
Director of Public Health
East Riding Health Authority
East Yorkshire HU10 6DT
UK

Dr T. Masud
Consultant Physician
Nottingham City Hospital
Hucknall Road
Nottingham NG5 1PB
UK

Professor P. Miller
Colorado Center for Bone
    Research
PC 3190 So
Wadsworth Boulevard
Suite 250
Lakewood
Colorado 80227
USA

Dr D.S. Simpson
School of Computing and
    Mathematics
University of Teesside
Middlesbrough
Cleveland TS1 3BA
UK

Dr J.G. Truscott
Division of Imaging and
    Radiotherapy Sciences
School of Healthcare
    Studies
Baines Wing
University of Leeds
PO Box 214
Leeds LS2 9UT
UK

1 Bone Mineral Density Measurement in the Management of Osteoporosis: A Public Health Perspective

R. Madhok and T. Allison

Introduction

The chapter starts with a description of the epidemiology of osteoporosis including the resource consequences of dealing with the associated fractures. It then outlines some guiding public health principles for osteoporosis services, including bone mineral densitometry (BMD), provision and describes the current situation for osteoporosis in regard to these. It then examines the salient features of a diagnostic test since these have a bearing on the use of BMD tests – their relevance to measuring BMD is also discussed. The chapter concludes with a brief discussion of the population screening versus use of BMD for case finding debate and outlines the current criteria for the use of BMD measurement.

Epidemiology of Osteoporosis[1,2]

Osteoporosis is a condition characterised by a reduction in the bone mass and disruption of bone architecture. The origins of osteoporosis are complex but in women it is generally agreed that the level of peak bone mass attained at puberty, the rate of fall in bone mass after menopause, and longevity are the three primary determinants.

The importance of osteoporosis lies in the fact that osteoporotic bones with their reduced bone strength are at a higher risk of fractures. These fractures have three distinctive features: they occur more commonly among women; the rates of these fractures increase with increasing age and hence are sometimes called age-related fractures; they have a tendency to occur in bones with a large trabecular or cancellous component such as hip, spine and distal forearm. These fractures cause considerable morbidity and are associated with increased mortality. The estimated remaining lifetime risk of osteoporotic fractures in Caucasian women at age 50 years, based on incidence rates in North America, is 17.5%, 15.6% and 16% for hip, spine and forearm respectively. The remaining life time risk of any osteoporotic fracture is almost 40% in white women and 13% in white men from age 50 onwards. Further details of the three common osteoporotic fractures follow together with a brief comment on other fractures.

Hip Fractures

Within the UK there were nearly 70,000 hip fractures in 1996. With each fracture costing the National Health Service (NHS) over £4800 the annual costs were estimated at £334 million.

As stated earlier these fractures are more common among women and the rates increase with rising age. Beyond 50 years of age, the incidence of hip fractures in women is twice that in men. However, because there are more elderly women than men, nearly 80% of these fractures occur among women.

The age-specific incidence increases from 1.8/10,000 in women in the age-group 50–54 years to 362/10,000 in women over 85 years of age. The corresponding figures for men are 1.3/10,000 and 147/10,000. The projected numbers are set to increase from 69,600 (55,700 in women and 13,900 in men) in 1995 to 81,300 (63,700 in women) in the year 2010 and 117,000 (89,500 in women) in the year 2030 in the UK.

Hip fracture rates vary substantially from one population to another, with non-Whites having a lower incidence. Within the European Union, Italy and Portugal have lower rates among women aged over 85 years compared with Denmark and Sweden. However, there is a considerable variation within populations of a given race and gender.

Hip fractures usually result after a fall from the standing position and although they show a marked seasonality, with substantial increases in the winter, the majority of them occur indoors. Of the falls that lead to hip fractures, about one-half are due to tripping or slipping, the rest are due to a loss of balance or syncope. One in 100 falls usually leads to a hip fracture – the likelihood of sustaining a fracture being dependent on protective reflexes and orientation of the fall.

The vast majority of hip fractures are treated surgically. Despite major advances in operative techniques and inplant technology, however, the outcomes for the patients are not always satisfactory with many patients unable to return to their prefracture status. Around 50% of hip fracture patients may become dependent on help from others and of those able to walk before fracture, half have difficulty in independent walking subsequently. In addition, hip fractures are associated with increased mortality – up to 20% excess mortality in the initial six months after the fracture.

Vertebral Fractures

Within the UK there were over 32,000 vertebral fractures in 1995. Routinely derived hospital discharge data for England and Wales suggest that as few as 2% of the incident vertebral fractures might be hospitalised. However, this is likely to be an under estimation.

Unlike hip fractures, comparatively little is known about the epidemiology of vertebral fractures due to two main reasons. Firstly, there is a lack of agreement on the definition of a vertebral fracture and secondly, due to the fact that a large proportion of them are asymptomatic.

Vertebral fractures are also more common among women and the incidence rates increase with rising age.

The age-specific prevalence rates (because of case ascertainment problems – prevalence rather than incidence rates are used for vertebral fractures; prevalence refers to new and existing fractures whereas incidence refers to newly arising fractures) increase from 699/10,000 in women in the age-group 50–54 years to 4340/10,000 in women over 85 years of age. The corresponding figures for men are 1350/10,000 and 2630/10,000. The projected numbers are set to increase from 32,300 (17,800 in women and 14,300 in men) in 1995 to 36,700 (19,700 in women) in the year 2010 and 47,200 (25,600 in women) in the year 2030 in the UK. One recent estimate of the age-adjusted incidence among American white women aged 50 years and over was 18 per 1000 person years.

Variations in vertebral fractures are less well studied but there is some evidence that they are less common in black than white women. As with hip fractures, vertebral fracture rates also vary within the European Union; Italy and Portugal have lower rates generally compared with Denmark and Sweden.

Vertebral fractures may occur in the absence of trauma or after minimal trauma such as bending, lifting or turning; falls account for a small proportion in women. One in three vertebral fractures in men occur as a result of severe trauma, for example, road traffic accidents.

Unlike hip fractures vertebral fractures are treated conservatively. Recent population based data show that overall survival among patients with vertebral fractures is worse than expected. At five years after fracture diagnosis, the estimated survival was 61% compared to an expected survival for those of like age and sex of 76%. As regards morbidity, physical functioning, self esteem and mood appear to be adversely affected in patients with vertebral fractures.

Forearm Fractures

Although a very common fracture relatively little is known about the epidemiology of osteoporotic forearm fractures, the most common type of which is the Colles' fracture, in the UK. The main reason for this is that the majority of these are treated as out-patients and within the NHS out-patient diagnostic information is not routinely collected. A multicentre study to ascertain the incidence phenomena is currently on-going within the UK (L. Edwards, Director of National Osteoporosis Society, personal communication).

Distal forearm fractures show a different pattern to hip or vertebral fractures. In white women, incidence rates increase linearly from age 40 to 64 years and then stabilise whereas the incidence remains relatively constant between ages 20 and 80 years in men. As a consequence, the majority of forearm fractures occur in women and the female predilection (age-adjusted female to male ratio of 4 to 1) is most marked for forearm fractures. The incidence of forearm fractures also varies from one geographical area to another and this generally parallels the hip fracture incidence rates – some of this variation is due to case ascertainment difficulties.

The falls leading to forearm fractures have been less well studied and in contrast to hip fractures occur outdoors and show a winter peak associated with icy conditions.

There is no excess mortality associated with forearm fractures but nearly half of all patients report only fair to poor functional outcome at six months. There is also the risk of neuropathies, algodystrophy and post-traumatic arthritis.

Other Fractures

Other sites are also affected such as proximal humerus, pelvis and proximal tibia.

Nearly 80% of proximal humerus fractures occur in people over 35 years of age and the majority are due to moderate trauma typically from a standing height. They are more common in women with poor neuromuscular function.

The rates of pelvic fractures also increase with increasing age and moderate trauma accounts for the majority of fractures of isolated pelvic bones and single breaks in the pelvic ring. Proximal tibia fractures, on the other hand, require severe trauma and the majority of these in older people are related to low bone mass.

In summary, osteoporotic fractures constitute a major public health problem. With increasingly ageing populations the disease burden is increasing. Patients with hip fractures currently occupy 20–30% of orthopaedic beds in the NHS, and this has a knock-on effect on elective procedures for which there are already long waiting lists. Within the European Union, the UK has a high incidence of osteoporotic fractures and as the availability of hospital beds is much lower, for example compared with Sweden, there are major implications for the NHS. The NHS costs per annum are already approaching the £1 billion mark.

Addressing Osteoporosis: Some Guiding Principles

The disease burden, and indeed given the changing demography with fewer providers caring for more pensioners in the future, the societal burden, due to osteoporosis is increasing. On the other hand, all health care systems including the British NHS are struggling to meet increasing demands and expectations within the finite resources available for health services.

From a public health view point, given increasing demands and finite resources it is essential to explore a new model for service planning and delivery. Obviously in the osteoporosis field, as in any other field, there are many stake holders and they all have a different perspective on the subject. However, health services discussions have too often been dominated by professional opinion, pressure groups or national policy makers – and to some extent this is right. These bodies have very valuable perspectives but equally it is necessary to ascertain the community's aspirations and local health needs assessment, and in subsequent service planning and delivery to reflect these to make the best use of the finite resources available (Fig. 1.1).

There are a number of other important principles which should guide the provision of relevant services for people with osteoporosis as follows; it is important to review these briefly before going into the specific issues around BMD measurement.

First, in terms of dealing with any condition, including osteoporosis, it is essential to look at the whole spectrum of the disease from health to death – the whole systems approach (Fig. 1.2). The necessary action can then be described in

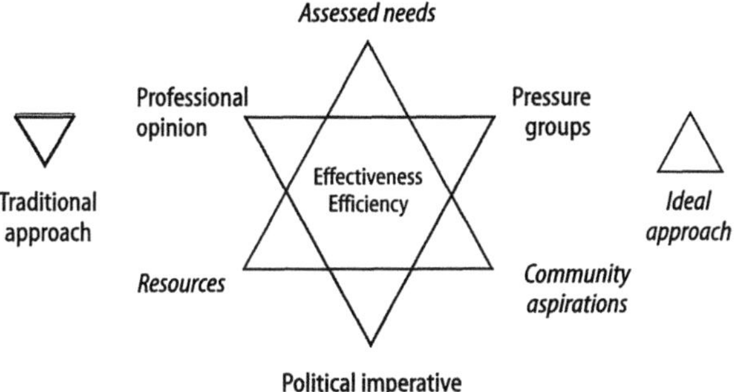

Figure 1.1 A model for planning services: improving services for people with osteoporosis.

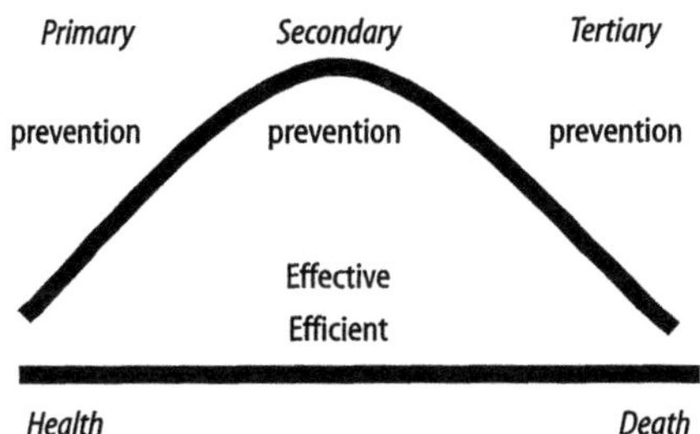

Figure 1.2 Whole systems approach to service provision.

terms of the three levels of prevention: (a) primary prevention, (b) secondary prevention, (c) tertiary prevention.

Primary prevention is the action taken prior to the onset of disease which reduces or removes the possibility that the disease will occur.

Secondary prevention is the action which halts the progression of a disease at its earlier stages and prevents complications through early detection and treatment.

Tertiary prevention includes treatment for established disease and its consequences and rehabilitation. The aim of tertiary prevention is to stop progression including complications and deal with any disability to ensure best quality of life for the patient.

Examining the whole spectrum of disease means that all age groups and all risk factors should be considered. Among the young, primary prevention is clearly most important, although there will be some young people who have specific clinical indications for further action. In older age groups, the importance of bone mineral density should not detract from potential interventions in other areas. Risk factors other than simple bone mineral density are associated with fracture, such as lack of exercise and poor vision.[3] The precise contribution of different risk factors to fracture is difficult to ascertain, but areas such as the prevention of falls in the elderly can be addressed as part of an osteoporosis strategy.

The second principle is that it is necessary to base any action on robust scientific evidence. There is now considerable emphasis on evidence-based medicine and clinical effectiveness and these considerations are assuming greater importance in the provision of services. Accordingly any action in the three levels of prevention should be subjected to two key tests.

1. Does this action result in improved outcomes for the patient? (effectiveness test);
2. How can this intervention be provided in the most cost effective and efficient manner? (efficiency test).

Thirdly, developing a service will mean investment and in many cases new money will be required. However, given that new money may not always be easily forthcoming, it may be necessary to critically examine the use of existing resources devoted to osteoporosis and other areas with a view to disinvestment from these. The released resources can then be redirected to the areas of most need based on effectiveness and efficiency considerations.

Thus, it may be necessary to consider disinvestment from other practices such as the use of drugs such as non- steroidal anti-inflammatory (NSAID) drugs (when there are other alternatives[4] and up to 10% of NSAID prescriptions are unused on unwanted and there are questions about the side-effects of some of the preparations); use of tests including X-rays (when the use of radiographs for example for ankle injuries is questionable[5]) and use of expensive implants for joint replacements and fracture treatment (when the lower cost hip replacement implants are also the ones with the most long term data and are most effective[6]).

Working Within Administrative Frameworks

Commissioning services designed to prevent and treat osteoporosis must be seen in the context of the relevant policy drivers. In the English NHS, following the production of the White Paper "The New NHS, Modern and Dependable", services are to be increasingly commissioned by primary care, either as primary care groups or primary care trusts. The large burden of disease caused by osteoporosis in primary care may influence their commissioning decisions. The overall local health policy will be set by the Health Improvement Programme, led by the Health Authority. This encompasses all areas of health care and so osteoporosis may not be high on its list of priorities in a given year. However, the government's strategy "Our Healthier Nation" may encourage more focus on osteoporosis. The Green Paper target of reducing accidents that result in hospital or family doctor consultation by at least one fifth by 2010 from a baseline at 1996 is combined with a whole systems approach to health promotion, commenting on national, local and personal action aimed at preventing osteoporosis.

The next section examines the state of the art in terms of the second and third guiding principles outlined above.

State of the Art: Evidence of Effectiveness for Osteoporosis Interventions

Three separate initiatives have examined the evidence base for various aspects of osteoporosis interventions:

1. A Working Party of the Royal College of Physicians of the UK
2. Eli Lilly National Clinical Audit Centre in the UK
3. A Working Group on behalf of the European Commission.

Working Party of the Royal College of Physicians[7]

This Working Party has recently reviewed the relevant research and summarised the evidence and made recommendations. The scientific evidence has been graded into the following levels depending on the type of trials or studies, with level I being the highest and IV being the lowest quality of evidence:

Ia   From meta-analysis of randomised controlled trials (RCT);

Ib   From at least one RCT;

IIa From at least one well-designed controlled study without randomisation;

IIb From at least one other type of well designed quasi-experimental study;

III From well-designed non-experimental descriptive studies, for example case–control studies, comparative studies and correlation studies;

IV   From expert committee reports or opinions and/or clinical experience of authorities;

I   From meta-analysis of observational studies.

The evidence is then summarised into three grades of recommendations: A, levels Ia and Ib; B, levels IIa, IIb and III; C, level IV. Table 1.1 shows some of the recommendations from this work.

These recommendations, in the main, however, concentrate on clinical and pharmacological interventions and do not go into the details of preventive measures. In addition, there is limited information about the likely costs and cost-effectiveness of these interventions. The choice between the population and high risk approaches is discussed and the document's main thrust is towards case finding.

Eli Lilly National Clinical Audit Centre[8]

The Eli Lilly National Clinical Audit Centre has also reviewed the evidence and produced a protocol for use by individual or group practices in primary care to audit their services. The protocol contains instructions to practices about organising the audits and has listed criteria which have been prioritised according to the strength of the research evidence and impact on outcomes. Two sets of audit criteria have been established: "Must Do" and "Should Do". "Must do" criteria are the minimum criteria as there is firm research evidence for them. "Should Do" criteria are additional criteria where there is some research evidence of their importance but where the impact on outcome is less certain; Table 1.2 lists all the criteria.

Working Group of the European Commission[2]

The recent report from the European Commission is the most comprehensive report on osteoporosis. Preventive strategies are described in two categories: non-pharmacological interventions and pharmacological interventions.

Table 1.1. Working Party of the Royal College of Physicians: selected recommendations for and evidence concerning the prevention and treatment of osteoporosis

Recommendation or evidence	Grade of recommendation
Prevention of osteoporosis	
For high risk strategies – there is some evidence that bone mass can be modified by calcium intake or other changes in lifestyle before the attainment of skeletal maturity	Grade A
Tibolone – an option for women in whom oestrogens are unacceptable or contraindicated	Grade A
Selective oestrogen receptor modulators such as raloxifene and tamoxifen exert some oestrogenic activity on bone	Grade A
Agents in the treatment of established osteoporosis	
Calcium supplements (1 g daily or more) decrease loss of bone in women with osteoporosis	Grade A
Pharmacological amounts of calcium decrease the risk of vertebral fracture	Grade A
but the effects on hip fracture are less certain	Grade B
HRT with or without opposed oestrogen prevents bone loss in women with osteoporosis	Grade A
Potential effect of HRT on hip and distal forearm fractures	Grade B
Calcitonin prevents bone loss in women with osteoporosis in a dose dependent manner	Grade A
Calcitonin decreases vertebral fracture frequency	Grade A
Protective effect of calcitonin on hip fracture risk	Grade B
Pain relief following crush fracture	Grade A
Bisphosphonates, etidronate and clodronate, prevent bone loss at the lumbar spine in women with osteoporosis	Grade A
Both decrease the risk of vertebral fracture	Grade A
Fluoride salts have a marked anabolic effect on cancellous bone mass at the spine	Grade A
When used with oestrogens or calcium they do not accelerate bone loss at other sites	Grade A
No protective effect has been shown on hip fracture risk	Grade B
Anabolic steroids prevent further bone loss in the elderly at all vulnerable sites and may decrease the risk of hip fracture	Grade A / Grade B
Calcitriol and alfacalcidol have been shown to decrease loss of bone in women with osteoporosis but the effects differ between studies	Grade A
Some, but not all studies have shown a decrease in vertebral fracture frequency	Grade A
No protective effect has been shown for hip fracture	Grade B
Exercise regimens have not consistently shown beneficial effects on bone mass	Grade B
Carefully structured exercises in women with established osteoporosis improve well-being, muscle strength and postural stability and may decrease the risk of further fractures	Grade B
Hip fracture risk can be decreased in the elderly by the use of hip protectors	Grade A

Table 1.1. *continued*

Recommendation or evidence	Grade of recommendation
Parenteral vitamin D (vitamin D_2 or D_3) with or without calcium supplements decreases the risk of hip and other fractures in the frail elderly	Grade A
The management of osteoporosis in men	
Intermittent cyclical etidronate may be useful in men with osteoporosis and vertebral fracture	Grade B
Alendronate may be beneficial when bone density is reduced at other sites	Grade C
Calcium and vitamin D supplementation may be useful, particularly in older men with osteoporosis	Grade C
In old or frail men with osteoporosis, consideration should be given to measures to decrease the risk of falling and reduce the impact of such falls	Grade C

Table 1.2. Eli Lilly audit criteria for osteoporosis services

'Must do' criteria

These are the minimum criteria that practices need to audit as there is firm research evidence to justify their inclusion. Every practice must include these criteria in the audit

1. The records show that a woman with an early menopause (before 45 years of age) has been offered hormone replacement therapy in the absence of contraindications
2. For women who have consulted within the last 12 months: the records show that, at least once between the ages of 44 and 55, (a) the menopausal status has been recorded and (b) hormone replacement therapy discussed
3. The records show that women on long-term corticosteroids have been assessed for the risk of osteoporosis and offered appropriate management
4. The records show that women with a history of current or previous fragility fracture of the hip, spine or wrist have been assessed for the risk of osteoporosis and offered appropriate management
5. The records show that women with fragility fractures of the spine have been considered for bisphosphonate treatment or hormone replacement therapy
6. The records show that elderly women in residential/nursing homes have been considered for calcium and vitamin D supplementation

'Should do' criteria

These are additional criteria for which there is some research evidence of their importance but where the impact on outcome is less certain.

7. The records show that (a) there has been an assessment of smoking habit and if necessary appropriate advice given; and that advice has been given about (b) exercise and (c) adequate dietary calcium intake
8. The records show that at least annually patients aged 75 and over have received advice about (a) exercise training, (b) fall prevention
9. The records show that women with risk factors for osteoporosis have been considered for bone mineral density (BMD) measurement

Reproduced with permission from the Authors.

Non-pharmacological interventions may reduce fracture risk by increasing peak bone mass, reducing age-related bone loss, decreasing the risk of falling, improving the protective neuromuscular responses associated with falling or reducing the impact of falls. There are three main non-pharmacological interventions: nutrition; prevention of, and protection against falls; and exercise.

Table 1.3. Some suggestions for preventing falls and avoiding environmental hazards

Individual factors
Plenty of liquids and good diet
Adjustment of prescription drugs
Physical exercise to increase strength and balance training from daily walking; learn to rise from a lying position and to dress and undress while sitting
Avoid long bathrobes and wide sleeves
Use good, comfortable footwear
Use correct glasses and a cane
Arrange contents of cupboards so that heavy objects are not too low and those commonly used are at a comfortable height

Environmental factors
Indoors
Loud doorbells; extra phone on side table
Light switches at all doors and use of high power bulbs (eg for people over 75 years old use 75 W bulbs)
Avoid elevated beds, slippery floors, loose carpets and wires, too much furniture, low chairs, dark entrances and corners
Handrails are important and doorsteps should be avoided
Change bath tub to shower with a chair
Outdoors
Good street lighting
Avoid uneven paving stones and steps
Clearly marked kerbs
Allow adequate time for traffic lights

Hip protectors
Currently for residents in institutions

Nutritional factors, particularly vitamin D and calcium, and physical exercise reduce the fracture risk by influencing peak bone mass, age related bone loss and increasing muscle strength. Table 1.3 lists some suggestions, from the European Commission Working Group, for preventing falls and avoiding environmental hazards.

Pharmacological interventions aim to reduce bone resorption and bone turnover or stimulate bone formation mainly and the following agents have been used.

1. Inhibitors of bone turnover: bisphosphonates, calcitonin, calcium, oestrogens;
2. Stimulators of bone formation: fluoride salts, parathyroid hormone;
3. Uncertain mode of action: anabolic steroids, ipriflavone, strontium, thiazide diuretics, vitamin D and metabolites.

However, it should be pointed out that although the above agents have been shown to be beneficial in terms of bone turnover and/or bone mineral density in post-menopausal women there are relatively few randomised controlled trials showing that these agents have prevented fractures. Furthermore, there are concerns that patients may not comply with treatment over prolonged periods of time.

The European Commission's Working Group has also estimated the annual costs of different preventive strategies, as follows: £5 for Vitamin D injection,

£30–150 for HRT, £75 for hip protectors in the elderly, £80–130 for vitamin D and calcium, £170 for etidronate, £350 for alendronate and £2000 for calcitonin.

Bone Mineral Density Measurement in the Management of Osteoporosis

Osteoporosis is a major public health problem for which effective action can be taken, as has been shown above. Early diagnosis is therefore essential to estimate the severity of disease, predict the subsequent clinical course and prognosis, and to trigger treatment.

Osteoporotic fractures which are the main clinical presentation of osteoporosis occur at a relatively late stage of the disease when there has been considerable bone loss. It is therefore necessary to explore whether there are other ways of identifying potential patients who can then be appropriately managed to reduce their chances of sustaining a fracture. This can be done in three ways:

1. Clinical risk assessment
2. Bone densitometry measurement
3. Assessment of biochemical markers of bone turnover

Clinical Risk Assessment

Many risk factors for osteoporosis have been identified. Some of these being endogenous, for example female gender, age, slight body build and Asian or Caucasian race, are not modifiable. Other risk factors are exogenous such as premature menopause, amenorrhoea or hypogonadism, glucocorticoid therapy, maternal history of hip fracture, low body weight, cigarette smoking, excessive alcohol consumption, prolonged immobilisation and low calcium and vitamin D intake. However, it is worth mentioning that most of these exogenous factors are not specific or sensitive and hence not very predictive of the risk to any individual (see below). The three main exogenous factors which are important are: male and female hypogonadism, glucocorticoid therapy and a past history of fractures.

Bone Densitometry Measurement

Since the main emphasis of this manual is on bone density measurement it is important to reflect on this in some detail. However, before deciding on the particular BMD test it is necessary to review some of the guiding principles for any diagnostic test. In choosing a particular test, the three important principles are:

1. Can the test measure the condition?
2. How good is the test in measuring the condition?
3. Will measuring the condition and detection of abnormality ultimately matter? In other words can effective treatment be instituted and, in case of osteoporosis, fractures prevented?

Some details about these three issues and their relevance for BMD measurements follow.

Can the Test Measure the Condition?

As stated previously there are two major causes predisposing to an osteoporotic fracture: bone abnormality whether mass or architecture, and trauma. In the context of this chapter the major issue is bone abnormality and particularly bone mass. However it is worth remembering that there is some debate about the relative contribution of bone architecture to subsequent fractures. Thus it is conceivable that although in a bone the bone content, and hence mass, may be sufficient overall, the quality of bone may be reduced rendering the bone more susceptible to fracture. Such thinking has led some proponents to argue that techniques including ultrasound and possibly computed tomography, which better reflect the architect of the bone, may be as important as measuring bone mass alone.

A number of methods for measuring BMD have been used at one time or another as follows.

1. Plain radiographs.
2. Dual X-ray absorptiometry (DXA)
3. Single photon absorptiometry (SPA)
4. Dual photon absorptiometry (DPA)
5. Quantitative computed tomography (QCT)
6. Ultrasound measurement such as speed of sound (SOS) or broad band ultrasonic attenuation (BUA)
7. Single X-ray absorptiometry (SXA).

In judging the relative values of these techniques the key question is whether the technique was developed appropriately and evaluated to ensure that it does measure BMD. In other words, is the test valid and reproducible? Validity or accuracy is the degree to which the results of the measurement correspond to the true state of the phenomena being measured and this can be done by comparing observed measurement with some accepted standard. Reproducibility is the extent to which repeated measurements of a relatively stable condition fall closely to each other. Reproducibility is also called reliability and precision. It is possible to have a technique that on average is valid but not as reliable because its results are imprecise by being widely scattered about the true value. On the other hand a technique may be reproducible but not valid. Presently, the expert opinion, reinforced by the Department of Health in the UK,[9] advocates DXA as the test of choice (see below).

How Good is the Test at Measuring the Condition?

In deciding on which method of bone mineral density measurement to choose from the range available it is essential to be aware of certain properties of the test as follows (Fig. 1.3):

		Disease	
		Present	Absent
Test	Positive	a	b
	Negative	c	d

$$\text{Sensitivity} = \frac{a}{a+c}$$

$$\text{Specificity} = \frac{d}{b+d}$$

$$\text{Positive predictive value} = \frac{a}{a+b}$$

$$\text{Negative predictive value} = \frac{d}{c+d}$$

Figure 1.3 Properties of a diagnostic test.

1. Sensitivity is the proportion of people with the disease who have a positive test for the disease and hence a sensitive test will rarely miss people with the disease.
2. Specificity is the proportion of people without the disease who have a negative test and hence a specific test will rarely misclassify people without the disease as having it.
3. Positive and negative predictive values can be calculated as shown in Fig. 1.3 and give an indication of how useful the test is in clinical practice.

Although there is little systematically collected information about the merits and demerits of various techniques based on these properties it has been estimated that the "accuracy of BMD measurements by DXA to predict fracture is as good as blood pressure to predict stroke, and significantly better than serum cholesterol to predict myocardial infarction".[7] It is also estimated that the use of

Table 1.4. Guides for deciding the clinical usefulness of a diagnostic test

1. Has there been an independent, "blind" comparison with a "gold standard' of diagnosis?
2. Has the diagnostic test been evaluated in a patient sample that included an appropriate spectrum of mild and severe, treated and untreated, disease, plus individuals with different but commonly confused disorders?
3. Was the setting for this evaluation, as well as the filter through which study patients passed, adequately described?
4. Have the reproducibility of the test result (precision) and its interpretation (observer variation) been determined?
5. Has the term *normal* been defined sensibly as it applies to this test?
6. If the test is advocated as part of a cluster or sequence of tests, has its individual contribution to the overall validity of the cluster or sequence been determined?
7. Have the tactics for carrying out the test been described in sufficient detail to permit their exact replication?
8. Has the utility of the test been determined?

From Sackett D.L., Haynes R.B., Guyatt G.H. et al. Clinical epidemiology: a basic science for clinical medicine. Little, Brown London.

BMD alone to assess risk has a high specificity but low sensitivity. The low sensitivity (approx 50%) means that half of all osteoporotic fractures will occur in women said not to have osteoporosis. For this reason the test is more useful for case finding and not population screening (see below).

In overall terms, in deciding which test to choose it is worth reflecting on the eight guides for deciding the clinical usefulness of a diagnostic test[10] (Table 1.4).

There has been some discussion about how osteoporosis is defined; the debate is complicated by the fact that diminishing BMD is a normal ageing phenomenon. At present the advice from the World Health Organisation (WHO) is that BMD measurements below 2.5 standard deviations (SD) of the young peak bone mass normal are clinically important. The WHO defines osteoporosis as "a disease characterised by low bone mass and microarchitectural deterioration of bone tissue, leading to enhanced bone fragility and a consequent increase in fracture risk".

The categories, based on BMD values, are as follows

Normal: a value for BMD within 1 SD of the young adult reference mean;

Low bone mass (osteopenia):   a value for BMD more than 1 SD below the young adult mean but less than 2.5 SD below the value;

Osteoporosis: a value for BMD 2.5 SD or more below the young adult mean.

Does Measuring the Condition Matter?

Even though there may be a valid and reproducible test which can diagnose osteoporosis it is essential to be certain that it can be made available to those in need and those who can benefit from early diagnosis in addition to ensuring that effective treatments are subsequently possible. It is important to be aware that not everyone who needs a test will demand it or that it will be available to those who do demand it. In health care, the "inverse care law" often applies whereby those in most need are also the most unlikely to receive the necessary and needed care. In addition, there are concerns that test results do not always subsequently influence patient management.

At present there is some controversy surrounding the use of BMD measurement[11,12] and not wishing to further polarise the debate it is important to reflect on the observations made in this chapter so that appropriate services can

Table 1.5. Criteria for population screening for presymptomatic disease

1. Is the disease important?
2. Is a safe and reliable test available?
3. Does the test discriminate well between normal and abnormal?
4. Can people with normal results be reassured?
5. Will people with false positive results be harmed due to anxiety or treatment?
6. Is the natural history of the disease known?
7. Is effective treatment available?
8. Is it possible to reach those who need the test?
9. Is the test affordable?

From   Committee on Health Promotion (1988). Population screening for pre-symptomatic disease. Guidelines for Health Promotion Number 4. Faculty of Public Health Medicine of the Royal College of Physicians of the United Kingdom, London.

be planned and delivered locally. In this regard it is appropriate to comment on the debate about population screening for osteoporosis. At present there is common agreement that there is no role for population screening to detect patients with osteoporosis because the current interventions available do not fulfil the necessary criteria for a population screening tool[13] (Table 1.5).

Overall, in terms of BMD measurements there is, currently, a minority who favour techniques other than DXA or do not advocate any diagnostic testing for osteoporosis. The majority including the Department of Health, however, favour the use of DXA in selective case finding. Accordingly, experts in the field have developed a list of clinical indications where it is appropriate to measure bone mineral density[14]

1. Selective case finding in states of premature untreated oestrogen deficiency
2. Confirmation of diagnosis in cases of clinical uncertainty where there is verte-bral deformity, multiple low trauma fractures or osteopenia on X-ray
3. Quantification of response in those receiving treatment for osteoporosis
4. Identification of those corticosteroid users who are fast bone losers
5. Quantification of bone loss in secondary osteoporosis states which include alcohol abuse, hyperparathyroidism, thyrotoxicosis, malabsorption syndromes, postgastrectomy and myeloma.

Additionally BMD measurement is considered of value in the assessment of individual women in whom knowledge that bone density was significantly reduced would be "critical" in decision making over the use of long-term HRT.

Assessment of Biochemical Markers of Bone Turnover

Biochemical markers of bone turnover use indices of bone resorption such as urinary excretion of hydroxyproline, pyridinoline and deoxypyridinoline, hydroxylysine glycosides and N-telopeptides or C-telopeptides of type 1 collagen, and indices of bone formation such as serum concentration of bone specific alkaline phosphatase and osteocalcin. Menopausal bone loss is associated with an increase in both bone markers: of resorption and formation. At present, bio-chemical markers are of limited clinical utility since they are poorly predictive of bone mineral density. However, there is at present, considerable on-going research in this field.

Summary of the Public Health Approach to Osteoporosis

The public health approach includes attention both to the population as a whole and to individuals and looks at the entire course of osteoporosis. Provision of primary prevention is important, including a focus on a good diet, exercise and cessation of smoking. Appropriate diagnosis and treatment should be provided for those at high risk of osteoporosis and effective services should be available for those who have suffered osteoporotic fracture. Robust scientific evidence should be used to justify all new or existing efforts aimed at managing osteo-porosis, whether preventative, diagnostic, as with bone mineral densitometry, or therapeutic. Finally, resources are essential; these may either be newly acquired or released by disinvestment.

Conclusion

This chapter has briefly described the epidemiology of osteoporotic fractures, which are the main manifestation of osteoporosis. There is potentially much that could be done to reduce the consequences of this disease both to patients and to the public purse. The hope is that early diagnosis followed by treatment may bring about a reduction in the incidence of fractures.

However, there are a number of issues which need consideration in deciding which test to choose and for which patients; given the likely resource consequences in view of the scale of the problem it is essential that the test that is chosen is both clinically and cost effective. The messages in this chapter are therefore important.

References

1. Cooper C, Melton LJ (1996) Magnitude and impact of osteoporosis and fractures. In: Marcus R, Feldman D, Kelsey J (eds) San Diego. Osteoporosis Academic Press Inc.
2. Director-General for Employment, Industrial Relations and Social Affairs (1998) Report on osteoporosis in the European Community: action for prevention. Official Offices for European Communities Publications, Malmo.
3. Cummings SR, Nevitt MC, Browner WS et al. (1995) Risk factors for hip fracture in white women. N Engl J Med 332:767–773.
4. Dieppe P, Frankel SJ, Toth B (1993) Is research into the treatment of osteoarthritis with non-steroidal anti-inflammatory drugs misdirected? Lancet 341:353–354.
5. Stiell IG, Greenberg GH, McKnight D et al. (1993) Decision rules for the use of radiography in acute ankle injuries. JAMA 269:1127–1132.
6. Murray D, Bulstrode C (1993) Designer hips: don't let your patient become a fashion victim. BMJ 306:732–733.
7. Royal College of Physicians of London. (1999) Osteoporosis. Clinical guidelines for prevention and treatment. RCP, London.
8. Lakhani M, Baker R, Khunti K (1998) Audit protocol: prevention and treatment of osteoporosis in women CT12. Eli Lilly National Clinical Audit Centre, Leicester.
9. Department of Health (1996) EL (96) 110: Improving the effectiveness of clinical services. NHS Executive, Leeds.
10. Sackett DL, Haynes RB, Guyatt GH et al. (1991) Clinical epidemiology: A basic science for clinical medicine. Little, Brown, London.
11. Barlow D, Cooper C, Reeve J (1996) Department of Health is fair to patients with osteoporosis. BMJ 312:297–298.
12. Sheldon TA, Raffle A, Watt I (1996) Why the report of the Advisory Group on Osteoporosis undermines evidence based purchasing. BMJ 312:296–297.
13. Committee on Health Promotion (1998) Population screening for pre-symptomatic disease. Guidelines for Health Promotion Number 4. Faculty of Public Health Medicine of the Royal College of Physicians of the United Kingdom, London.
14. Advisory Group on Osteoporosis (1994) Department of Health, London.

2 Measurement of Bone Density: Current Techniques

J.G. Truscott

Introduction

Since the discovery of X-rays by Röntgen in November 1895 there has been interest in utilising them for the examination of bone. In fact as early as January 1896 the first paper appeared which contained a radiograph. There can be little doubt as to the utility of radiographs in the examination of the skeleton, in particular for the location of fractures and dislocations. Plain radiographs also have a role in the assessment of bone mineral density; advanced osteopenic change or established osteoporosis can easily be detected using, for example, lateral views of the thoracolumbar spine. However, many problems have been found in using this approach. Many attempts have been made to quantify bone mineral from images on radiographic film starting in the 1930s with the work of the American dentist Hodge. Together with his co-workers he examined many variables likely to affect the measurement of bone mineral content (BMC) using direct radiographic methods.[1] In the late 1930s a system which shone a collimated beam of light through a radiograph was used by Pauline Mack to obtain quantitative values from radiographs.[2] This system, albeit modified, was in use into the early 1970s when it was used for measuring the bones of astronauts who had undergone weightlessness during space flight. In 1951 it was pointed out by Ardran that bone destruction could not be shown on radiographs as the images appeared normal until a loss of BMC of the order of 20–30% was present.[3] He also demonstrated the poor reproducibility of the plain film methodology. A need was established for an imaging modality, which was capable of producing not just useful images of the bone anatomy, but also quantitative data that was not subject to the limitations of work based around the use of radiographs. In 1963 a direct method of measuring BMC was developed by Cameron and Sorenson[4] and was used to quantify the loss of bone due to osteoporosis in the forearm bones. This technique known as single photon absorptiometry made the reproducible measurement of bone mineral content a reality. This technique and others that were developed from it is examined in more detail in the section that follows.

Techniques of Bone Measurement

Single Photon/X-Ray Absorptiometry

This technique utilises a well-collimated beam of photons of a single energy. Such a beam may be used to measure the attenuation offered by objects placed in its path. In order to obtain bone mineral content it is necessary to place the region to be scanned in a water bath. At the energies chosen, water and soft tissue offer similar attenuation to the photon beam and if the overall thickness of water, plus subject is kept constant, any variations in attenuation may be considered to be due to variations in bone mineral. In early systems of this type the forearm was the preferred site for measurement which was achieved by passing a monochromatic beam of radiation through the water bath and the forearm to a photomultiplier detector located coaxial with the source of radiation. In the system shown in Fig. 2.1

$$I_x = I_o e^{-\mu l}$$

Where: I_o is the flux output from source; I_x is the flux arriving at the detector; μ is the effective overall attenuation coefficient and l is the effective absorber thickness.

However, by manipulating the equation and using a water bath it is possible to obtain values for $l_{x,b}$ (the effective bone thickness at point x) because the attenuation coefficients for both bone mineral and water are known. In order to carry out a scan both source and detector were moved synchronously across the forearm and a trace such as that shown in Fig. 2.2 obtained. The level marked as background in this figure is equivalent to the transmission through water or soft tissue alone and as can be seen a reduction in transmitted intensity is obtained through both the ulna and radius. The shaded area in the diagram is proportional to bone

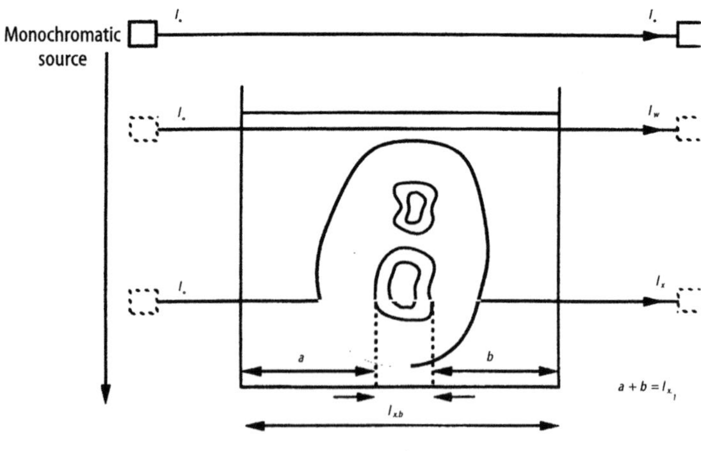

Figure 2.1 The underlying principle of single photon absorptiometry (SPA). (From Truscott et al.[20] with permission.)

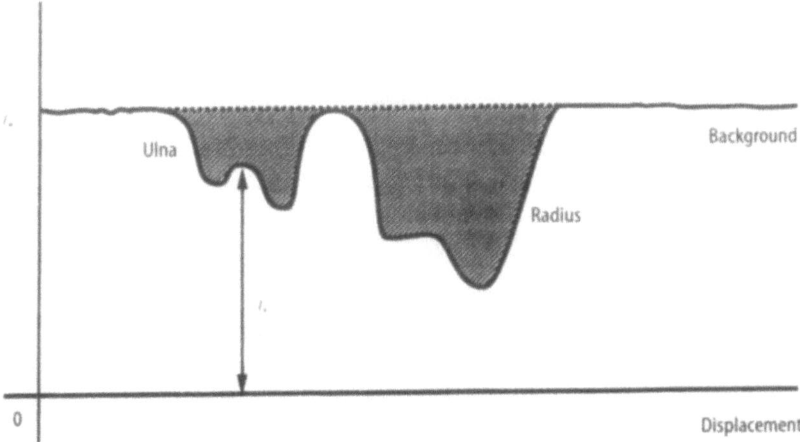

Figure 2.2 The method for recovering bone mineral content (BMC) from single slice single photon absorptiometry (SPA). (From Truscott et al.[20] with permission.)

mineral content from a single passage of the scanner beam through the forearm. By acquiring a number of adjacent scan lines it is possible to build up a bone mineral content image of the region of interest. A value for bone mineral density (g cm^{-2}) may then be obtained by dividing the total BMC by the overall area of the region of interest.

Because of the need for a water bath this methodology has realistically been restricted to the appendicular skeleton notably the distal portions of the radius and ulna. Some systems have been built which carried out scans of the os-calcis but these have not seen major clinical use.

Dual Photon/X-Ray Absorptiometry

In 1966 Reed[5] demonstrated the possibility of using two photon beams of differing energies in order to compensate for the differences in soft tissue thickness and hence to be able to measure BMC without using a water bath. This development meant that the axial skeleton could now be measured as bone mineral content could be obtained whilst measuring the subject in air rather than in a water bath. This was considered to be particularly important as the majority of osteoporotic fractures occur in the spine and hip and these regions are not amenable to water-bath techniques of measurement.

A system for dual photon absorptiometry is shown in Fig. 2.3 and the two energies, high and low, required by the technique are denoted by the superscripts H and L, respectively. Two equations like that given above, one for each energy, may be solved as simultaneous equations to allow for the calculation of bone mineral density (BMD).

The original technique was known as dual-photon absorptiometry (DPA) and the two energies required were obtained from isotope sources. Due to the limited radiation from such sources the technique was slow in obtaining an image and had very limited spatial resolution. Isotope sources reduce in activity as they

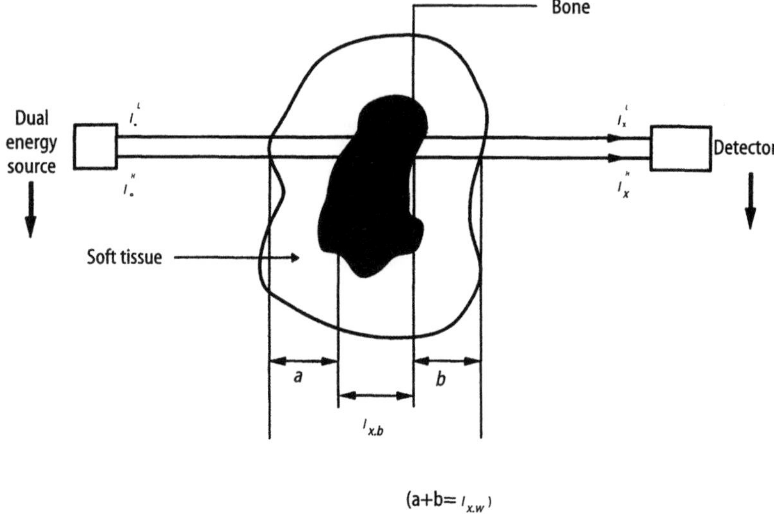

$$(a+b = I_{x.w})$$

Figure 2.3 The underlying principle of dual photon absorptiometry (DPA). (From Truscott et al.[20] with permission.)

decay with time and there was also a requirement for the operator to make allowances for this when calculating results.

In 1970 Krokowski[6] suggested an improvement to this technique by demonstrating that an X-ray source could be used in place of the isotope sources. This gave an immediate increase in the flux of photons passing through the subject in a given time and hence a reduction in scan time. The relative permanence of X-ray generators compared to isotope sources also produced a saving in running costs. The equations are solved in exactly the same manner as for dual photon absorptiometry but because X-rays are used this technique is known as dual-energy X-ray Absorptiometry (DXA).

Materials display absorption characteristics, which are energy dependent. Prominent among these are the K-edges of the atomic structure of these materials which preferentially absorb various energies. By judicious choice of these materials it is possible to construct a "K-edge filter" which will produce the two energies required for DXA when illuminated by a fixed voltage X-ray tube. Another way in which two X-ray energies may be obtained is by switching the voltage to the X-ray tube to produce two different output energy spectra. This is referred to as "energy switching".

These systems are identical in use, each having a bed on which the subject lays. An X-ray source is held beneath the bed and the detector, carried on a scan arm is above the patient. These two move in a rectilinear pattern over the regions of interest to produce an image. Within these images various regions can be chosen for analysis to produce quantitative values for BMC and BMD.

Quantitative Computed Tomography (QCT)

Because both the single and dual energy absorptiometric techniques are projection methods it means that measurements take place through both cortical and trabecular bone resulting in a mean value for BMC and BMD which encompasses the two components. This means that in regions where the cortical bone density is high relative to the trabecular component, changes in the content of trabecular bone, which is the most metabolically active, may be masked in such an overall measurement. Such effects may be particularly noticed in the lumbar spine where spinal processes, which have a high cortical bone density, may effect the ability to detect deterioration in the trabecular content. This could be overcome by a method capable of producing a cross sectional view through the site of interest.

Computed tomography (CT) is very good at giving such slices but because the equipment in routine clinical use derives a broadband of radiation energies from an X-ray source it is necessary to calibrate such systems with a bone equivalent phantom so that values for BMC and BMD may be calculated. This is normally achieved by placing a calibration phantom under the region of the lumbar spine so that it is reconstructed in the slice through the spine which is used for analysis.[7] In these slices the cortical and trabecular regions are immediately obvious but the spatial resolution of the system is not good enough to reveal individual trabeculae. A typical vertebral slice is shown in Fig. 2.4 where the difference between the outer cortical and inner trabecular bone regions may readily be seen.

However, the general pattern of the structure may be observed and region of interest software used to obtain BMC and BMD values in selected regions. Although highly accurate in examining the anatomy and density in these regions within the spine and the fact that CT systems are available in many centres the need for a calibration phantom, the increased radiation compared to DXA and the cost per scan on such systems make its use as a routine measurement technique less practical.

In order to reduce both cost and dose, densitometric QCT systems have been developed which utilise single-energy techniques to measure the peripheral skeleton (primarily radius and ulna, but tibia and fibula are possible). The cortical and

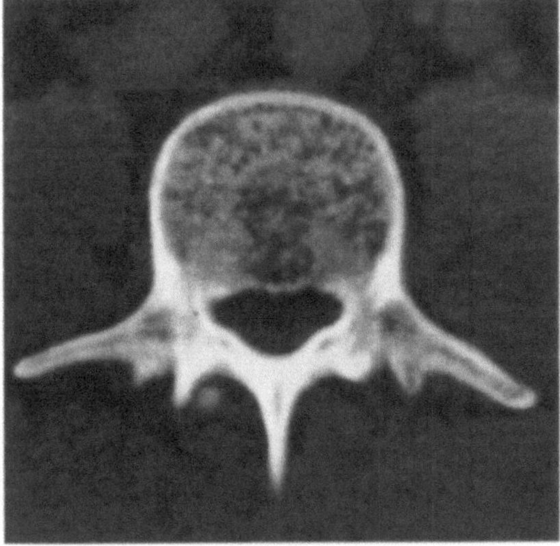

Figure 2.4 A computed tomogram of a lumbar vertebra. The mass of the vertebral body can be measured. (From Woolf and Dixon[21] with permission.)

trabecular bone compartments can be separated to allow determination of subtle changes in trabecular BMD. In the forearm it has been demonstrated[8] that the distal portions of the radius and ulna can have a relative trabecular content of as high as 75%. These areas are attractive as scan sites because Colles' fracture occurs in these regions and such fractures are proposed as early indications of osteoporosis. Selection of the wrist also means that peripheral QCT systems can be compact, compared to the whole body systems, which is another factor in keeping costs to an acceptable level. Such systems are, however, liable to inaccuracy in BMD estimation due to changes in fat content in the marrow space; this factor has restricted their role primarily to research.

Ultrasound Measurements

The previous techniques have all involved the use of ionising radiation, albeit at a very low dose. Systems that could obtain similar information to those above, but without the use of ionising radiation, would be very attractive. Current interest in such systems is centred on the use of ultrasound in the measurement of bone.

There are two key ultrasound measurements used in the assessment of bone; speed of sound (SOS) and broadband ultrasonic attenuation (BUA). The site of measurement has been in the main, the os-calcis, with a transmitter at one side of the heel and a receiver at the other. An ultrasound pulse is generated at the transmitter and coupled to the heel either by means of a water bath or by surface contact. The wave passes through the heel and is detected by the receiver. By examining the transmit and receive waves the two quantities, SOS and BUA, can be calculated.

SOS is intuitively the simplest measurement to understand. The time interval between transmission of the wave and its reception can be measured as can the distance between these two transducers. Dividing the distance the wave has travelled by its time of flight will give the speed of sound, in this case for the os calcis.

BUA is a little trickier to understand. The pulse generated at the transmitter is rich in frequencies (hence broadband). The amplitude of the generated signal, passed through a water bath alone, can be measured over a range of frequencies (e.g. 200–1000 kHz). If the heel is then introduced into the beam path a similar measurement can be made. Two such traces, A_W and A_H respectively, are shown in Fig. 2.5.

The attenuation offered to the passage of ultrasound can be calculated across the frequency range subtracting A_H from A_W. (hence broadband ultrasonic attenuation). The attenuation is frequency dependent and non-linear. Resort to logarithms produces a quantity of log attenuation per unit frequency that is expressed in decibels (a logarithmic unit) per megahertz ($dBMHz^{-1}$), which is the slope of the graph of attenuation with respect to frequency (Fig. 2.6). This graph has a higher slope in normal subjects than in osteoporotics and is thus clinically useful.

The proposed relationship between these numbers and the bone itself are as follows. When considering the speed of sound it is well established that the denser a material, the faster sound will travel in it. (Remember the hero in those old films pressing his ear to the railway line to hear the train coming before it could be heard in air – the railway line was denser so the sound got there sooner). Thus the denser the bone the higher is SOS. High values are good. When con-

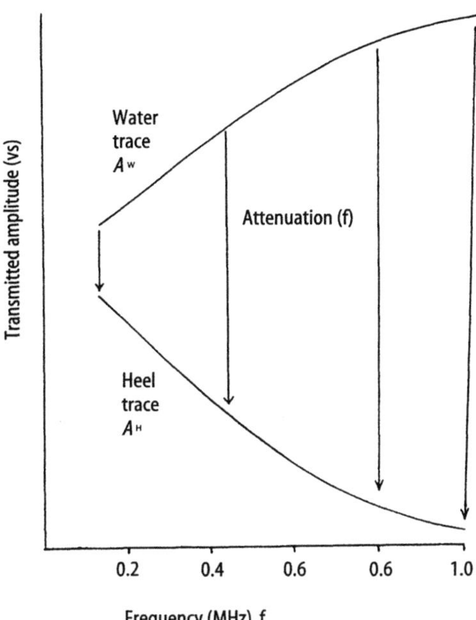

Figure 2.5 Description of water and heel amplitude spectra. (From Palmer and Langton[22] with permission.)

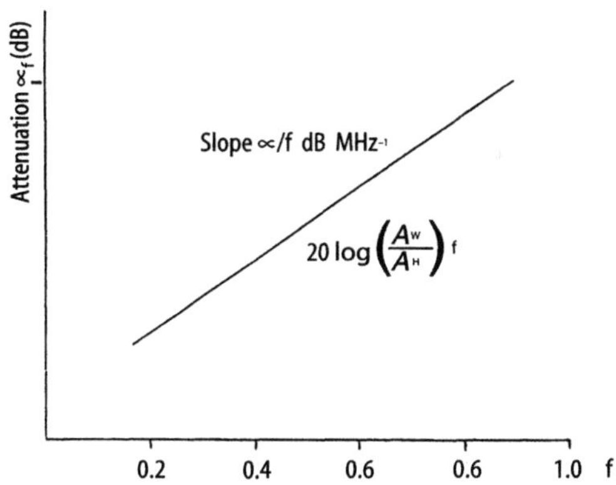

Figure 2.6 The resultant attenuation trace from Fig. 2.5. (From Palmer and Langton[22] with permission.)

sidering BUA the method of attenuation must be allowed for. At similar bone density values (as measured by DXA) cancellous bone has been shown to be considerably more attenuating than cortical bone. This is thought to relate to the structure component which is high in dense trabecular bone, reducing as the structure is removed (osteopenia?) and negligible in cortical bone (virtually structure free) where density plays a greater part. It has been shown[9] that the BUA value for normal subjects is higher than that for osteoporotic patients when measured in the os-calcis (a highly trabecular site), the implication being that there is a loss of structure due to removal of trabeculae and structural degeneration. Once again high values are good.

Magnetic Resonance Imaging (MRI)

This is another technique that does not use ionising radiation. It is capable of producing high-resolution three-dimensional images of selected regions of the body. As little signal is produced in bone but relatively large signals in bone marrow and surrounding soft tissue it means that although it is difficult to quantitate bone it is possible to produce high resolution images of trabecular regions. Such images may then be quantified in terms of morphological parameters such as the space occupied by the trabeculae relative to the volume of interest being considered. Significant correlation has been shown between such parameters and changes in BMD values in the calcaneus.[10] Preliminary results show that high resolution MRI may have a potential use in the quantitative assessment of trabecular structure. Because of the extremely high cost of such techniques it is unlikely that they will be incorporated into routine clinical use and are more likely to remain as a research tool for investigating the structural changes that occur in osteoporotic bone.

Radiation Protection

It should be borne in mind that if a radiative system is used the person directing or ordering the examination should have been on an educational course for the Protection of Persons Undergoing Medical Examination or Treatment (POPUMET) which explains the regulations pertinent to the administration of radiation. Such courses also describe the hazards associated with the use of radiation for both subjects and operators. Anyone using these types of system should contact their local Radiation Protection Service for advice about set-up and use of such systems and the availability of POPUMET courses in their area. At the time of going to press these regulations are being replaced by a Europe-wide concordat on radiation protection, which is currently being framed into legislation in the member countries. Consultation should be complete and the law in force by 2000. It is important to check with local Radiation Protection Services to determine what effects these new regulations may have on current or proposed bone measurement services.

The Measurement Sites

Routine radiography for osteoporosis has for many years relied on contact radiographs of the hand together with anterior posterior views of the pelvis and proximal femora. Lateral views are also made of both the lumbar and thoracic spine. The hand radiographs were subject to metacarpal radiogrammetry as described above. The films of the spine are examined for progressive radiolucency indicative of a reduction in bone mineral content but subject to the constraint noted above that 20–30% must have been lost before such lucencies are apparent. Of more interest in these films is the examination of individual vertebrae for shape change such as wedging or crushing of the vertebrae. These types of fractures are characteristic of osteoporosis. It is possible by making measurements of the heights and widths of vertebrae on the radiographs obtained to convert this rather qualitative method into a quantitative scale. Radiographs of the hip can be examined for trabecular orientation and organisation in the femoral neck region. This general examination has been put on a more rigorous footing by use of the Singh index[11] where patient radiographs are compared to standardised sets of radiographs and classified in grades one to seven with one being the worst case and seven having both mineralised and highly organised trabeculae.

These methods are generally qualitative and at best quantitative but on limited scale values (i.e. 1–7 for the Singh grade). As noted above it is possible to use films of the phalanges to undertake radiographic photodensitometry and although measurements are available on a continuous scale using such systems, the variations in film development, X-ray energy, soft tissue coverage and beam filtration all affect both precision and accuracy. The use of such systems has been largely superseded by photon absorptiometry.

Single photon absorptiometry is confined to the peripheral skeleton, mainly the distal forearm and os calcis. These sites are chosen because of their high trabecular content and it is felt that measurements at such sites would reflect the bone loss due to the high metabolic activity at such sites. The os calcis is a load bearing bone and the BMC will be reflective of general activity, a factor that made the site attractive for ultrasonic bone assessment. Single photon absorptiometry gives a direct measurement of BMC at the site of interest and is reflective of systemic bone activity. The relationship between sites of common osteoporotic fracture, the hip and spine, and measurements made in the forearm and heel have been demonstrated in many studies. The wrist is the site of Colles' fracture which often occurs in osteoporotic subjects before other fractures.

Dual photon absorptiometry has allowed the direct measurement of sites of osteoporotic fracture. The femoral neck and lumbar spine are common sites for dual energy measurements. In fact the World Heath Organisation has adopted such measurements as the best measure of future fracture risk.[12] The relationship between declining bone density and fracture risk is considered to be approximately the same as that between blood pressure and the risk of stroke. From such measures the WHO recommend the diagnosis of osteopenia as being more than 1 standard deviation (SD) below the young normal mean value for BMD and osteoporosis as being more than 2.5 SD below this value. DXA of the forearm and os calcis is also now being used for the reasons stated above. New sites have recently been evaluated for the study of bone loss with the hand being used in arthritis, as early changes occur in this region in both osteoarthritis and rheumatoid arthritis. Whole body scanning reveals generalised bone loss and may have a place in monitoring systemic disease. Other pathologies and their relationship to bone changes are discussed in Chapter 5.

Current Systems

This review of available bone measurement systems will concentrate on the newer systems produced by each of the main manufacturers. Earlier systems, which form the bulk of those currently in use, are thoroughly explored in Wahner and Fogelman's encyclopaedic work[13] to which readers are directed for a thorough study of all the technical aspects of absorptiometry. In terms of cost (this of course varies with time, manufacturer and model) a rough guide would put the peripheral DXA and ultrasound systems at between £10 000 and £20 000; the pencil beam DXA systems at between £30 000 and £50 000; and the fan beam systems at between £60 000 and £100 000. Peripheral QCT systems are in the same price bracket as pencil beam DXA systems.

Pencil Beam DXA Systems

All systems have the facility to measure at the lumbar spine (AP view) and proximal femur and to compare current scans with those carried out previously. All systems have reference databases for these sites. The ability of each scanner to measure other sites of interest is considered in the overview of each instrument.

Hologic

The QDR 4000 is the current pencil beam system from Hologic and uses a switched pulse X-ray system to obtain the two energies required for the technique. The in vivo precision for the AP lumbar spine is 0.8% in normals and 1.1% in osteoporotics and in the neck of femur is 1.4% for normals and 1.7% for osteoporotics. Doses for these examinations range from 3 mR to 5 mR. Optional scan modes include decubitus lateral spine BMD, forearm, small animal and general region of interest. Also available is a scoliotic spine analysis, which tailors vertebral BMD to spine curvature. The manufacturer quotes two scan modes, fast and precision with fast scans taking 2.4 min for the spine and 3.6 min for the hip with precision mode scans taking twice as long. The system is controlled by a Pentium computer running Windows 95 and having a 2 GB hard disk drive for storage and a 1 GB JAZ cartridge disc system for archival storage. A CD ROM reader is also included as is a HP colour Deskjet printer. Hardware options include a Magneto-Optical disk storage system.

Lunar

Lunar produces two systems in this area of the market, DPX-MD and DPX-IQ with the MD variant being upgradable to IQ. These systems use K-edge filtration to obtain the two energies required. Both systems have a choice of scan bed length of 240 or 180 cm. The smaller bed size will permit both AP spine and femur scans, which are standard on both systems, but not whole body scanning which requires the larger bed and then comes as standard with both systems.

The DPX-MD carries out both spine and femur scans with a precision of 1% each examination carrying a radiation dose of 1 mR and taking approximately 4 minutes. Optional scan modes include lateral spine, forearm/hand, paediatric, orthopaedic and small animal. A Pentium computer running Windows 95 controls this system. Other formalities such as storage devices, printers and network compatibility can be supplied to specific requirements or budget.

The DPX-IQ is a faster and more precise variant of the MD utilising a higher output flux to achieve these benefits. In this system the AP spine acquisition takes 1 min at a precision of 0.5% and the femoral neck takes 2 min with 1% precision. Both examinations carry doses of <3 mR. Software and hardware options are as for the DPX-MD system.

Norland

Norland offers three systems, the Compact Eclipse and the full-sized XR-36, both of which are fully described by Wahner and Fogelman.[13] They are both capable of carrying out spine and femur scans in 2 and 3 min respectively with a dose of ~2.5 mR. The precision for AP spine scanning is 0.7–1.0% and for the femoral neck 0.9–1.2%. The systems use K-edge filtration to obtain the two energies required by DXA. Computer systems can be supplied to the user's requirements and additional facilities available include forearm, lateral spine and total body options although the latter, which includes body composition, is only available on the XR-36.

Recently, Norland have introduced the EXCELL densitometer. This system has faster scan times than the previous systems with AP spine and femur taking <1.5 and <2 min respectively. Precision is similar but with dose reduced to <1 mRem in high speed mode.

Fan Beam DXA Systems

Both Hologic and Lunar produce fan beam DXA systems which use solid state arrays of detectors and C-arm configurations to produce scans, which although incurring marginally higher doses, take considerably less time than pencil beam systems. The C-arm system allows rotation of the source-detector to facilitate imaging at different angles, notably lateral spine scans with the patient in the supine position.

An effect occurs due to fan beam geometry that is not present in pencil beam systems. Due to the fan of radiation both magnification and geometric distortion can take place. Fig. 2.7 shows that objects of the same size produce a larger image the nearer they are located to the source. It can be shown mathematically that although this has an effect on the measurement of both BMC and area the value of BMD is relatively unchanged.[13]

Reports generally have estimates of BMC and area calculated from knowledge of the bed position between source and detector and these measurements should be used with this effect in mind. BMD is relatively insensitive to this effect and manufacturers report in vivo precision values of 1% or less for its measurement. The available systems are outlined below.

Hologic

Hologic offer the QDR 4500 Acclaim series of fan beam densitometers which includes four models each with the option to upgrade to more advanced systems. All systems produce energies by the switched pulse system. The series starts with the QDR 4500C which is a compact system with a 86 cm by 51 cm imaging area

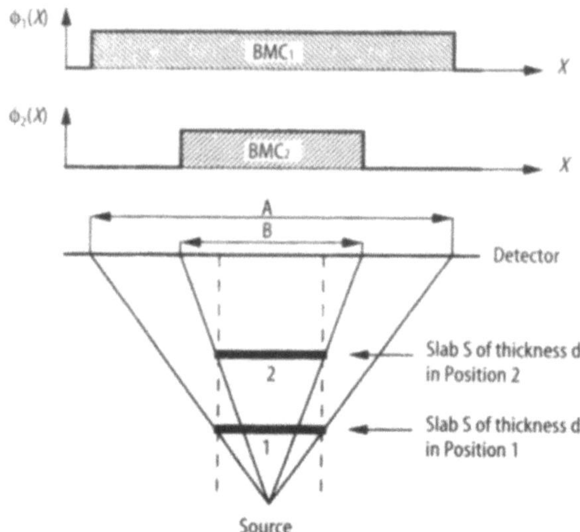

Figure 2.7 The effect of geometric distortion caused by fan-beam geometry on BMC and BMD. While BMC (represented by the hatched area) is proportional to the source-to-object distance, BMD is computed by dividing BMC by projected area and is not affected. (From Wahner and Fogelman[13] with permission.)

and capable of scanning both lumbar spine and hip. Spine and femur scans take approximately 15 seconds.

Next in this family is the QDR 4500 W offering a 195 cm × 66 cm scanning area with facilities of lumbar spine and hip scanning as before but also with whole body scanning in 6 min to measure bone mineral and body composition.

Third in the series is the QDR 4500 SL with a 96 cm × 65 cm scanning area. This system does not have total body scans but does have both lumbar spine and hip scans with an improved acquisition time of 10 seconds. The system does however carry out densitometric scans of the lumbar vertebrae with the patient in the supine position in a time of 2 min. It features the 'side by side' display of spatially synchronised PA and lateral views of the spine which helps in the identification of deformity and in the assessment of the validity of PA scan results.

The final system, the QDR 4500 A, has a scanning area of 195 cm × 65 cm, can carry out PA spine and femur scans in 10 seconds, whole body scans in 180 seconds and lateral spine densitometry scans in 120 seconds. A further research scan of the whole of the spine in the lateral aspect may be obtained with the patient in the supine position in 7.5 seconds using a single energy mode. This image is for morphometric analysis only, to identify wedge and crush fractures in the spine.

All systems have the option of forearm acquisitions in a time of 30 seconds.

Lunar

Lunar make the EXPERT XL fan beam densitometry system having a scan area of 198 cm × 64 cm and producing its two energies by filtration. Standard software allows AP spine and total femur acquisitions in 6 seconds. Additional software modules enable forearm/hand acquisition in 10 seconds, lateral spine densitometry with the subject supine in 24 seconds and total body acquisition in 160 seconds (both bone and body composition analysis). In the optional single energy mode a full lateral spine acquisition may be obtained in 38 seconds for morphometric analysis to show vertebral heights and deformations.

New in 1999 is the Lunar PRODIGY fan beam system. This system is a blend of pencil beam scanning and fan beam technology. The narrow fan beam lies along the axis of the patient and is scanned over the body in a rectilinear fashion. The use of a cadmium zinc-telluride array detector improves sensitivity considerably allowing faster scan times than pencil beam systems but with reduced patient dose levels compared to current fan beam systems. Typically an AP spine or femur scan takes 30 seconds with 5 min for a total body scan. A new facility introduced on this system is the ability to scan both femurs in a single acquisition.

Peripheral QCT

Norland produce the Stratec XCT 2000 peripheral QCT system. This is a single energy system working at a mean photon energy of 38 keV. Because the system is tomographic a single energy may be used to obtain bone density values with the subject in air. The system has a measurement diameter of 140 mm and although forearm acquisitions are the norm it does mean that the lower leg is accessible. Scans of the forearm take approximately 140 seconds and give a pixel size ranging from 100 μm to 800 μm. The images allow separate analysis of cortical and trabecular regions and thus small changes in trabecular content may be detected.

Compact Densitometry Systems

Two systems are currently available using DXA techniques but differing technology.

Lunar

Lunar offer peripheral DXA in a compact form with the PIXI (Peripheral instantaneous X-ray Imager) which utilises cone beam geometry and an optically coupled solid state imaging detector to acquire either forearm or heel scans in 5 seconds with a resolution of 0.2 mm $\times$ 0.2 mm per pixel. The two energies are obtained by dual energy supply (55 and 80 kVp) and imaging is carried out by capturing complete images at each energy in rapid succession. The manufacturers report short -term precision of 1% for the forearm and 0.8% for the os-calcis. This system is only just becoming available and few are in clinical use at the time of writing.

Norland

This company offers the pDEXA system for peripheral densitometry of the forearm. The system uses a scanning technique to acquire the forearm image in

Table 2.1. Characteristics of some current DXA systems

Maker	System	Site	Manufacturers Quoted		
			Time	Precision	Dose
Pencil Beam Systems					
Hologic	QDR4000	AP Spine	2.4 min	0.8–1.1%	3 – 5 mR
		Femur	3.6 min	1.4–1.7%	
Lunar	DPX-MD(IQ)	AP Spine	1–4 min	1%(0.5%)	1 mR(<3 mR)
		Femur	2–4 min	1%(1%)	
Norland	XR-36/Eclipse	AP Spine	2 min	0.7–1.0%	~2.5 mR
		Femur	3 min	0.9–1.2%	
	EXCELL	AP Spine	<1.5 min	1%	<1 mR
		Femur	<2.0 min	1.2%	<1 mR
Fan beam systems					
Hologic	QDR4500	AP Spine	10–15 s	1%	C and W 5 mR
		Femur	10–15 s	1%	SL and A 7 mR
Lunar	EXPERT-XL	AP Spine	6 s	1%	27 mrem
		Femur	6 s	1%	27 mrem
	PRODIGY	AP Spine	30 s	1%	3.7 mrem
		Femur	30 s	1%	3.5 mrem
Compact systems					
Lunar	PIXI	Forearm	5 s	1%	–
		Heel	5 s	0.8%	–
Norland	pDEXA	Forearm	5 min	2%	–

the distal third region in approximately 5 min. The system energies of 28 keV and 48 keV are derived by the use of a tin filter on a 60 kVp X-ray source. Pixel resolution is 1 mm × 1 mm. The accuracy of the technique is typically within 2.0%.

The information on current DXA systems is summarised in Table 2.1. These data concentrate, mainly on spine and femur measures as they are the two most commonly used in clinical practice.

Ultrasound Systems

Because of the appeal of portable, non-radiative systems a number of ultrasound systems are now being manufactured. As previously noted these systems do not measure bone density directly but SOS and BUA and as this chapter is concerned with bone density measurement, only a cursory review of these systems is given. The systems are divided into those using water bath and skin-contact techniques and the measurements carried out by each system noted. Further information may be obtained from the manufacturers.

Water Bath Systems

All systems measure both BUA and SOS and are designed to make measurements at the heel.

DMS UBIS5000 is a scanning system with in vivo precision of 0.5% for BUA and 0.25% for SOS and imaging resolution of 1 mm which may be improved to 0.125 mm. The system produces a scan image in the region of 85 mm × 85 mm in a time of 2 min.

LUNAR Achilles+ is a fixed transducer system with in vivo precision of 1.5%, which reports a quantity known as 'Stiffness', a combination of BUA and SOS, offering improved correlation with DXA results. Scans are completed in 4 min. A new FDA approved version of this system, Achilles Express, which maintains fixed separation transducers but uses fluid-filled contact pads, rather than a water bath, has just been introduced. The removal of the water bath has had two immediate effects; the system is considerably lighter (10 kg) and there is no water settling time, hence scans can be completed in 1 min. The system again measures 'Stiffness' but with a slightly poorer precision (2%) possibly due to the contact to the heel being made through silicon membranes. This system is completely stand-alone having no need for a controlling computer and a built in thermal printer gives a report, which includes a small reference graph.

Osteometer DTU-one is a scanning system offering in vivo precisions of 0.2% (SOS) and 1.6% (BUA). The imaging resolution is 0.5 mm on a scan region of 60 mm × 80 mm. Scans are of 4 min duration.

Contact Systems

Hologic Sahara measures BUA and SOS in the heel and by combination of these two quantities also calculates a qualitative ultrasound index (QUI) which can be a more diagnostically sensitive measurement of bone status and has a precision of 2 units. Scans take some 60 s and the system is portable having a weight of 7.5 kg plus a computer. This system is approved by the American Food and Drug Administration (FDA).

IGEA DBM sonic 1200 measures only SOS in the phalanges of each hand with a precision of 0.4%. This calliper-based system is highly portable with a weight of 6.5 kg and can be run without a computer as it has its own built-in controller and display. As each finger is measured the measurement time is longer than that for other systems at approximately 5 min. A new version of this system with built in data logging is just becoming available.

McCue CUBA Clinical measures both velocity of sound and BUA in the os calcis in a time of approximately 2 min. These quantities are reported with precisions of 0.03% and 0.68%, respectively. The transducers are positioned on the heel by means of servo-motors, thus ensuring a reproducible contact pressure. This portable system weighs 15 kg.

Myriad Soundscan Compact measures SOS in the tibia with a precision of 0.3%. Scan times are of the order of 2 min and the system uses a single multiple element transducer unit containing both transmitter and receiver. The system is portable weighing 5 kg and operating from a lap-top computer. The American FDA approves this system.

Sunlight Omnisense measures SOS at up to 70 skeletal sites including os calcis, neck of femur and vertebra. The manufacturers report reproducibilities of between 0.5% and 1.5% depending on measurement site. A single transducer unit is used and measurements can be obtained, again depending on site, in between 30 s and 3 min. The system is designed for desk-top use and weighs 11 kg.

Metra Biosystems QUS2 is a novel contact system that carries out a scan of the heel. This allows a region of interest to be placed on the calcaneus hence improving reproducibility. The system reports an ultrasound bone index based on the BUA to a precision of better than 2%. The system is highly portable, weighing only 3.2 kg, and is capable of operation from a rechargeable battery.

Quality Assurance

All the techniques that have been discussed here, in their various implementations by their manufacturers, generally include both a quality assurance phantom and software for the analysis of measurements made using the phantom. The initial purpose of such test objects and software is to assure that the measurement system is fully functional. Measurement and analysis of these objects usually takes place at the beginning of the day's measurement session and is valid for a period of 24 h. After this period it is generally necessary to repeat the quality assurance procedure in order to assess the condition of the measurement system. Significant variations from the previous day's values will usually meet with an error message.

The error bounds that the manufacturers' set for variations in day to day performance are generally sufficient to detect system failures. However, drift over a period of time, such as several months, may not provoke an error message as changes from day to day are generally so small that the quality assurance tests are all passed. It is important that operators of systems are aware of these problems and take measures to monitor the long-term behaviour of their measurement systems. Instructions for implementing such quality checks may be found in Pearson and Cawte[14] and Garland et al.[15]

The use of phantoms to achieve intersystem calibration is currently being evaluated and involves measuring a single standard phantom on a number of machines in order to compare the values obtained on each. The initial motivation for such comparison was for standardisation of results acquired during multi-centre drug trials. Having obtained these values from a standardised calibration object it is then possible to calibrate results obtained from the measurement of patients and of volunteers. If collection of reference data is carried out using systems at different sites, which have been calibrated using the same reference object, this would make possible the collection of standardised reference ranges and its use would confer a number of advantages. The first advantage would be the ability to compare measurements made on the same individual but on different machines. Such a situation may occur if a patient moved from one district to another and was subsequently measured on a different system. The second benefit is that the collection of such reference data would allow the identification of regions within a country where BMD values within the population were different from those in the general population. This may well have significance in the framing of health policy and in the allocation of resources to the regions.

Discussion

For many years researchers have compared BMD measurements at various sites in the body. Unsurprisingly significant correlations were found between, for example, the BMD value in the lumbar spine and the BMD value in the hip. Although significant these correlations were not strong enough to be predictive. Similar work has recently been done comparing ultrasonic measurements made in the os-calcis with bone mineral density measurements made at the spine and hip. As with the inter-site density comparisons, highly significant correlations were found which once again failed to reach predictive strength. These results tend to confirm the suspicion that if one wants to know the condition of bone at a particular site then the measurement should take place at that site.

More recently rather than looking at the correlation between values measured at different sites and by different modalities research has been directed towards assessing the ability of a particular measurement to predict risk of future fracture. Two large studies, one involving 6189 postmenopausal women of over 65 years age[16] and one involving 5662 elderly women of mean age 80.4 years,[17] have both shown that ultrasonic measurement of the os-calcis predicts the risk of hip fracture in this group of women as well as does DXA measurement of the hip. These interesting findings may well have influenced the American FDA to start approving ultrasound systems for the clinical measurement of bone. It is worth adding that this sort of analysis of the data appears to be far more clinically relevant than attempts to predict bone mineral density values at other sites from a single measurement made at one specific site.

Work is currently being carried out to determine the role for ultrasonic measurements in the clinical repertoire. Although much work still remains to be carried out the general feeling at this time seems to be that its place may be in primary care. This view may be reinforced by the fact that the systems making these measurements carry no radiation burden, are generally light and are also portable making them ideal for use in the community. As can be seen from the two major studies previously mentioned the ability to predict future fracture risk has only been validated in postmenopausal women older than 65 years. Until further research work has been carried out it may be difficult to justify the use of such systems to measure women in younger age groups, particularly women who are perimenopausal.

Currently there is little doubt that DXA measurement of the lumbar spine and femur is the "gold standard" for identifying patients with osteoporosis. This view was both confirmed and encouraged by the 1994 WHO report on the assessment of fracture risk.[12] However, the cost of such systems makes it unlikely that they will be seen on a regular basis in primary care. All things considered one of the pencil beam systems is likely to be the instrument of choice for use in osteoporosis clinics in district general hospitals. Fan beam systems are currently relatively expensive compared to other modalities and are likely to be confined to research establishments in the near future. Clinicians may be better served by considering the ability of a given system to predict future fracture rather than to define osteoporosis, which will automatically limit them to the DXA systems. As noted above, although the different modalities seem to identify different "at risk" populations they all seem to have the ability to predict future fracture in these populations implying that each is telling us something different about our subjects. Recent work using modalities together has shown increased power to predict fracture when both modalities give "low" values. This synergy should be exploited, where possible, to further benefit the patient. In these terms it seems unwise to rate one modality as inherently "better" than any other as they seem to offer different and complementary information. Similar arguments may be used when considering the use of axial or peripheral measurements. There is little doubt that site specific fracture risk prediction is best served by measurement at that particular site. However, general fracture risk prediction, independent of site, can be achieved by measurement at either peripheral or axial sites. Again, it seems likely that multiple sites may give incremental rather than conflicting information.

The interpretation of bone mineral density measurements is considered in Chapter 4, however there is much current debate about the use of reference data in which to set the individual result. Differences in reference data have been noted between the three major DXA manufacturers; Hologic, Lunar and Norland, and a method for standardisation of spinal BMD results has been suggested.[18] It has been suggested that femoral BMD values could be normalised to the National Health and Nutritional Examination Surveys (NHANES) III data set as presented by Looker et al.[19] Although neither of these suggestions has as yet been universally adopted) there is an obvious need for results to be interpreted in both a rigorous and reproducible manner. The newest scanners from Hologic, Lunar and Norland all give the user the opportunity to base reports on the NHANES III data.

Current practice involves reporting of BMD values compared to the mean BMD value for a young normal subject. If a reference value is selected to accord with local conditions it should be borne in mind that both the mean value and the standard deviation about it may vary from both manufacturers reference values and the reference values obtained in the locations. Such changes, particularly in the standard deviation, can lead to quite different values of T-score being obtained by the use of different reference values. Such problems lead once again to the conclusion that rigorous and reproducible methods of reporting bone mineral density are required. To this end, Bona Fide an associate of the Lunar Corporation has recently produced a slide rule system to convert measurements made on Hologic systems into a standard T-score expressed as a function of Lunar, Hologic or NHANES III data.

More interest is being directed towards the healthy growth and mineralisation of bone in children. Currently this is predominantly an area for research. Several points are, however, evident. Firstly, the use of T-score reporting is entirely inappropriate as it does not take developmental age into account. Secondly, reference ranges for both boys and girls are required. Such ranges should take into account both body habitus and pubertal status. Thirdly, but by no means finally, there will be concerns about applying even the very small radiation doses associated with DXA to children. Under these circumstances ultrasonic evaluation may be the only socially acceptable way forward.

Body composition measurements are becoming more common, driven by an interest in the balance of fat and lean in individuals with eating disorders or with diseases known to affect body composition balance such as acquired immunodeficiency syndrome (AIDS). Various therapies are also suspected of causing changes in body composition and frequently a measurement of body composition will be required as an outcome measure in a study of therapy. If such measures are required then the choice will be DXA.

I hope that this brief introduction to the various technologies will give the reader a flavour of what is available and the relative benefits of each technology. The starting point for all of us should be to consider what patient groups confront us and what measurements we would find useful before we purchase a measurement system. Sometimes this is very obviously not the way purchasing decisions have been made with either novelty or the power of many functions attracting the buyer rather than the ability to address a specific problem. This has led to many research systems languishing, mainly unused or unusable, in clinical departments when a simpler, more suitable device would have been in full-time use.

References

1. Hodge HC, vanHuysen G, Warren SL (1935) Factors influencing the quantitative measurement of the Roentgen ray absorption of tooth slabs. Am J Roentgenol 34:523–528.
2. Mack PB, Vogt FB (1939) A method for estimating the degree of mineralisation of bones from tracings of roentgenograms. Science 89:467.
3. Ardran GM (1951) Bone destruction not demonstrable by radiography. Br J Radiogr 24:107.
4. Cameron JR, Sorenson J (1963) Measurement of bone mineral in-vivo: an improved method. Science 142:230–234.
5. Reed GW (1966) Measurement of bone mineralisation from the relative transmission of ^{241}Am and ^{137}Cs radiation. Phys Med Biol 11:174.
6. Krokowski E (1970) Calcium determination in the skeleton by means of X-ray beams of different energies. In Jelliffe AM, Strickland B (eds) Symposium ossium, Livingstone, Edinburgh.
7. Cann CE, Genant HK (1980) Precise measurement of vertebral mineral content using computed tomography. J Comput Assist Tomogra 4:493–500.
8. Schlenker RA, vonSeggen WW (1976) The distribution of cortical and trabecular bone mass along the lengths of the radius and ulna and the implications for in-vivo bone mass measurements. Calcif Tissue Res 20:41–52.
9. Langton CM (1987) Critical analysis of the ultrasonic interrogation of bone and future developments. In: Palmer SB, Langton CM (eds) Ultrasonic studies of bone, IOP Publishing, Bristol, pp 73–89.
10. Ouyang X, Selby K, Lang P, et al. (1997) High resolution magnetic resonance imaging of the calcaneus: age related changes in trabecular structure and comparison with dual X-ray absorptiometry measurements. Calcif Tissue Int 60:139–147.
11. Singh M, Nagrath AR, Maini PS (1970) Changes in trabecular pattern of the upper end of the femur as an index of osteoporosis. J Bone Joint Surg 52A:457–467.
12. WHO (1994) Assessment of fracture risk and its application to screening for postmenopausal osteoporosis. WHO Technical Report Series 843, WHO, Geneva.
13. Wahner HW, Fogelman I (1999) The evaluation of osteoporosis: dual energy x-ray absorptiometry in clinical practice. Martin Dunitz, London.
14. Pearson D, Cawte SA (1997) Long-term quality control of DXA: a comparison of Shewart rules and Cusum charts. Osteoporosis Int 7:338–343.
15. Garland SW, Lees B, Stevenson JC (1997) DXA longitudinal quality control: a comparison of inbuilt quality assurance, visual inspection, multi-rule Shewart charts and Cusum analysis. Osteoporosis Int 7:231–237.
16. Bauer DC, Gluer CC, Cauley JA et al. (1997) Broadband ultrasound attenuation predicts fractures strongly and independently of densitometry in older women. A prospective study. Arch Int Med 157:629–634.
17. Hans D, DArgent-Molina P, Scott AM et al. (1996) Ultrasonographic heel measurements to predict hip fracture in elderly women. The EPIDOS prospective study. Lancet 348:511–514.
18. Genant HK, Grampp S, Gluer CC et al. (1994) Universal standardisation for dual X-ray absorptiometry: Patient and phantom cross-calibration results. J Bone and Miner Res 9:1503–1514.
19. Looker AC, Wahner HW, Dunn WL et al. (1995) Proximal femur bone mineral levels of US adults. Osteoporosis Int 5:389–409.
20. Truscott JG, Devlin J, Emery P (1996) Imaging techniques. 2 Modern methods. Baillieres Clin Rheumatol 10.
21. Woolf AD, Dixon AStJ (1988) Osteoporosis: a clinical guide. NMartin Dunitz: London.
22. Palmer SB, Langton CM (1987) Ultrasonic studies of bone. IOP Publishing: Bristol.

3 Methodological and Reporting Considerations

D.S. Simpson and J.G. Truscott

Introduction

Reference data have a major impact on our daily lives in many ways. Clinical measurements of various sorts are used to assess our health: are we too heavy; is our blood pressure too high; is our blood cholesterol normal? All these judgements are based on comparison of the measurement to accepted reference data sets.

Two simple examples will serve to illustrate some of the factors we may wish to consider when using reference data. First let us consider the reference value for driving speed in a built up area – where the speed limit is 30 mph. This reference level has been determined by an outside body as being applicable to certain roads. Several considerations in the application of this limit will be considered which have similarities with dual-enery X-ray absorptiometry (DXA) bone mineral densiometry (BMD) ranges.

Firstly how is the data point measured? We have a speedometer in our car, but how accurate is it? also how reproducible is it? will it register different values on different occasions when we are travelling at 30 mph? If a radar speed gun is used by a policeman at the kerb side will it give the same answer as the car speedometer? If not, is the difference significant? If it is, which system is giving the "correct" answer? [Of course it is always the police system! (This is the concept of the "gold standard").] This illustrates the sort of problems that are associated with the measurement systems.

Another set of problems is associated with interpretation. Here context is of vital importance. Usually whether we drive at 29 or 31 mph in a 30 mph area is unimportant – particularly if the system for measurement is relatively insensitive to such differences. However, few people would dispute that driving at 60 mph in this zone would be dangerous. However, driving at the permitted speed may also be dangerous if the conditions were those of a wet, foggy, dark evening in late winter, driving past a school when children are leaving. These sorts of conditions mirror the judgements which must be made, in context, by a clinician faced with the results of a bone density scan.

The second example which will be dealt with in the next section, concerns the obtaining of reference data. Here the example above is inappropriate as the reference value of 30 mph is imposed by an external body.

We also need to consider, when we carry out a DXA scan, what a BMD measurement will be used for. If we are unsure we should perhaps examine our need for the scan in the first place. If we need to diagnose osteoporosis or osteopenia, then we will need to compare our scan to a reference data set which is appropriate. If we wish to assess fracture risk we will need to examine the scan value in the context of both the reference range and the known relationships between BMD values and fracture incidence.

If, however, we wish to monitor the changes in BMD in an individual with either disease or therapy then reference ranges may not be necessary as we can gain the information we need by performing a number of scans over a period of time and assessing their behaviour relative to one another.

What Are Reference Ranges?

The introduction referred to a reference value, the speed limit, rather than a reference range. So how do the two differ? Reference ranges are designed to somehow reflect what is "normal" in the population under consideration. This means that in order to construct such ranges an underlying definition of "normality" is needed. Because populations have diversity we need to determine what members of the "normal" population are suitable for inclusion in or exclusion from the proposed reference range. We also need to consider whether the quantity we are measuring varies with age, in which case age-related reference ranges must be established by measuring sufficient people across the age range where changes are likely.

Similarly hormonal changes may influence the measured value and conditions such as puberty or menopause may need to be considered in the collection of data for the reference range. Data may need to be collected for a specific system if

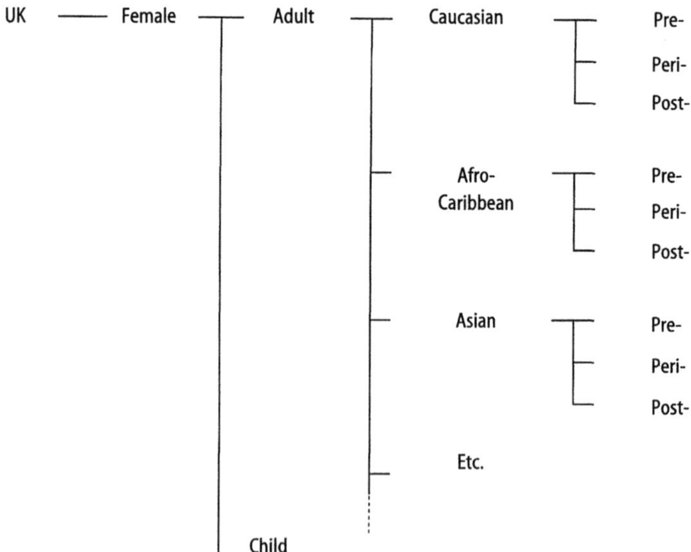

Figure 3.1 Potential UK female populations requiring reference ranges.

differences between systems exist. Also ranges for each sex and each ethnic group will possibly be required. This means that the number of ranges that are likely to be needed will soon proliferate as is shown in Fig. 3.1.

Further to all these considerations we must establish whether the quantity is likely to change with time. An example of this would be the height of 16 year olds, which has been steadily increasing over the last 100 years. The rate at which these changes occur will govern how frequently it will be necessary construct new reference ranges.

In summary, the reference range will define the diversity existing within the "normal" population. This it will do by means of a representative sample drawn from this population. Quantitative limits should be produced about any "normal" value which will allow us to judge the significance of any measured value which departs from this reference.

From the above, very general outline it can be seen that the establishing of such ranges is by no means a trivial undertaking and a good deal of thought about both the necessity for and the gathering of new data needs to be done before embarking upon such an undertaking.

Some Simple Mathematics Used in the Interpretation of DXA Measurements

This section deals with the terms which are frequently used when DXA systems, or indeed many of the other bone measurement techniques, are interpreted. Some of the terms refer to variability in system performance (precision and accuracy), some refer to the interpretation of an individual's result compared to reference data (T-score v Z-score) and one refers to the ability to detect the change in an individuals BMD over a period of time (least significant difference). These terms will be explained in context and simple methodologies given for their calculations.

Precision

The terms precision and reproducibility are used interchangeably in the interpretation of DXA scans and mean the same thing. In bald terms they refer to the ability of a DXA system to produce the same result when measuring the same thing, time after time. As an analogy imagine an archer shooting arrows repeatedly at a target. If all the arrows land closely together then the precision or reproducibility is good, if they are scattered all over the target then the precision or reproducibility is poor.

As scientists, however, we require a quantitative method of measuring precision which will allow the performance of various systems to be compared rather than the qualitative terms "good" and "poor" mentioned above. There are many ways of calculating the precision of a system but just one simple way for in vivo precision measurement is outlined below.[1] The formula may at first glance look intimidating but it is little more than a recipe for carrying out the calculation.

The methodology is to make the same measurement on an individual, twice, at the same visit (e.g. two femur scans) using exactly the same set up. Call these measurements a and b. We should make these paired measurements on a number of individuals (n), ideally more than 10, usually 20 or so will be sufficient to ensure a reasonably representative value. The reproducibility may then be calculated as the coefficient of variation (CV) which is expressed as a percentage.

$$CV\% = 100 \sqrt{\frac{\sum_{i=1}^{i=n}(a_i - b_i)^2}{2n}} \bigg/ \frac{\bar{a}+\bar{b}}{2}$$

where $\bar{a}$ is the mean value of all the first measurements and $\bar{b}$ is the mean of all the second measurements. a_i and b_i indicate the first and second measurements on person number i, respectively. The symbol Σ indicates that we should take the sum of the squared differences for all the people measured. Typical values for precision on DXA systems range from 0.5% to 3% depending on instrument and measurement site. Because each pair of measurements is obtained at the same visit this is often referred to as short-term precision.

The scheme cannot be used to measure long-term precision because of the biological variation of people over time. We could, however, use the same scheme to calculate the in vitro precision over time by measuring inert phantoms of known BMD at various intervals and calculating the CV% which would be indicative of system variability over that period. The short-term in vivo precision (P_s) and long-term in-vitro precision (P_l) may then be added in quadrature, according to the theory of error propagation to give an estimate of long-term precision in vivo (P) as follows:-

$$P = \sqrt{P_s^2 + P_l^2}$$

which is a good indicator for most purposes and it will be found that in good quality systems P_s will predominate.

Accuracy

The term accuracy refers to the ability of a system in making a measurement, to produce an answer which is close to the 'real' value of the quantity being measured.

By revisiting the analogous archer and examining the target once again we may note where his arrows cluster relative to the "bulls-eye". If they are close to it or in it then they are accurate, otherwise they are not. Again a quantitative rather than qualitative method is sought to express accuracy.

A method that has frequently been used is to measure a range of bones of varying densities in a water bath to obtain a set of calculated BMD values. The bones are then defatted to remove the marrow and then baked in an oven to reduce them to ash. The mass of this bone ash is then accepted as the "real" value of bone mineral. The system is then calibrated so that the measured BMD is as near as possible to the "real" BMD. The variability which is left about the calibration curve then defines the accuracy of the system.

It is unusual to embark on this sort of calibration exercise for a commercial system as the experiment will already have been performed by the manufacturer. The measurement of reference materials in daily quality assurance routines enables small drifts in the equipment to be compensated for thus maintaining the system accuracy over long periods of time.

Z-Score

In the reference range construction, detailed below, the collected data are summarised in the form of a mean value and the standard deviation (SD) about that value for each age, or band of ages, included in the range.

The Z-score quantifies how far a BMD measurement, on a subject, departs from the mean value for that subject's age. This departure is quantified in terms of the number of SDs from the mean value as follows:

$$Z-score = \frac{subject\ BMD\ -\ age\text{-}matched\ mean}{age\text{-}matched\ SD}$$

with a negative Z-score indicating a BMD lower than the mean for that particular age. This implies that the same BMD value could give different Z-scores depending on the subjects age. This is because the reference mean value changes with age, and in some cases so may the SD. This type of scoring system is felt to be particularly appropriate for BMD values in children and the elderly. The reasons for this are explained later.

Traditionally a Z-score between +1 and –1 has been considered "normal" between –1 and –2 as "osteopenic" and below –2 as "osteoporotic". Although fairly well accepted these cut-off levels are somewhat arbitrary.

T-Score

Like the Z-score the T-score expresses a difference between reference values and subject value in terms of SDs. In this case, however, the mean used is that for "young normal" data which is composed of reference data for 20–39 year olds. A single value of mean and SD is calculated for this entire group and is used for calculation as follows:

$$T-score = \frac{subject\ BMD\ -\ young\ normal\ mean}{young\ normal\ SD}$$

A negative T-score indicates a BMD level below that of the mean. With this reference system a certain value of BMD should always give the same T-score, irrespective of age, as the mean and SD used for calculation are invariant. The implications of this factor are discussed later in this chapter.

Both the WHO[2] and the UK Advisory Group on Osteoporosis[3] agreed on the interpretation of T-scores in diagnosis. A T-score above –1 is treated as normal, between –1 and –2.5 as being indicative of bone loss (osteopenia) and below –2.5 as constituting osteoporosis.

An obvious problem with the use of the T-score is that it classifies nearly all women over the age of 70 as being either osteopenic or osteoporotic and thus fails to help in the clinical management of these subjects.

Least Significant Difference

Our ability to detect changes in BMD in an individual over a period of time is intimately tied up with the reproducibility of our systems. One could envisage a problem occurring when we have measured a difference over, for example, a one-year period of 1% and must decide whether such a difference is significant or not. Remembering that precision measures the variability within the system's ability to reproducibly measure the same BMD, we may conclude that the difference we have measured is due solely to system variability and not to a time change in BMD.

The concept of the least significant difference (LSD) that can be detected may be defined as:

$$\text{LSD} = 2 \times \sqrt{2} \text{ (System precision)}$$

which is expressed as a percentage. Under this definition we may have 95% confidence ($p < 0.05$) that a difference in measured BMD which exceeds the LSD is a true change in mineral content. Thus in the example given above the LSD would be $2 \times \sqrt{2} \times 1\% = 2.83\%$. This gives us a quantitative method for assessing the significance of observed BMD changes in an individual over time.

How BMD Reference Ranges be Developed

In broad terms, the requirements that might be necessary for the construction of reference ranges were examined earlier. This section looks at the specific ways in which these broad principles could be implemented in the collection of reference data for the construction of BMD ranges.

A patient's BMD, rather than their bone mineral content (BMC), is normally used in establishing reference ranges. Engelke et al.[4] in looking at the factors influencing the precision of DXA measurements describe why they believe the use of BMD is advantageous compared with BMC.

Densitometry Systems

The first restriction will be that of system availability. It is not currently possible to produce ubiquitous ranges using a single manufacturers equipment and we are restricted to producing reference data for a specific type and make of equipment (e.g LUNAR DPX series or HOLOGIC QDR).

Ethnic Groupings

The next consideration should be the selection of the ethnic grouping for whom we wish to develop a reference range. Britain is a multicultural, multiethnic society and thus it is unlikely that a single reference range will accommodate the entire population. Data are rarely collected for African or Afro-Caribbean populations as this ethnic grouping has generally high BMD values and is perceived as being at low risk of fracture. Of the groupings a large amount of data are available on Caucasians although both regional and national variations have been noted. Asian and oriental data are relatively poorly represented particularly where these ethnic groups are not living in their country of origin. As an example we may like to consider whether separate ranges may be required in the UK for Asians born in the subcontinent and those born in the UK.

The findings in the USA have led to Indian Asians born in the US being included in the Caucasian reference ranges. This highlights the point that we must be very specific in defining exactly what we mean by any ethnic classification.

Sex (Gender)

The next point is relatively straight forward: do we wish to develop ranges for males or females individually or will combined ranges be suitable?

Age Range

The next consideration is the age range we wish to cover in our reference data. The simplest data to gather could be young 'normal' data upon which T-score reporting is based. This comprises the mean BMD value for 20–39-year olds (where BMD is assumed to be relatively invariant with age) and the standard deviation about that mean.

The age range 40–70 years includes the menopause in females and Fig. 3.2 shows what happens in the age range about the mean age at menopause (51 years). Here the variability in the data is quite marked and can be attributed to the wide range of ages at which the menopause occurs. Menopause is accompanied by a rapid bone loss phase and it is the differences in age of onset of this phase that is chiefly responsible for this increased variance in the data.

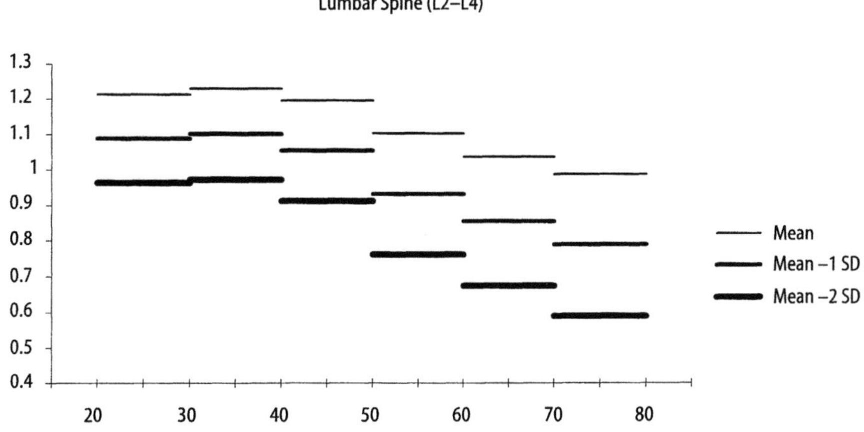

Figure 3.2 Typical plot of decade lumbar spine (L2–L4) BMD. (Source of data is that used for three year moving averages for lumbar spine BMD in Truscott et al.[8]

Similarly, puberty is associated with a rapid increase in BMD due to hormonal activity. Once again the onset of puberty occurs at a range of ages as does the achievement of any of the pubertal stages. This implies that a range based on age alone would have a high degree of variability in this group.

In the age range above 70 it may be difficult to find sufficient subjects who meet our criteria for normality. A small sample size will result in a wide degree of variability in the data.

Currently large amounts of data have been collected for the young normal and peri-menopausal periods in females. Current interest is centred on men, older women (where data are sparse), and children for whom measurement software has only recently become available.

Regional, National or International Ranges

It is hoped that by now the reader may be aware of the pitfalls involved in trying to produce international reference ranges. The types of range which currently exist are examined below where it is noted that there are also likely to be differences between regions within the UK. Where such differences exist, regional rather than national reference ranges should be considered. The interesting Catch-22 to this argument is that regional ranges need to be established in order to cater for regional variations, the need for which can only be initially established by comparing regional data with national data!

Inclusion and Exclusion Criteria

The topics discussed above define the broad inclusion criteria for our reference data. Our definition of normality within these inclusions is usually based on a proscriptive list of exclusions. Several are listed here that are in regular use, interested readers may care to construct their own lists: Endocrine disorders, adrenal disorders, malignancy, chronic gastrointestinal or liver disease, Paget's disease, diabetes, rheumatoid arthritis, renal stones, steroid therapy, anticonvulsant drugs, sodium fluoride, heparin, thyroxine, hysterectomy, oophorectomy, prolonged bedrest or hip/spine/wrist fracture. This list is by no means exhaustive and consideration could be given to early/late menopause and whether or not use of hormone replacement therapy (HRT) is now considered 'normal'.

The numbers of subject measurements which are needed for each section of the range is also a consideration. Many statistical techniques are available (e.g. power calculations) to determine the required numbers to an apparently high degree of accuracy. The bottom-line is that "enough" subjects are needed in each band however many that might be. We would suggest, as a rule of thumb, that enough data have been acquired when both the mean and more importantly the standard deviation are virtually invariant to the addition of further data.

Construction of Reference Ranges

Having collected all the data subject to the conditions given above, what do we do with it? Fig. 3.2 has shown one way of dealing with the data – that of decade means. Here the data are banded in 10-year intervals and the mean and SD calculated and plotted as shown. As noted before there is an increase in SD about the menopause. This would imply that in order to be declared osteoporotic using a Z-score the actual loss of BMD would need to be larger than that required in other age bands. This is one of the reasons why the WHO criteria for diagnosis are based on the T-score. Reducing the age band from 10 years to 5 years goes some way towards mediating this effect. An improved method involves the use of the 'moving average'. In this technique the mean and SD values are calculated, for example, in a three year band centred around a certain age (e.g. for a centre age

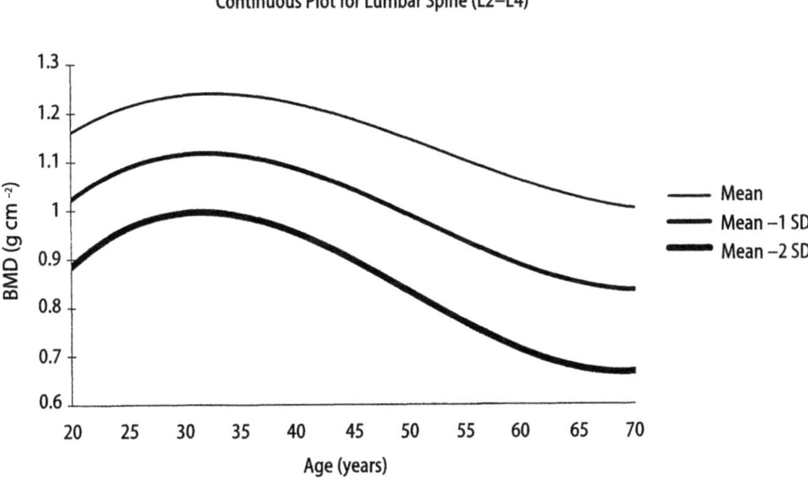

Figure 3.3 Typical continuous plot for lumbar spine (L2–L4) BMD (Source of data is that used for three year moving averages for lumbar spine BMD in Truscott et al.[8]

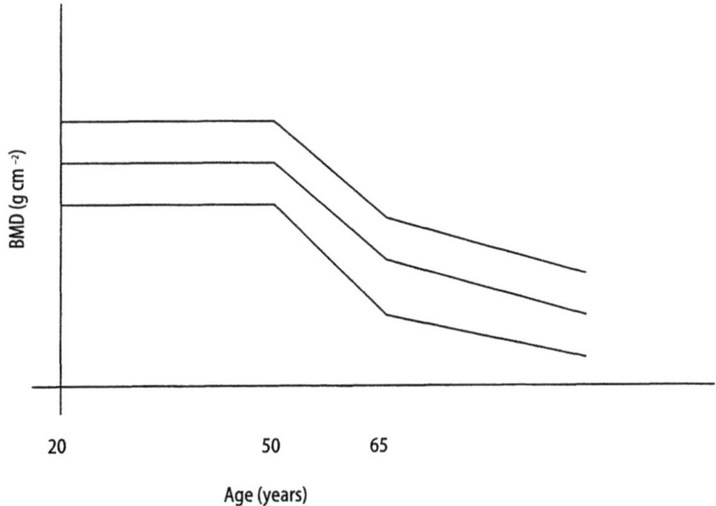

Figure 3.4 Piecewise linear fit to female data.

of 30 years, data for 29 and 31 would also be included). The centre age is moved by one year and a new mean and SD for the three-year band is calculated. This has the effect of smoothing out major jumps in the data caused by sampling noise. This can be further reduced by fitting curves to the data for means and standard deviations as shown in Fig. 3.3. Another method, favoured by some manufacturers, is the piecewise linear fit, such as shown in Fig. 3.4. This necessitates fitting three straight lines to the data, for women, one for young normal, one perimenopausal and one postmenopausal. Usually a single value for SD is assumed and fitted throughout.

Codicil

Currently, BMD values are reported to three decimal places. There is a danger that if any machine reports a value to three decimal places then the user believes the answer has to be 'correct', that all figures have a significance and the values are not to be questioned. Taking into account the reproducibility of the scanner (1–2%), and any possible operator error, what can be said about this precise figure is that there is a very high probability that it is precisely wrong. Remembering the concept of least significant difference presented on p. 42 the reader may safely discard the third decimal place and certainly should not use it as a basis for clinical decision making. A start towards encouraging this in future would be to produce our reference data to only two places of decimals.

Reference Ranges Currently Available to DXA Users

A quick review of the literature should reveal to the reader a large number of studies purporting to contain 'normal' data. Closer examination will, however, show that the majority of these studies contain small numbers of subjects and that these subjects were often chosen as controls for clinical studies where the criterion for normality was solely absence of the study target disease. For our purposes these data should be discarded in favour of the larger prospective studies designed specifically to obtain reference data. Several studies of this nature have been reported and representative ones from each category; local, multicentre and national, will be examined. Firstly, however, we will look at a typical range developed and distributed by a DXA manufacturer.

Reference Data Supplied by the DXA System Manufacturer

Over the years all of the DXA system manufacturers have collected reference data. Initially data were collected prospectively by the manufacturers themselves. Some of these data had been collected using the older dual photon absorptiometry (DPA) systems and converted, by cross-calibration, for use on DXA systems. Some of the data were collected by them directly on DXA systems utilising all the criteria for collection listed above. Further to this, data have also been supplied by users and researchers around the world for inclusion in the reference databases which are supplied with the DXA systems.

Individual databases are now supplied for both males and females and also for a wide range of ethnic groupings which were initially classified by terms such as Caucasian, Asian, etc. but which now are, in the case of Lunar systems, defined by the country of origin of the data (Australia to USA). These reference data have grown over the years and have been tailored in response to the needs of the users in each country.

Initially, the reference data were collected for women in the age ranges about the menopause, as those were the subjects most frequently measured by such systems. In fact these systems were initially produced in response to the problem of perimenopausal bone loss and the consequent associated increase in fracture risk.

The utility of these systems in the measurement of other subjects was soon recognised and many other groups were included relatively quickly. Such groupings encompassed older women (where fracture incidence is high), men (where osteoporosis is becoming more prevalent), young adults (where peak bone mass is an indicator of future fracture risk) and currently children (where failure to mineralise properly is indicative of future bone problems), This means that in the very near future we can expect to have supplied, with any system we purchase, reference data which are specific to our country and covering any age range for which we are interested, from the cradle to the grave.

Locally Collected Reference Data

When DXA systems first became available the reference data supplied were mainly based on samples from the US population. The reason for this was that these systems were, and in the main still are, manufactured in the US.

In response to this, users in the UK started to accumulate their own reference data. The majority of these data were gathered prospectively and based around the criteria discussed above. Typical of these types of data collection are the Leeds Female Caucasian reference data[5] based on 329 normal women, gathered by one of the authors. Many similar studies have been performed both in the UK,[6] and Continental Europe.[7] These references are not meant to be exhaustive or indeed representative but just offer examples of the type of study one may encounter.

In many cases the data from these local studies have been incorporated into the manufacturers' databases to give national data.

Another reason for gathering local data has been to obtain local ethnic data. Examples of reasons for this may include determining whether Asians born in the UK have different bone mineralisation from those born on the Indian sub-continent, or whether Caucasian women living in Birmingham are different from those living in Dundee. If differences are found in these data they may well have implications for interpretation of an individual DXA scan and also if a specific geographical region has reference data which are significantly different from those of surrounding regions there may be public health implications of such findings to be considered.

In the current situation, more and more, the clinical interpretation of results may be based on data gathered from the country provided by the manufacturers. However, for the reasons stated above, gathering regional reference data is a legitimate research exercise both for identifying secular population trends and for public health issues.

Combination of Reference Data from Multiple Centres

Often, in order to create reference range data which can be used on a national basis, the data obtained from several sites have been combined. However, before such combination is undertaken it is necessary to ensure the following. First, the subjects must all have been chosen in the same way; that is that all the criteria listed on p. 44 have been fulfilled.

Secondly any variation between the DXA machine at each of the sites must have been allowed for. This is usually done by performing scans on a single reference test object at each of the sites, and using the BMD values from these scans to calibrate the systems to some notional norm. All DXA results on a system will be converted using the appropriate calibration factor. Having removed the variability in the data due to system variation, the data obtained on each system should be checked against that from all other systems before pooling the data. Any group of data that is significantly different, although interesting, should be excluded.

A very simple plan for this type of data combination has been proposed by the authors[8] but many other ways are proposed in the literature and we recommend a thorough survey to identify a methodology which would best suit the data available.

As mentioned earlier, there are a whole series of factors that have to be taken into account when determining reference ranges and, as a consequence, there is a need to standardise the data. The European Community's COMAC-BME group and the International DXA Standardisation Committee have proposed different methods. Simmons et al.[9] compared two methods on a group of 2000 patients. The difficulties of standardising data are illustrated very clearly when they report "Considering the effects of both reference data and standardisation techniques together, there was a wide variation of patient classification, with the number of patients classified as osteoporotic varying from 9.6% to 21.1% for the postero-anterior spine L2-L4 region and from 2.3% to 27.6% for the femoral neck". These findings illustrate how important it is that a BMD measurement should only be used as one factor, albeit an important one, in determining a patient's management.

A further complication in the determination of reference ranges is the apparent difference in normal BMD ranges between different parts of the country. In England a number of studies have been published which indicate local/regional variations.[6,8] As these studies tried to eliminate calibration error, there is either a true local/regional variation or bias may have been introduced due to different selection criteria or subject responses at the various sites. It is known that there are regional variations in the frequency of heart disease, for example, so a regional variation in BMD may similarly exist.

Whether these differences are due to variation in socioeconomic, environmental or other factors is still to be determined. When using regional ranges care is needed in interpretation of longitudinal results for patients who move from one region to another.

Whether these combined ranges of data are suitable for general use is still a matter for debate, however, the very act of collecting such information may well reveal regional differences in BMD which may have public health implications, making the exercise useful in itself.

NHANES Reference Data

The National Centre for Health Statistics (NCHS)[10] in the United States, has for many years undertaken National Health and Nutritional Examination Surveys (NHANES), the purpose of which is "the collection and dissemination of health and nutrition data, obtained best or only by direct physical examination, clinical and laboratory tests, and related measurement procedures". Part of these studies has involved bone densitometry measurements. The first NHANES involved over 32,000 individuals and was conducted between 1971 and 1975 with the latest survey (NHANES III) undertaken between 1988 and 1994. A number of epidemiological follow-up studies (NHEFS) have also been conducted. An indication of the complexity of these surveys can be gauged by the "Analytic and Reporting Guidelines" of NHANES III which stretched to some 50 pages.

Papers containing reference data based on the NHANES III data have been published[11] containing data about mineralisation in adults from various ethnic groupings. The densitometry was performed using three Hololgic QDR 1000 densitometers in mobile installations.

Initially these data were only suitable for use on Hologic systems in the USA. Work by Genant et al.[12] demonstrated a method of universal standardisation suitable for comparing results from the three major densitometry manufacturers: Hologic, Lunar and Norland. Notwithstanding this Faulkner et al.[13] pointed out that there were still differences between the normative data supplied by the manufacturers leading to different reporting for a comparable BMD obtained in each of the systems. Because of this problem the manufacturers are attempting to introduce NHANES reference data for use on their machines, which should lead, in time, to standard reporting in the USA.

Although there are similarities between US and European reference data there is a reluctance, on the part of the UK bone densitometry community, to base reporting on US data. A need for a UK, or European, equivalent to the NHANES databases is clear and it is important to work towards the acquisition of such data which could then be used on any or all densitometry systems.

What Reference Data Would We Really Like?

In some ways this question has already been addressed in the section on the construction of reference ranges. However, to reinforce these ideas we should look at a potential shopping list of reference data. Within the UK there is no equivalent to the NHANES type of study which covers both ethnic groupings and adult male and female data. A study of this type, not confined to a single machine manufacturer, would be invaluable in allowing consistent reporting to uniform data sets. Also, such a study would reveal regions where BMD was predominantly different from those in the rest of the country.

Within such a study an attempt could be made to document the changes in BMD around the menopause, perhaps by producing ranges of BMD in terms of years since menopause rather than chronological age. Such a study should also give consideration to obtaining sufficient data on older people to make these ranges reliable.

The recent increase in interest in bone mineralisation in early life has made the development of reference ranges for children a matter of some urgency. Poor diet and increasing inactivity in young people is leading to a failure to achieve the maximum potential bone mass at maturity. This in turn is increasing the risk of fractures in later life. It is essential that reference ranges are developed, especially for puberty where large bone mineral changes are occurring, against which we may judge an individuals bone development. These assessments in early life give an opportunity to influence peak bone mass, by adjusting life style and diet, and may help to prevent fractures later in life. There is little doubt that we can make a major impact at this stage and the development of such ranges is a matter of some urgency.

Presentation of Results

Tabular/Graphical Approach

Apart from recording the BMD values, one of the main functions of reporting should be to help the clinician interpret the figures. One important aspect of this is how the reference range is presented. All the common methods of reporting BMD (tabular, Z-scores, T-scores, percentiles) rely to a large extent on the mean and SD of a selected age range. As a rule of thumb, if a person's BMD is not less than 1 SD below the mean then no action is taken, if it is between 1 SD and 2 SD below the mean then action is most probably required and if it is more than 2 SD below the mean then action is almost certainly required.

A typical tabular form consists of two tables; one for the lumbar spine (L2-L4) and one for the femoral neck. Each line of the table would represent one decade and give the mean, mean –1 SD and mean –2 SD for that decade, e.g.

20–29   Mean   Mean –1 SD   Mean –2 SD

The clinician would then compare their patient's BMD with the appropriate entry in the table and use that in helping to determine treatment or investigation.

One particular difficulty with this approach concerns the 50–60 age range. This range naturally contains pre-, peri- and postmenopausal women. As the menopause, and the approach of the menopause, is known to affect a woman's BMD it is not surprising that the SD for this age range is larger than that for the 20–30 age range. If the values in the table are plotted then a graph similar to Fig. 3.2 will be derived.

A well-known problem of using decade data are that of discontinuities at the boundaries. In Fig. 3.2 it can be seen that if a woman has a scan the day before her 40th birthday and her BMD was 0.95 g cm^{-2} then she would be below the mean –2 SD for her age. If she had the scan a day later, on her 40th birthday, then she would be between the mean –1 SD and the mean –2 SD.

These discontinuities become more pronounced the larger the SD. These difficulties are not so apparent to the clinician if the BMD value and the normative data are represented in a purely tabular, as opposed to a graphical, form.

Provided the reference group is large enough, using five-year intervals rather than decades can partially relieve the problem of discontinuities. If the reference group is not large then there is the danger that the discontinuities increase due to a greater variability in the standard deviations. The effect of using decades when the reference group is not very large is that it smoothes out some of the variability in the standard deviation.

Z-Scores

Z-scores, which measure how far the subject's BMD is away from the age matched mean in terms of standard deviations, are another way of recording the findings. For example, if a subject's BMD value is 0.85 g cm^{-2} and the mean for that - particular age is 1.0 g cm^{-2} with a standard deviation of 0.1 for the relevant age matched population, then the Z-score would be -1.5; that is, Z-score = (0.85–1.0)/0.1. Z-scores do however, suffer from a similar difficulty to that of the tabular reporting method in that for the same BMD value a subject's Z-score can change substantially when moving from one age range to another due to the differing standard deviation for each age. If the next age range had a mean of 0.95 g cm^{-2} and a standard deviation of 0.11 then the Z-score for the same BMD would be -0.9. This should not be too surprising as the Z-score and tabular approach are really expressing the same thing in two different ways.

Even if Z-scores did not have this variability when moving from one age range to another, the question that has to be asked is "Is it a meaningful figure for the referring clinician or the patient?". If one considers a subject with two scans, a year apart, with no change in BMD, then, if the two scans fall within the same age range the Z-score will be the same but if they span two age ranges then the Z-score could be substantially different. Conversely, the subject may have a substantial change in BMD between two scans but if the scans fall in different age ranges the Z-score may not change.

T-Scores

To try to alleviate the problems encountered with Z-scores, the WHO has recommended that T-scores are used. As noted above T-scores are similar to Z-scores except that they use the mean and standard deviation values for the young adult band. Hence the same BMD value will give the same T-score regardless of the age of the subject.

A difficulty with T-scores for a clinician is that the same T-score may require to be interpreted in a significantly different way depending on the subject's age. In the elderly there is an increasing incidence of degenerative diseases and Blake and Fogelman[14] argue that there are problems relating to the use of T-scores in the elderly and argue that the decisions about treatment are generally best made on the basis of the Z-score. With respect to the elderly, it is worth noting that the NHANES data do not contain any information for the population over the age of 74.

Percentiles

The tabular, Z-scores and T-scores approaches all rely on discrete age groupings whereas in fact changes in an individual's BMD value, like weight and height, are continuous processes. Clinicians are familiar with weight and height charts in paediatrics so a similar system for BMD values should be easily understood.

Truscott et al.[8] suggest a methodology for the construction of reference ranges from which percentiles can be developed. This approach requires a relatively large number of subjects in order to provide good coverage across the age range but it does offer the clinician a better appreciation of the subject's position relative to the reference range. In addition the results of any previous scans can be incorporated onto the chart so both the subject's current position and how they have changed relative to their earlier position can be seen.

A scheme for the conversion of Z-scores into percentile values, based on the use of the normal distribution, is given by Wahner and Fogelman.[15] The choice of which of these two forms to use is one of individual preference.

Conclusions

We may be forgiven for thinking that the choice, use and development of reference ranges is a minefield into which we should not venture. This feeling is probably due to the fact that we have, in this chapter, concentrated on the short-comings of the current reference ranges, the potential difficulties in the creation of new ranges and the problems of reporting within the ranges we have. This may well give the impression of "doom and gloom" which is far from the truth. In pointing out these relatively minor problems we should not lose sight of the huge advantages that DXA measurement systems have brought to the diagnosis and monitoring of osteoporosis.

Despite variability between machines, operator error, differences in standardisation methods, the need for different ranges, potential regional variation and different methods of reporting, "bone densitometry remains the best current predictor of future fracture risk".[16] The more variables there are the greater is the need to educate the clinician who is going to have to interpret the findings and the greater is the danger that the clinician comes to rely on the BMD value alone and not the other factors that have to be taken into account.

As with other reference data the context within which a particular result is considered should include any previous BMD scans. The treatment of two women of the same age and background with the same BMD values, for example, may be significantly different if one woman has falling BMD readings whereas the other has constant values. A further complication is that when the lumbar spine is considered a patient may be diagnosed as osteoporotic following the WHO guidelines but fall outside the definition when the femoral neck BMD is considered. This highlights the immense importance of clinical judgement in diagnosis which should never be abdicated to the use of levels set by some external body, however profound their deliberations.

A report of how one service has attempted to help referring clinicians can be found in the paper by Fordham.[17] Kanis et al.[18] offers a practical guide for the use of bone mineral measurements in the assessment of treatment of osteoporosis.

A lot of work has been undertaken on reference ranges for BMD but a lot more still needs to be done. Further work will take more of the variability out of the process. In addition to the development of the ranges themselves it is important that clinician education continues to ensure that the correct interpretation of the figures is made. Despite all the potential problems, it is important that normative ranges are developed to help clinicians identify those patients for whom further investigation or treatment may be necessary and to help guide management of osteoporotic patients.

References

1. Nilas L, Hassager C, Christiansen C (1988) Long term precision in dual photon absorptiometry in the lumbar spine in clinical settings. Bone Miner 3:305–315.
2. WHO study Group (1994) Assessment of fracture risk and its application to screening for postmenopausal osteoporosis. WHO Tech Report No 843. WHO, Geneva
3. Advisory Group on Osteoporosis (1994) Report, Department of Health, London.
4. Engelke K, Gluer CC, Genant HK (1995) Factors influencing short-term precision of dual x-ray bone absorptiometry of spine and femur. Calcif Tissue Int 56:19–25.
5. Truscott JG, Oldroyd B, Simpson M et al. (1993) Variation in lumbar spine and femoral neck bone mineral measured by dual energy x-ray absorption: a study of 329 normal women. Br J Radiol 66:514–521.
6. Petley GW, Cotton AM, Murrills AJ et al. (1996) Reference ranges of bone mineral density for women in Southern England: the impact of local data on the diagnosis of osteoporosis. Br J Radiol 69:655–660.
7. Rico H, Revilla M, Hernandez ER et al. (1991) Total and regional bone mineral content in normal premenopausal women. Clin Rheumatol10:423–5.
8. Truscott JG, Simpson D, Fordham JN. (1997) A suggested methodology for the construction of national bone densitometry reference ranges: 1372 Caucasian women from 4 UK sites. Br J Radiol 70:1245–1251.
9. Simmons A, Simpson D, O'Doherty MJ et al. (1997) The effects of standarization and reference values in patient classification for spine and femur dual energy x-ray absorptiometry. Osteoporosis Int 7:200–206.
10. US Department of Health and Human Services, Centres for Disease Control and Prevention, National Centre for Health Statistics; 6525 Belcrest Road, Hyattsville, Maryland. 20782–2003. USA http//www.cdc.gov/nchswww/
11. Looker AC, Wahner HW, Dunn WL et al. (1995) Proximal femur bone mineral levels of US adults. Osteoporosis Int 5:389–409.
12. Genant HK, Grampp S, Gluer CC et al. (1994) Universal standardisation for dual X-ray absorptiometry: patient and phantom cross-calibration results. J Bone Miner Res 9:1503–1514.
13. Faulkner KG, Roberts LA, McClung MR (1996) Discrepancies in normative data between Lunar and Hologic DXA systems. Osteoporosis Int 6:432–436.
14. Blake GM, Fogelman I (1997) Interpretation of bone denstiometry studies. Semin Nucl Med 27:248–60.
15. Wahner HW, Fogelman I (1994) The evaluation of osteoporosis: dual energy X-ray absorptiometry in clinical practice. London, Martin Dunitz.
16. Cooper C (1996) Rationale and clinical indications for bone-density measurements. Osteoporosis Int Suppl 2:S6–8S.
17. Fordham JN. (1996) Providing a primary care open access clinic for osteoporosis. Osteoporosis Int Suppl 2:S26–S27.
18. Kanis JA, Devogelaer J-P, Gennari C (1996) Practical guide for the use of bone mineral measurements in the assessment of treatment of osteoporosis: a position paper of the European Foundation for osteoporosis and bone disease. Osteoporosis Int 6:256–261.

4 Definitions and Interpretation of Bone Mineral Density in a Clinical Context

R. Eastell

Introduction

Bone measurements have a central role in the management of the patient with osteoporosis. They are used for the diagnosis of osteoporosis, to predict who is likely to fracture in the future and for monitoring changes in bone in response to therapy. X-ray based techniques such as dual-energy X-ray absorptiometry have been most used in clinical practice.

The Diagnosis of Osteoporosis

Definitions for osteoporosis have usually been conceptual, and so difficult to relate to individual patients. An example was produced by a Consensus Development Conference[1] as ".. a systemic skeletal disease characterised by low bone mass and microarchitectural deterioration with a consequent increase in bone fragility and susceptibility to fracture." This definition is elegant but difficult to apply to an individual patient.

An operational definition of osteoporosis has been proposed by a Working Group of the World Health Organisation.[2] This defines osteoporosis by the patient's bone mineral density in relation to the mean value in normal young subjects.

Low bone density is defined as a T-score less than –1. This means that the bone mineral density (BMD) is less than one standard deviation (SD) below the mean for young adults. This category includes about 40% of all women over age 50, based on measurement at the total hip.[3]

Osteoporosis is defined as a T-score less than –2.5. This category includes about 17% of all women over age 50, based on measurement at the total hip.[3]

Established osteoporosis is defined as a T-score less than –2.5, and the presence of an osteoporosis-related fracture, such as wrist, hip or vertebral fracture.

This approach was originally used to evaluate the prevalence of osteoporosis. It may be used in the individual, particularly when there is a question about the current risk of fracture, such as:

1. Is the fracture related to osteoporosis?
2. Should high impact activities be avoided?
3. Is the radiological appearance of low bone density confirmed?

This approach has been considered for decisions about initiating therapy.[4] This is counterintuitive, as at age 50 almost nobody has a T-score of –2.5, whereas at age 90 almost everybody has a T-score below –2.5. Nonetheless, in a cost–utility analysis, a T-score of about –2.5 was an appropriate threshold for treatment between the ages of 55 and 75 years.

The T-score approach has a number of limitations for the definition of osteoporosis. It elevates a risk factor for fracture to the status of a diagnostic criterion, it ignores the importance of other determinants of bone strength, it ignores higher fracture risk associated with a certain level of bone mineral density in older women, and it does not specify the technique or the site at which bone mineral density should be measured (except that it should be made at the spine, hip or radius). The use of a single cut-off is also problematic. Some patients with vertebral fracture may have values above a T-score of –2.5, and in patients below this threshold, the lower the BMD the greater the risk of subsequent fractures. The better approach is to consider that the lower the BMD the greater the risk of fracture (see below).

Prediction of Fracture Risk

The future risk of fracture needs to be calculated in order to best prevent osteoporosis. A number of factors have been identified that predict the risk of fracture, including clinical risk factors, bone mineral density, quantitative ultrasound measurements and biochemical markers of bone turnover.

Many clinical risk factors have been identified that are associated with increased risk of osteoporosis (Table 4.1). These factors have the advantage that they are often easily identified, e.g. patients taking corticosteroids. However, most of them are uncommon. The National Osteoporosis Foundation have proposed four risk factors that are common and easy to identify.[4]

1. Low or moderate trauma fracture after age 40;
2. Parent with fracture of hip, wrist or vertebra after age 50;
3. Lowest quartile of weight (less than 58 kg);
4. Current cigarette smoker.

These risk factors may themselves be associated with low BMD, but they also have an association with fracture that is independent of BMD.

Low BMD is a predictor of fracture. In a number of prospective studies (summarised by Marshall et al.[5] a decrease in BMD (at the spine, hip, forearm and heel) was associated with an increase in fracture risk at many skeletal sites. The strongest association was between the femoral neck and the risk of hip fracture, with a 1 SD decrease in BMD being associated with a three-fold increase in the risk of fracture.

Low ultrasound measurements of the heel (by Lunar Achilles or Walker Sonix UBA 575) are predictive of fracture.[6,7] A decrease of 1 SD in speed of sound (SOS) or broadband ultrasonic attenuation (BUA) of the heel was associated with a two-fold increase in the risk of fracture. This increase in risk was independent of the association of low ultrasound and low BMD measurements. Thus, it may be possible to combine ultrasound and BMD measurements.

Table 4.1. Risk factors for osteoporosis in postmenopausal women[20]

Genetic factor	
	First-degree relative with low-trauma fracture
Environmental factors	
	Cigarette smoking
	Alcohol abuse
	Physical inactivity
	Thin habitus
	Diet low in calcium
	Little exposure to sunlight
Menstrual status	
	Early menopause (before age 45 years)
	Previous amenorrhoea (e.g. due to anorexia nervosa, hyperprolactinaemia)
Drug therapy	
	Glucocorticoids (7.5 mg/day of prednisolone or more for more than 6 months)
	Antiepileptic drugs (e.g. phenytoin)
	Excess substitution therapy (e.g. thyroxine, hydrocortisone)
	Anticoagulant therapy (e.g. heparin, warfarin)
Endocrine diseases	
	Primary hyperparathyroidism
	Thyrotoxicosis
	Cushing's syndrome
	Addison's disease
Haematological diseases	
	Multiple myeloma
	Systemic mastocytosis
	Lymphoma, leukaemia
	Pernicious anaemia
Rheumatological diseases	
	Rheumatoid arthritis
	Ankylosing spondylitis
Gastrointestinal diseases	
	Malabsorption syndromes (e.g. coeliac disease, surgery for peptic ulcer)
	Chronic liver disease (e.g. primary biliary cirrhosis)

Biochemical markers can be used to assess bone formation and bone resorption (Table 4.2). High levels of biochemical markers of bone resorption (e.g. deoxypyridinoline and C-telopeptide of type I collagen) have been associated with increased risk of hip fracture in prospective studies.[8] Values above the reference range for young women (i.e. a T-score of more than 2) were associated with a two-fold increase in the risk of fracture. This increase in risk was independent of the association of high biochemical marker levels with low BMD. Again, it may

Table 4.2. Biochemical markers of bone turnover

Bone formation	
	Serum alkaline phosphatase (bone isoform)[a]
	Serum osteocalcin[a]
	Serum C- and N-propeptides of type I collagen
Bone Resorption	
	Urinary excretion of pyridinium crosslinks of collagen (e.g. deoxypyridinoline)[a]
	Urinary excretion of C- and N-telopeptides of collagen[a]
	Urinary excretion of galactosyl hydroxylysine
	Urinary excretion of hydroxyproline
	Serum tartrate-resistant acid phosphatase

[a]Specific to bone and particularly useful in osteoporosis[20]

be possible to combine measurement of markers with measurement of BMD or ultrasound.

The above studies usually give the relative risk of fracture. It is more important in the individual to give absolute risk. One approach to this is to calculate the lifetime risk of fracture. This can be estimated if the relationship between BMD and fracture risk at different ages is known, if the expected lifespan can be accurately predicted and the current BMD is known. It could be improved if the rate of bone loss could be predicted, e.g. using biochemical markers of bone turnover. The lifetime risk of fracture has been predicted in this way from forearm BMD[9] and the remaining lifetime fracture probability from the heel BMD.[10] Ideally, such an approach would be calculated from BMD, ultrasound, biochemical markers and lifestyle risk factors.

Patients in the lower quartile of the reference range for hip bone density have a risk of fracture that is eight times higher than those in the upper quartile.[5] Patients who are in the lower quartile are at risk of significant bone loss (e.g. menopausal woman) should be considered for treatments that prevent further bone loss. The lower quartile includes patients whose spine or hip BMD is less than a Z-score of less than –1, or about 88% of that expected for their age. This Z-score approach can be used to answer the following questions.

Is the lifetime risk of fracture high? Prevention of further bone loss may be considered necessary if the Z-score is less than –1.

Is secondary osteoporosis present (e.g. thyrotoxicosis)? This might indicate the need for a thorough set of investigations, especially if the Z-score is less than –2.

This was chosen because of ease of communication. The cut-off points of –1 and –2 were chosen as they represent (approximately) the lower 25 and 2.5 percentiles for spine and hip BMD. A Z-score of –1 actually defines the bottom 16% of the distribution, but here we are measuring two sites, spine and hip, and their BMD is correlated; about 25% of women have either a spine or hip Z-score of less than –1. The cut-off points relate to the intervention as follows.

1. If the treatment is inexpensive and has other health benefits (e.g. HRT) then a threshold of a Z of –1 is recommended. This and the other intervention thresholds can be altered in the light of other risk factors, e.g. family history of osteoporosis-related fracture, slender stature, current cigarette smoking, previous fracture of wrist, hip or vertebra.[4]
2. If rapid bone loss is expected, e.g. high-dose corticosteroid therapy, a higher threshold should be used (e.g. a Z-score of 0, so as to include 50% of patients or a T-score of –1.5).
3. The further investigation of patients with a Z-score less than –2 of expected could be carried out by the referring physician.

Monitoring

Concept of Response

It is difficult to define a responder in the treatment of osteoporosis because it is not ethical to observe the rate of bone loss in a period prior to therapy. The definition needs to be based on information from clinical trials. Information from the placebo group can then be used to define a responder. For example an increase in lumbar spine BMD that is more than 2.77 times the standard deviation of BMD measurement above the placebo group mean would indicate response (at $p = 0.05$). The information from an alendronate trial was used to calculate this as 5.4%.[11] The least significant change for femoral neck was 8%. These estimates of least significant change were made in a clinical trial setting and are likely to be higher in the clinic setting where quality assurance may not be so stringent.

In practice, there are two issues about these cut-off points. The first is whether a $p = 0.05$ is too stringent. We are often happy to be "fairly sure", and so using a $p = 0.15$ may suffice. The critical change for the spine would then be 4.0%. For a treatment like alendronate or HRT about half of patients would be considered responders (greater than 4%), and so a measurement at one year would be worthwhile. For a treatment with a smaller BMD effect (raloxifene, calcitonin) it may be better to wait for 2 years to make a repeat measurement.

A similar approach can be used to calculate least significant change for biochemical markers of bone turnover. Bone resorption markers were measured in postmenopausal women and a figures of 25% for free deoxypyridinoline by immunoassay and 55% for n-telopeptides of type I collagen by immunoassay were found.[12] These estimates of least significant change are rather high and may be too much given the current treatments we have for osteoporosis which often result in a 5–10% change[13,14] over 3 years in BMD and 20–60% decrease over 3 months in bone resorption markers. It would be better to detect response by making multiple measurements of BMD or markers, or by using a less stringent p-value.

Bone Mineral Densitometry

This is the most useful way of monitoring treatment response. It is important to examine for treatment response to identify poor compliance, patients who do not absorb the drug or patients who do not respond for unknown reasons. Compliance can be improved by encouragement. Poor absorption of an orally administered drug may indicate malabsorption syndrome. Poor response would indicate the need to change the dose or the type of treatment.

The best bone density measurement would show a large response to treatment and have good precision. The lumbar spine measurement comes closest to this ideal with the femoral neck, total body, forearm and ultrasound measurements all being poor. An alternative to lumbar spine is the total hip measurement. Another alternative is to use biochemical markers of bone turnover.

As mentioned above the strict figure for a response at the lumbar spine is 5.4%. This will be the average response of most patients to HRT or bisphosphonates at two to three years. The ideal timing for the second measurement would be 2 years if dual-energy X-ray absortiometry (DXA) were a scarce resource.

The changes over time are not always due to the effect of the treatment. An increase in BMD can occur as a result of degenerative changes in the lumbar spine region L1–L4, particularly endplate sclerosis. A fracture within this region will result in an increase in BMD, and the fractured vertebra should be excluded from all analyses. A change in the reference range may falsely indicate an increase, if the percentage of expected rather than the actual BMD is used to calculate the change. Over the age of 60 years degenerative change in the spine is common, and here total hip measurements are more useful. There is a need for alternative methods of monitoring therapy.

Biochemical Markers of Bone Turnover

These markers reflect bone formation or bone resorption (Table 4.2). The bone formation markers include osteocalcin, the bone isoform of alkaline phosphatase and the propeptides of type I collagen (PICP, PINP). These are all measured in the serum, the latter three are stable and do not require immediate freezing and they all show low day to day variability. The response to therapy is slower than for the resorption markers and is maximal at 6 months with HRT and bisphosphonates. The mean decrease after these treatments is 20–40%.[12,13] The ratio of response to variability will probably result in these markers being most useful for monitoring therapy.

The bone resorption markers include deoxypyridinoline and related telopeptides, galactosyl hydroxylysine and hydroxyproline. These are all measured in the urine. They are stable and do not require immediate freezing but they all show high day to day variability, especially hydroxyproline. The response to therapy is faster than for the formation markers and is maximal at 3 months with HRT and bisphosphonates. The mean decrease after these treatments is 30–70%.[12,13] The ratio of response to variability will probably result in these markers being most useful for identifying early response.

At present, these markers are only used in selected cases when the lumbar spine BMD cannot be used to monitor response.

Description of Bone Density Results

There are several different units for describing bone density results. These each have advantages and disadvantages.

The Absolute Value For Bone Mineral Density ($g\ cm^{-2}$).

This approach is difficult to interpret as most doctors do not have a feel for the normal range for BMD results. However, this result is crucial for comparing with a follow-up result. (Note that the result for Lunar machines is about 16% higher than for Hologic and Norland machines.) The Inernational Committee for Standards in Bone Measurement has recommended that standardised BMD be reported for all machines using published equations.[15,16] The results from these standardised measurements are given in $mg\ cm^{-2}$ and so can be distinguished from those reported conventionally.

Percentage of Expected (%)

This approach expresses the BMD result as a percentage of expected (usually for age, although it can be used for comparison to young normal). The approach has the advantage that there is no requirement to memorise the reference range and it is a simple way to communicate results to people unfamiliar with statistical concepts. However, there is no "feel" for the normal spread of results. For example, the lower limit of the reference range is 75% of expected for lumbar spine yet it is 85% of expected for total body BMD measurements.

Standard Deviation Units (T-score and Z-score)

This approach expresses the BMD result in standard deviation units such that the average value is zero and the reference range is between +2 and –2. It can be used to compare to age-matched controls (Z-score) or to young normals (T-score). It has the advantage that it relates to the relative position within the reference range. It has the disadvantage in that it requires the referring physician to have some knowledge of statistics and it assumes that the reference range is normally distributed.

Percentiles

This approach is similar to the standard deviation approach in that the average person with be at the 50th percentile and the reference range will extend from 2.5 to 97.5 independent of the measurement being made. It has the advantage that doctors are familiar with this approach from using growth charts for children and that it relates to the relative position within the reference range and does not assume a normal distribution. The information (in relation to the reference range) is not provided by any manufacturer. It is not useful for follow-up measurements as a change from the 10th to the 20th percentile is much bigger than the change from the 40th to the 50th percentile.

A Practical Approach to Reporting BMD

Table 4.3. The recommended report form includes lumbar spine (particularly useful for treatment monitoring) and total hip (particularly useful for fracture prediction, and recommended by the International Committee for Standardisation of Bone Measurement[21]

Result	Lumbar spine	Total hip[a]
BMD, (g/cm^{-2})		
T-score, SD units		
Z-score, SD units (%)		

[a]The report should be based on the lower of the two BMD sites.

A working party of the National Osteoporosis Society in the UK (R. Eastell, I. Fogelman, J. Adams, C. Cooper, J. Fordham and F. Ring) prepared the following recommendations about reporting BMD measurements (Table 4.3). The following options can then be ticked by the doctor preparing the report.

1. The result is above the expected level for age. The patient is at relatively low risk for fracture.

2. The result is between a Z-score of 0 and –1 (88% and 100% of expected for age). The patient has a small increase in the risk of fracture. Recommend modification of lifestyle (adequate calcium intake, weight-bearing exercise, avoidance of smoking and of excess alcohol). Calcium and vitamin D supplements are likely to be particularly effective in the housebound elderly.

3. The result is less than a Z-score of –1 (88% of expected for age). Prevention of bone loss is recommended, e.g. hormone replacement therapy in a post-menopausal woman.

4. The result is less than a Z-score of –1 (88% of expected for age) **and** the T-score is less than –2.5. Treatment of osteoporosis is recommended, e.g. bisphosphonates, hormone replacement therapy, calcitriol, calcitonin.

5. The result is less than a Z-score of –2 (75% of expected for age). Recommend referral to the Metabolic Bone Clinic or thorough investigation for secondary causes of osteoporosis.

6. The patient has a vertebral fracture as a result of low trauma (based on spinal radiographs). Recommend referral to the Metabolic Bone Clinic or thorough investigation for secondary causes of osteoporosis.

It is recommended that a clinical interpretation be added to each report.[17] This would take into account the information in the referral letter and the patient questionnaire (if available). BMD measurements can be difficult to interpret and so should be reported by a competent and experienced clinician.

Issues Arising with the Use of BMD in Clinical Practice

Measurement of Multiple Sites

The prevalence of osteoporosis in women over 50 years at the total hip is 17%. If the spine and forearm are also measured the prevalence increases to 40%. Thus, the more sites that are measured, the more likely is it that a woman will have osteoporosis by BMD criteria. There is no simple resolution to this issue. Furthermore, there is no evidence that a second bone density measurement can provide any additional information to the first measurement about the risk of fracture.

A practical approach to using spine and hip BMD is to consider only lumbar spine (L1–4, or L2–4) and total hip (and not femoral neck, Ward's triangle, or trochanteric regions) and to take the lower of these. The spine is commonly artefactually elevated because of degenerative changes. This approach allows for this problem.

Source of Reference Ranges

Reference ranges need to be based on large numbers of subjects. There is argument over whether this population should be unselected ("community based") or selected. It is common to take a partially selected approach in which women taking HRT, corticosteroids or whom are known to have vertebral fractures are excluded. Each approach has its limitations.

An example of a database based on a large number of subjects is the NHANES III database from the US. This can be used for the proximal femur, but lumbar spine was not measured, and it is usual to use the instrument manufacturer's database for this. The reference range could be based on a sample of the local population, but this is an expensive approach, and the difference between US and UK populations is not large. For non-Caucasian populations, separate databases are required, but there is no information on how to interpret T- and Z-scores in these populations.

Reference Ranges for Men

The original WHO guidelines did not address the issue of osteoporosis definition. There have now been a number of studies indicating that the appropriate reference range for men is young men and the T-score cut-offs should be the same as for women.[18]

Use of Risk Factors with BMD

Some of the risk factors for fracture do not work through BMD, e.g. family history of fracture. It would be useful to combine risk factors with BMD to predict fracture risk. In the National Osteoporosis Foundation guidelines, based on the paper by Eddy et al.[4] an approach has been recommended. Thus if one risk factor (given above) is present then the threshold for intervention is raised by 0.5 SD, and if two or more are present the threshold for intervention is raised by 1 SD. This is a rather formal approach, but in practice incorporating risk factors is likely to be part of a clinician's judgement.

Use of Peripheral Bone Measurements

Quantitative ultrasound and peripheral bone density could be used along with spine and hip measurements. For example, if the result from these peripheral devices is below a critical value (e.g. a T-score of –2) then intervention may be indicated, if it is above a certain threshold (e.g. a T-score of 1) then reassurance may be given. In the intermediate region (T-score of –2 to 1), then spine and hip measurements could be made.[19]

Value of BMD Measurements at Different Ages

Bone density measurements have been evaluated as predictors of fracture in women in the age range 50–80 years. Below this age there is little information about the use of BMD as a predictor for fracture. It would be very difficult to carry out a prospective study to examine the risk of fracture in this population as the absolute risk of fracture is so low. In women over 80 years, there is still predictive value of BMD for fracture; indeed the relationship between BMD and fracture may even be stronger in these older women. However, spine BMD measurements are likely to be unreliable, because of the high prevalence of spondylosis.

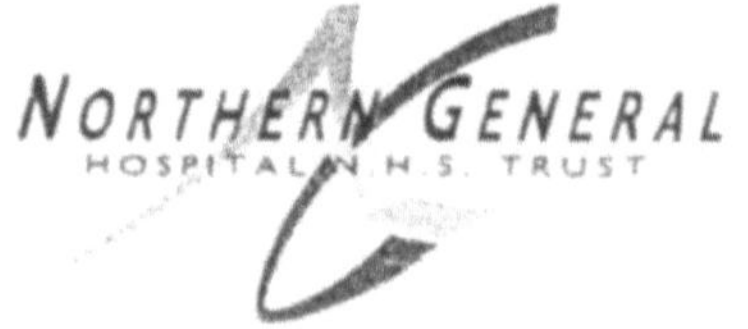

BONE MINERAL DENSITY REPORT

OSTEOPOROSIS CENTRE
NORTHERN GENERAL HOSPITAL
HERRIES ROAD
SHEFFIELD
S5 7AU

Telephone: (0114) 271 5340 or 271 4783

Consultants: Professor R Eastell, Dr NFA Peel, Dr P Lawson
Centre Manager: Sister PR Bainbridge

Name   ....   Hospital number ....

Date of birth   ....   Date of measurement ....

Referred by   ....

Bone mineral density (BMD) was measured by dual-energy x-ray absorptiometry using the **Hologic QDR 4500/A** densitometer based at the Osteoporosis Centre, Northern General Hospital. Results should not be compared with those from either the Lunar DPX or the Hologic QDR 1000/W densitometers.

The graphs show the BMD in comparison to an age-and sex-matched reference range (*female*).

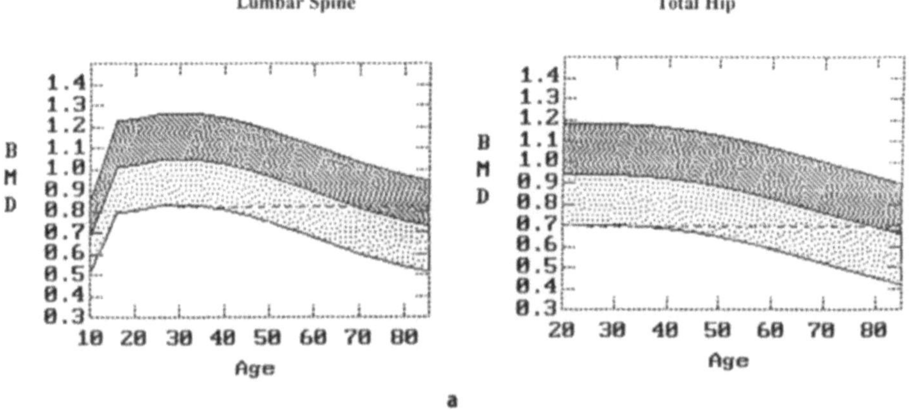

Figure 4.1a,b Report forms used at the Osteoporosis Centre, Northern General Hospital, Sheffield

RESULT	LUMBAR SPINE	TOTAL HIP
BMD, g/cm^2		
T-score, SD units		
% expected for age		

INTERPRETATION

☐ The result is above 100% of expected for age. The patient is at relatively low risk for fracture.

☐ The result is between 88 and 100% of expected for age. The patient has a small increase in the risk of fracture. Recommend modification of lifestyle (adequate calcium intake, weight-bearing exercise, avoidance of smoking and of excess alcohol). Consider calcium and vitamin D in individuals over 65.

☐ The result is less than 88% of expected for age. Prevention of bone loss is recommended, eg hormone replacement therapy in postmenopausal women, calcium and vitamin D in individuals over 65.

☐ The result is less than 88% of expected for age *and* the T-score is below -2.5. Treatment of osteoporosis is recommended, eg hormone replacement therapy, bisphosphonates, calcitriol, calcitonin.

☐ The result is less than 75% of expected for age. We therefore suggest that further investigations may be appropriate. *Unless we hear from you to the contrary*, we will arrange a metabolic bone clinic appointment.

☐ The patient has a vertebral fracture as a result of low trauma. We therefore suggest that further investigations may be appropriate. *Unless we hear from you to the contrary*, we will arrange a metabolic bone clinic appointment.

COMMENTS

....

b

Example of BMD Reporting in Practice

The report forms we use are shown in Fig 4.1. These are not meant to be followed to the letter, they incorporate both T- and Z-scores, and some authorities prefer to base all decisions on T-scores. The most important point is that in addition to the BMD interpretation, there is space for the reporting physician to comment.

Acknowledgement

I am grateful to my colleagues Dr N. Peel and Dr P. Bainbridge for their helpful contributions and to members of the NOS Working Group for their advice (I. Fogelman, J. Adams, C. Cooper, J. Fordham and F. Ring).

References

1. Anonymous (1997) Consensus development statement. Who are candidates for prevention and treatment for osteoporosis? Osteoporosis Int 7:1–6.
2. WHO Study Group (1994) Assessment of fracture risk and its application to screening for post-menopausal osteoporosis. WHO technical report series 843. WHO, Geneva.
3. Looker AC, Orwoll ES, Johnston CC et al. (1997) Prevalence of low femoral bone density in older US adults from NHANES III. J Bone Miner Res 12:1761–1768.
4. Eddy DM, Johnston CC, Cummings SR et al. Osteoporosis: review of the evidence for prevention, diagnosis and treatment and cost-effectiveness analysis. Introduction. Osteoporosis Int 8(Suppl 4):S7–8.
5. Marshall D, Johnell O, Wedel H (1996) Meta-analysis of how well measures of bone mineral density predict occurrence of osteoporotic fracture. Br Med J 312:1254–1259.
6. Bauer DC, Gluer CC, Cauley JA et al. (1997) Broadband ultrasound attenuation predicts fractures strongly and independently of densitometry in older women. a prospective study. Study of osteoporotic fractures research group. Arch Intern Med 157:629–634.
7. Hans D, Dargent-Molina P, Schott AM et al. (1996) Ultrasonographic heel measurements to predict hip fracture in elderly women: the epidos prospective study. Lancet 1348:511–514.
8. Garnero P, Hausherr E, Chapuy MC et al. (1996) Markers of bone resorption predict hip fracture in elderly women: the epidos prospective study. J Bone Miner Res 11:1531–1538.
9. Suman VJ, Atkinson EJ, O'Fallon WM et al. (1993) A nomogram for predicting lifetime hip fracture risk from radius bone mineral density and age. Bone 14:843–846.
10. Wasnich R (1998) Bone mass measurement: prediction of risk. Am J Med 95:6S–10S.
11. Eastell R. (1966) Assessment of bone density and bone loss. Osteoporosis Int 6:S36–S37.
12. Hannon RA, Blumsohn A, Naylor KE et al. (1998) Response of biochemical markers of bone turnover to hormone replacement therapy: impact of biological variability. J Bone Miner Res 13:1124–1134
13. Garnero P, Shih WJ, Gineyts E et al. (1994) Comparison of new biochemical markers of bone turnover in late postmenopausal osteoporotic women in response to alendronate treatment. J Clin Endocrinol Metab 79:1693–1700.
14. Liberman UA, Weiss SR, Broll J et al. (1995) Effect of oral alendronate on bone mineral density and the incidence of fractures in postmenopausal osteoporosis. N Engl J Med 333:1437–1443.
15. Genant HK, Brman ME, Hangartner T et al. (1995) Letter to the Editor: standardisation of spine BMD. Bone 17:435.
16. Felsenberg D, Fuerst T, Genant HK et al. (1997) Letter to the editor: standardisation of femur BMD. J Bone Miner Res 12:1316–1317.
17. Miller PD, Bonnick SL, Rosen CJ et al. (1996) Clinical utility of bone mass measurements in adults: consensus of an international panel. Seminar in Arthritis and Rheumatism 25:361–372.
18. Melton LJ 3rd. Atkinson EJ. O'Connor MK et al. (1998) Bone density and fracture risk in men. Bone Miner Res 13:1915–1923.
19. Baran DT, Faulkner KG, Genant HK et al. (1997) Diagnosis and management of osteoporosis: guidelines for the utilization of bone densitometry. Calcif Tissue Int 61:433–40.
20. Eastell R (1998) Treatment of postmenopausal osteoporosis. Engl J Med 338:736–746.
21. Hanson J (1997) Standardization of femur bond [letter]. J Bone Miner Res 12:1316–1317.

5 The Use of Bone Density Measurements in Male and Secondary Osteoporosis

R.M. Francis

Introduction

The increasing interest in the management of osteoporosis has been stimulated by awareness of the socioeconomic cost of osteoporotic fractures, the development of techniques for the diagnosis and monitoring of the condition and the introduction of effective treatments which prevent bone loss and decrease the risk of fractures. The development of dual energy X-ray absorptiometry (DXA) techniques in particular, has allowed the accurate and precise measurement of bone mineral density (BMD) at the major sites of fracture, such as the spine and hip. DXA bone density measurements are therefore being used increasingly for the diagnosis of osteoporosis and monitoring the response to treatment.

There is a strong inverse relationship between BMD and fracture risk, with a 2–3-fold increase in fracture incidence for each standard deviation reduction in BMD.[1] Other factors may affect fracture risk independently of BMD, including trabecular architecture, skeletal geometry, bone turnover, postural instability and propensity for falling.

BMD measurements may be expressed as standard deviation (SD) units above or below the mean value for normal young adults or relative to the mean value for control subjects of the same age, to give T- and Z-scores, respectively. The T-score reflects current fracture risk, whereas the Z-score predicts lifetime fracture risk, but the relative merits of T- and Z-scores in clinical practice remain controversial.[2]

The World Health Organisation (WHO) has defined osteoporosis as a BMD 2.5 SD or more below the mean value for young adults (T-score < –2.5), whereas the term severe or established osteoporosis indicates that there has also been one or more fragility fracture.[3] BMD measurements between 1.0 and 2.5 SD below the young normal mean value (T-score –1 to –2.5) have been classified as osteopenia or low bone mass.[3] Although the WHO definition is useful for the diagnosis of osteoporosis, it does not necessarily represent a threshold for treatment. This is important as 70% of women above the age of 80 years have a T-score of less than –2.5, but only a proportion of these will sustain an osteoporotic fracture. For these reasons there has been a trend to use Z-scores in interpreting BMD measurements in older people, to identify individuals whose bone density is lower than expected for their age and who are at greater risk of osteoporotic fractures.

The WHO criteria were defined for women, so may not necessarily be appropriate for the diagnosis of osteoporosis in men. Furthermore, the relationship between BMD and fracture incidence may be different in secondary and postmenopausal osteoporosis, as women on oral corticosteroids fracture at a higher BMD than women with postmenopausal osteoporosis.[4]

Osteoporosis in Men

Although osteoporotic fractures are generally considered to be a problem afflicting older women, it is increasingly recognised that osteoporosis also occurs in men (Fig. 5.1). The lifetime risk of symptomatic fracture for a 50-year-old white man in the US has been estimated to be 2.5% for the forearm, 5% for the vertebra, and 6% for the hip, whereas the corresponding figures for a 50-year-old woman are 16%, 15.6%, and 17.5%, respectively.[5] Currently about 15% of symptomatic vertebral and 20% of hip fractures in the UK occur in men. These fractures are associated with excess mortality, substantial morbidity and health and social service expenditure.[6]

Overall mortality is increased by about 18% after symptomatic vertebral fractures, but this may be due to coexisting conditions rather than the fracture itself. Men with vertebral fractures have substantially less energy, poorer sleep, more emotional problems, pain and immobility than expected. The overall mortality

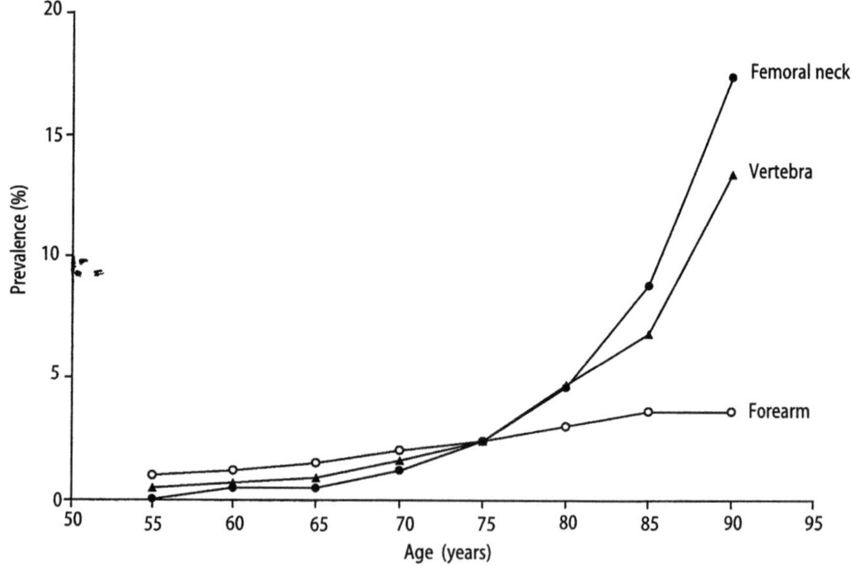

Figure 5.1 Cumulative prevalence of osteoporotic fractures with age in men. Prevalence calculated by F.H. Anderson and R.M. Francis from the incidence data of Melton et al.[5]

after hip fracture is higher in men than women, at 5.4% below the age of 75 years and 20.7% in older subjects, compared with 1.2% and 7.5%, respectively, in women. There is also considerable morbidity after hip fracture in men, with only 21% living independently in the community a year later, whereas 26% receive home care and 53% live in an institution. The annual cost of osteoporotic fractures in the UK has been estimated at £942 million, of which 20–25% is attributable to fractures in men.[6,7]

Pathogenesis of Osteoporosis and Osteoporotic Fractures in Men

Bone density and therefore the risk of fracture at any age is determined by peak bone mass, the age at which bone loss starts and the rate at which it progresses. Although peak bone mass is higher in males than females, because of their larger skeletal size, bone density at maturity is similar in both sexes. Peak bone mass is mainly determined by genetic factors, but age at puberty, physical activity and dietary calcium intake during childhood and adolescence are also important. The adolescent rise in bone mass occurs at an older age in males than females, because of their later onset of puberty. Young men with a past history of constitutionally delayed puberty have reduced bone density in the forearm and lumbar spine, when compared to normal men matched for duration of exposure to post-pubertal levels of testosterone. The magnitude of the effect of pubertal age on bone density may be sufficient to place men with constitutionally delayed puberty at increased risk of osteoporotic fractures later in life.[6,7]

Bone loss starts at about the age of 35 in both sexes, with men losing 15–45% of trabecular bone and 5–15% of cortical bone with advancing age, whereas women lose 35–50% and 25–30%, respectively. The greater bone loss in women is mainly related to the phase of rapid bone loss in the decade after the menopause. Although there is no dramatic reduction in sex steroid concentrations in middle aged men, there is a small decrease in serum testosterone and a proportionately larger increase in sex hormone binding globulin (SHBG) in later life, such that biologically active free testosterone declines with age. As hypogonadism is a significant cause of osteoporosis in males, this reduction in unbound testosterone is likely to contribute to age-related bone loss in men. There is also increasing evidence that the effects of testosterone on the male skeleton may be mediated in part by aromatisation to oestradiol.[8] Other potential causes of bone loss in men include physical inactivity, tobacco and alcohol consumption, declining vitamin D metabolite concentrations, secondary hyperparathyroidism and decreased calcium absorption.[6,7]

Case–control studies of men with symptomatic vertebral fractures show a significantly increased risk of fracture with smoking, alcohol consumption and underlying secondary causes of osteoporosis.[6,9] Secondary causes of osteoporosis may be found in over 50% of men with symptomatic vertebral fractures, the most common of which are hypogonadism, oral steroid therapy, gastric surgery and alcohol abuse.[10,11] Case–control studies show that the risk of hip fracture in men is increased by secondary causes of osteoporosis, such as past history of gastric resection, thyroidectomy and hypogonadism, and by conditions associated with falling, such as cerebrovascular disease, Parkinsonism and dementia.[6] A prospective study of elderly men showed a higher risk of hip fracture with low femoral neck bone density, quadriceps weakness, increased body sway, falls in past year, previous fractures, low body weight and short stature.[6]

Investigation of Osteoporosis in Men

As mentioned earlier, the WHO criteria for the diagnosis of osteopenia and osteoporosis were only established for women, so may not necessarily be appropriate in men. Nevertheless, there is a similar relationship between BMD and fracture risk in both sexes,[12] suggesting that the WHO criteria may potentially be applicable in men and women. In a recent case–control study, we found lumbar spine BMD T-scores of < 2.5 in 56% of men with symptomatic vertebral fractures,[9] compared with only 3% in male control subjects (Fig. 5.2). A further 33% of the men with vertebral fractures had evidence of osteopenia (T-score < –1.0 to –2.5). This study showed not only a significant reduction in BMD in the lumbar spine, but also at all sites in the hip in patients with symptomatic vertebral fractures (Fig. 5.3).

BMD measurements have been advocated for the assessment of men with fractures after minimal trauma, apparent reduced bone density on X-ray or underlying secondary causes of osteoporosis, such as hypogonadism and prolonged oral steroid therapy.[7] Unfortunately, there is no agreement on the threshold BMD value at which treatment should be considered in men. In male subjects with a history of previous fracture but normal BMD measurements (T-score > –1.0), the fracture is most likely to be due to antecedent trauma. Men presenting with a fragility fracture and evidence of either osteopenia or osteoporosis, should be considered for treatment to prevent further bone loss. In men with no history of fragility fractures, treatment should probably be reserved for those with definite

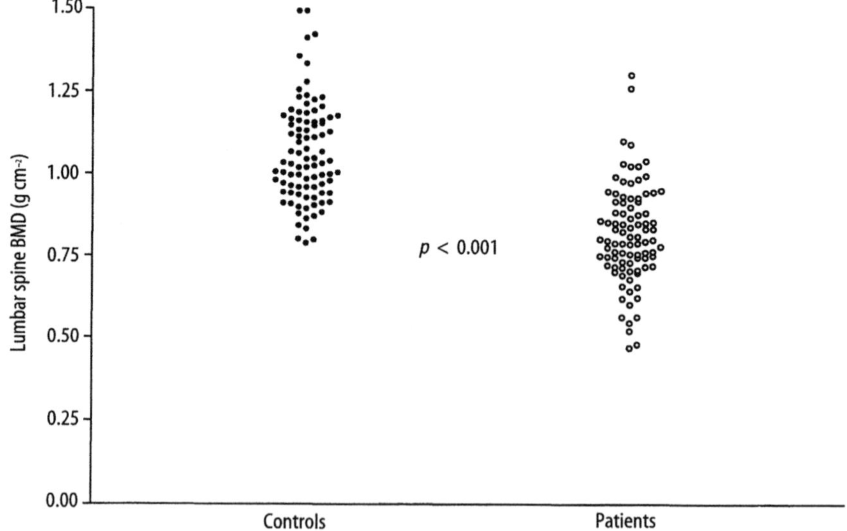

Figure 5.2 Lumbar spine BMD in patients with symptomatic vertebral fractures (o) and control subjects (●). Data derived from Scane et al.[9]

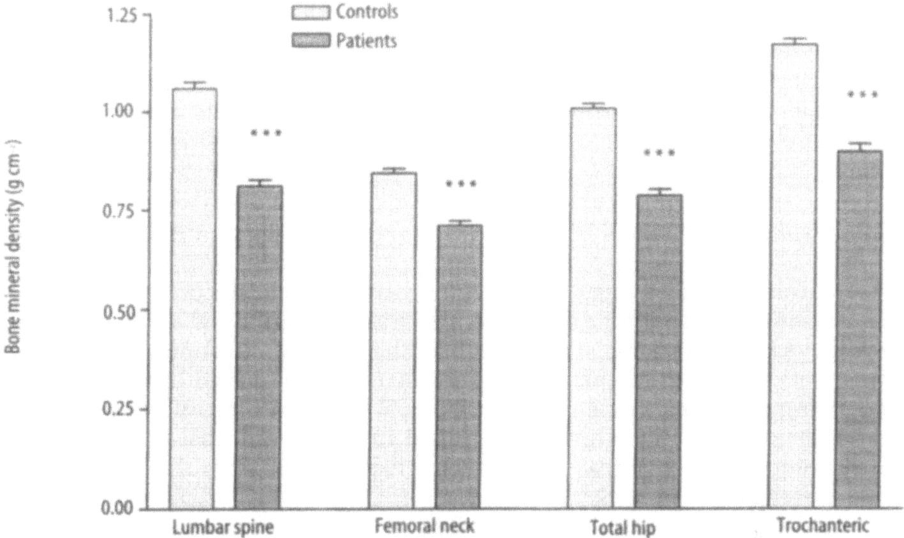

Figure 5.3 Lumbar spine, femoral neck, total hip and trochanteric BMD measurements (mean ± SEM) in patients with symptomatic vertebral fractures and control subjects. The statistical significance of differences between patients and control subjects is indicated (***, $p < 0.001$). Data derived from Scane et al.[9]

osteoporosis (T-score < -2.5) and greater than expected reduction in BMD for their age (Z-score < -1.0).[7] If there is an underlying secondary cause of rapid bone loss, such as oral corticosteroid therapy or organ transplantation, treatment may be appropriate at a higher BMD.

Secondary causes of osteoporosis should be sought in men presenting with fragility fractures and/or low BMD by careful history, physical examination and appropriate investigation, as treatment of underlying conditions such as hyperthyroidism, hypogonadism and hyperparathyroidism may reverse the osteoporotic process and increase bone density. Investigations should include full blood count, erythrocyte sedimentation rate (ESR), biochemical profile, thyroid function tests, serum testosterone, SHBG, gonadotrophins, prostate specific antigen and serum and urine electrophoresis.[10]

Management of Osteoporosis in Men

All men with osteoporosis or fragility fractures should be given advice about lifestyle measures to decrease bone loss. These include eating a balanced diet rich in calcium, stopping smoking, moderating alcohol consumption and maintaining regular physical activity and exposure to sunlight throughout life. Where there is a history of falls, attempts should be made to identify underlying intrinsic and extrinsic causes, in the hope that these may be modified and the risk of further falls and fractures decreased. There is also growing interest in the use of hip protectors, which are available in appropriate sizes for men and women, which may decrease the risk of femoral neck fractures in frail elderly patients with recurrent falls.

There is no well established treatment for osteoporosis in men, as few controlled studies dealing exclusively with the effects of treatment on bone density and fracture incidence in men with osteoporosis have been published. Nevertheless, therapeutic options for the treatment of osteoporosis in men include bisphosphonates, testosterone supplementation, fluoride salts and calcium and vitamin D.[6]

Bisphosphonates

Observational studies suggest that intermittent cyclical etidronate therapy increases lumbar spine bone density in men with idiopathic and secondary osteoporosis.[6] An observational study examined the effect of 24 months' intermittent cyclical etidronate in 36 men with spinal osteoporosis, seven of whom had an underlying secondary cause of osteoporosis. There was a significant increase in bone density of 8% in the lumbar spine and 10% in the femoral neck with treatment, compared with annual rates of bone loss of 1.3% from the spine and 3% from the femoral neck in 12 patients monitored without treatment before starting the study.[6] In an uncontrolled observational study in 42 men with vertebral fractures followed for a median of 31 months, intermittent cyclical etidronate therapy increased spine BMD by 3.2% annually, and femoral neck bone density showed a non-significant rise of 0.7% per year.[13] Four other uncontrolled studies show similar increases in spine bone density in men with osteoporosis treated with cyclical etidronate.[6] It would therefore appear that cyclical etidronate has comparable effects on bone density in men and women, although the effect on fracture incidence in men remains unclear. Nevertheless, a postmarketing surveillance study using the UK General Practice Research Database investigated the effect of cyclical etidronate in 7977 patients, 733 of whom were men.[6] There was a significant reduction in the risk of vertebral fractures (relative risk 0.44; 95% confidence intervals 0.20–0.97) in osteoporotic men treated with cyclical etidronate compared with untreated osteoporotic men (van Staa TP, personal communication), but this was not the case for non-vertebral fractures (relative risk 0.92; 95% confidence intervals 0.52–1.63). Controlled studies of other bisphosphonates such as clodronate, alendronate and risedronate in men with osteoporosis are either under way or planned.

Testosterone

Testosterone replacement therapy in hypogonadal men with osteoporosis increases bone density, particularly if the epiphyses are still open. Testosterone supplementation may also have a beneficial effect on bone density in eugonadal men with osteoporosis. An uncontrolled study[14] of testosterone treatment in 14 eugonadal men with vertebral fractures showed an increase in spine bone density of 6.1% after three years treatment (Fig. 5.4). An observational study of testosterone treatment in 21 eugonadal men (age range 34–73 years) with vertebral osteoporosis showed a significant increase in spine bone density of 5% in six months, although no change in hip bone density was seen.[15] Subsequent analysis of the biochemical markers of bone turnover showed a reduction in bone resorption with testosterone, which may have been mediated by conversion into

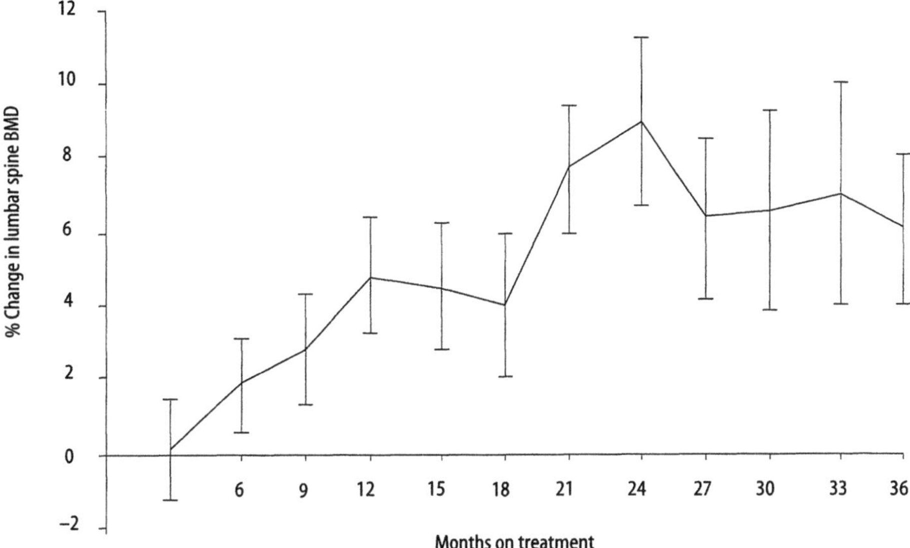

Figure 5.4 The effects of testosterone supplementation on lumbar spine BMD in a group of eugonadal men with vertebral fractures. Data from Scane et al.[14]

oestradiol.[15] Testosterone treatment may cause changes in body composition which could potentially lead to spurious elevation in bone density, but this is unlikely to account for the magnitude of the observed increase in bone density.[15] A randomised controlled crossover study in 15 men on long-term corticosteroid treatment showed an increase in spine bone density of 5% after 12 months treatment with testosterone, whereas no change was observed during the control period of 12 months observation.[16] Although the overall effect of testosterone treatment on cardiovascular risk factors appears neutral, at least in the short term, information is still required on the longer-term effects on the risk of heart and prostatic disease. A multicentre randomised controlled trial of testosterone treatment in eugonadal men with spinal osteoporosis is required, to investigate the effects on bone density and vertebral fracture incidence, as well as body composition, cardiovascular risk factors and the prostate.

Fluoride Salts

A German randomised controlled trial (RCT) suggests that low-dose intermittent monofluorophosphate and calcium may be useful in the management of osteoporosis in men.[17] A total of 64 men with generalised osteoporosis were randomised to receive cyclical monofluorophosphate (15 mg fluoride day) for three months out of four and continuous calcium (950–1000 mg day^{-1}) or 1000 mg calcium daily alone for three years. Monofluorophosphate increased spine bone density by 8.9%, whereas patients receiving calcium alone lost 2.4% (Fig. 5.5). There was a smaller increase in hip bone density measurements with monofluorophosphate and a 66% reduction in vertebral fractures.[17] Although the

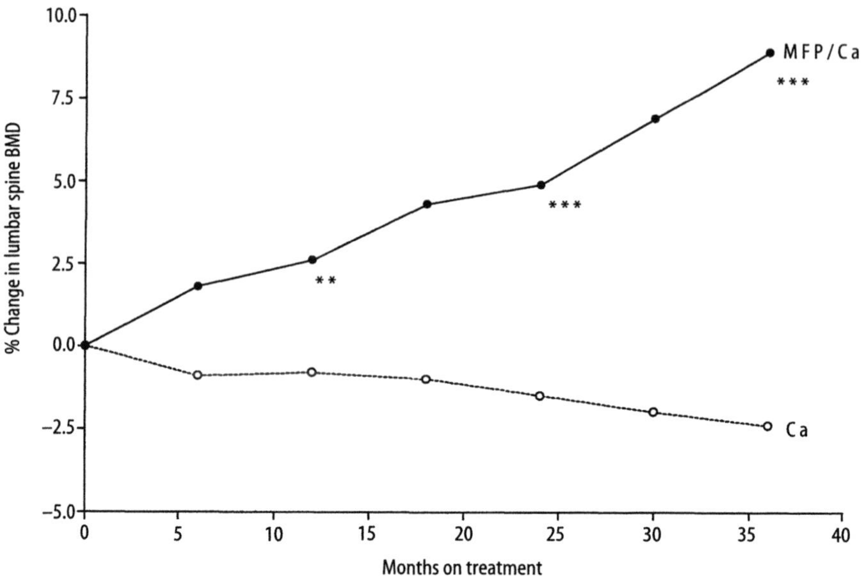

Figure 5.5 The effects of treatment with intermittent monofluorophosphate and calcium (MFP/Ca) and calcium alone (Ca) on lumbar spine BMD in men with osteoporosis. Data from Ringe et al.[17]

results of this study appear promising, previous experience in women suggests that the therapeutic window for fluoride treatment is narrow.

Calcium and Vitamin D

The role of calcium and vitamin D supplementation in the management of osteoporosis in men remains unclear.[6,7] In a randomised controlled trial in normal men aged 30–87 years, supplementation with 1000 mg calcium and 1000 iu of vitamin D daily had no effect on bone loss from the forearm or spine. In contrast, an American study in older men and women (mean age 70 years) living at home demonstrated that 700 iu vitamin D_3 and 500 mg elemental calcium daily had a modest beneficial effect on bone density and decreased the incidence of non-vertebral fractures. A controlled study of elderly men and women in Finland also demonstrated an overall reduction in total number of fractures with an annual intramuscular injection of 150,000 or 300,000 i.u. vitamin D. However, the Dutch randomised controlled trial of vitamin D supplementation (400 iu daily) in elderly men and women showed a small beneficial effect on hip bone density, but no reduction in the incidence of hip fractures.[6]

Choice of Treatment

The effects of cyclical etidronate, testosterone and intermittent monofluorophosphate on lumbar spine BMD in men with osteoporosis are broadly comparable (Fig. 5.6). Other potential treatments for osteoporosis in men include

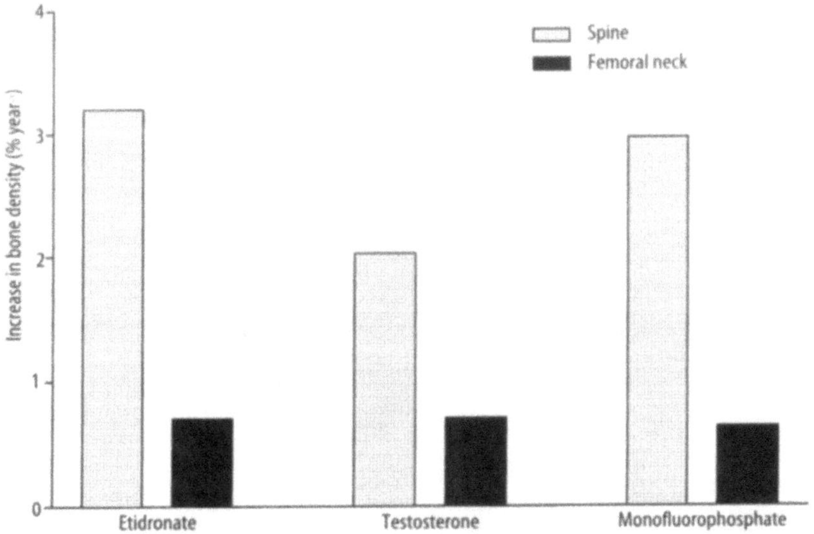

Figure 5.6 The effects of treatment with cyclical etidronate,[13] testosterone supplementation[14] and intermittent monofluorophosphate[17] on lumbar spine and femoral neck BMD in men with osteoporosis.

calcitonin, anabolic steroids, parathyroid hormone and growth hormone, but there is relatively little published information on their use in men.[7] A UK Consensus Group has suggested that bisphosphonates are the treatment of choice at present,[7] with advantages for cyclical etidronate (low cost), alendronate (greater increases of BMD at the hip BMD) and intravenous pamidronate (particularly in men with high bone turnover). Calcium and vitamin D supplementation is most likely to be useful in housebound or frail elderly men with osteoporosis. In view of the lack of an established treatment for osteoporosis in men, consideration should be given to referring men with osteoporosis to specialist centres, for investigation of underlying causes and monitoring the effect of empirical treatment on BMD. It has been suggested that bone density measurements are repeated every one to two years in men on treatment for osteoporosis.[7]

Secondary Osteoporosis

Secondary causes of osteoporosis may be found in up to 35% of women and 55% of men with symptomatic vertebral fractures (Fig. 5.7). The most frequently encountered causes are oral corticosteroid therapy, skeletal metastases, myeloma, gastric surgery, anticonvulsant therapy, hyperthyroidism and male hypogonadism.[10,18] Secondary causes of osteoporosis may also increase the risk of hip fractures in men and women.

Secondary causes of osteoporosis should be sought by careful history, physical examination and appropriate investigation, as treatment of underlying conditions may reverse the osteoporotic process and increase bone density. Investigations may include full blood count, ESR, biochemical profile, thyroid

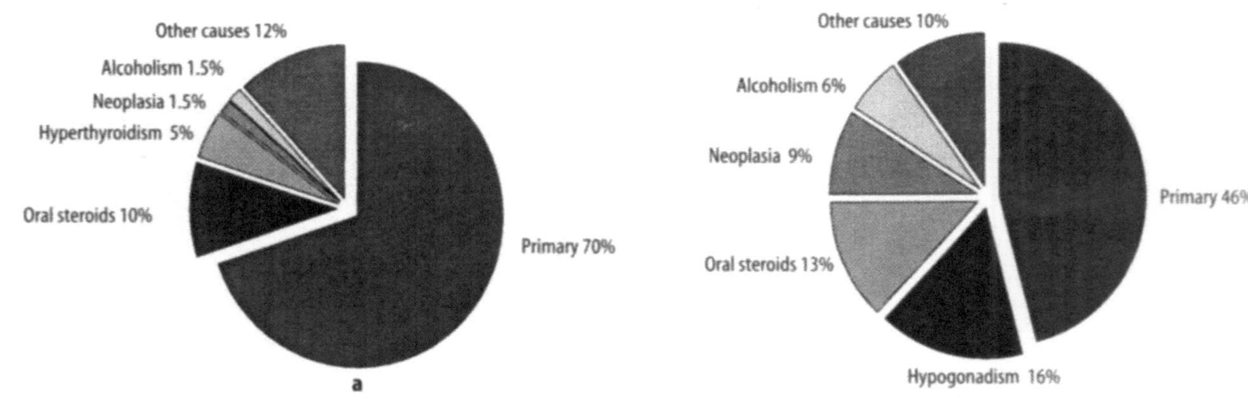

Figure 5.7 Prevalence of secondary causes of osteoporosis in (**a**) women and (**b**) men with symptomatic vertebral fractures attending the Bone Clinic in Newcastle upon Tyne. Data derived from Caplan et al.[18] and Baillie et al.[10]

function tests and serum and urine electrophoresis, together with serum testosterone, SHBG, gonadotrophins and prostate specific antigen in men.

As secondary causes of osteoporosis are common in patients with fragility fractures and there are potential differences in the relationship between BMD and fracture risk and in the response to treatment in these conditions, it is appropriate to consider the use of bone density measurements in the management of patients with secondary osteoporosis.

Cushing's Syndrome

The association between Cushing's syndrome and osteoporosis was first recognised in 1932, when Harvey Cushing first described the clinical features of endogenous hypercortisolism.[19] He recognised that the majority of patients with this condition had spinal osteoporosis. The reduction in bone density is more marked in the trabecular bone of the spine, ribs and femoral neck than in the cortical bone of the appendicular skeleton. The decrease in trabecular bone density in Cushing's syndrome is in the region of 20%, and is associated with an increased risk of fractures of the ribs and vertebrae. Successful treatment of Cushing's syndrome leads to a gradual increase in bone density, such that it may be normal ten years later.[19] Bone densitometry may therefore be useful in monitoring the response to treatment of patients with Cushing's syndrome and assessing the need for additional antiresorptive therapy.

Oral Corticosteroid Therapy

Since corticosteroids were first used therapeutically in 1948, it has become apparent that exogenous hypercortisolism is also associated with the development of osteoporosis. Although Cushing's syndrome is a relatively rare cause of osteoporosis, corticosteroid therapy is the commonest cause of secondary osteoporosis, occurring in up to 20% of patients with symptomatic vertebral fractures.[10,18] Oral corticosteroids lead to a rapid loss of bone in the first year of treatment, with an overall loss from the lumbar spine or hip of 15–20%. This leads to a doubling of the incidence of forearm and hip fractures and a five–six fold increase in the risk of vertebral fractures.[20] Most studies suggest that 10–20% of patients receiving oral corticosteroids develop fragility fractures, but one study shows that up to 32% of asthmatics on such treatment develop vertebral or rib fractures.

Pathogenesis of Corticosteroid-Induced Osteoporosis

The pathogenesis of corticosteroid-induced osteoporosis is different from postmenopausal osteoporosis, in that the major histological and biochemical abnormality is a reduction in bone formation, although there is less convincing evidence of increased bone resorption. Patients with corticosteroid-induced osteoporosis may also sustain fractures at a higher bone density than individuals with postmenopausal osteoporosis.[4]

A number of changes in bone metabolism are observed with oral glucocorticoid therapy, which may contribute towards the development of osteoporosis. These include malabsorption of calcium, secondary hyperparathyroidism, decreased sex steroid production in men and women and raised urinary calcium excretion. The underlying condition for which a patient takes corticosteroids may also itself influence bone loss, as a result of factors such as immobility and the inflammatory process.[20]

There is general consensus that doses of prednisolone of 7.5 mg daily and above are associated with the development of osteoporosis. Although inhaled corticosteroids influence the biochemical markers of bone turnover, there is little evidence that their use increases the risk of osteoporosis and fractures.[20]

Management of Corticosteroid-Induced Osteoporosis

The potential causes of bone loss with corticosteroid therapy provide a rationale for the use of calcium supplements, vitamin D and its metabolites, hormone replacement therapy (HRT) and antiresorptive and anabolic agents. As the mechanisms of bone loss are different in corticosteroid-induced and post-menopausal osteoporosis, caution should be used in extrapolating the results from one situation to the other. In order to confirm the efficacy of any treatment for corticosteroid-induced osteoporosis, long term RCTs are required which are large enough to detect not only an increase in bone density, but also a reduction in fracture incidence. Although studies are now examining the prevention and treatment of corticosteroid-induced osteoporosis, most are relatively short term and lack the statistical power to accurately assess the effect of intervention on fracture incidence.

Calcium and Vitamin D

Although calcium supplementation may decrease bone loss to some extent, rapid bone loss has been reported in patients starting oral corticosteroids, despite the coadministration of calcium supplements. Whereas a non-randomised controlled study showed no apparent effect of calcium and vitamin D on corticosteroid-induced bone loss, a more recent two year RCT demonstrated that calcium (1000 mg day^{-1}) and vitamin D (500 iu day^{-1}) prevented bone loss from the spine and femoral trochanter in patients on long term, low dose corticosteroids (mean daily dose of 5–6 mg prednisolone) for rheumatoid arthritis.[20]

Calcitriol

In a controlled trial in 103 patients starting oral corticosteroids, a year's treatment with calcitriol and calcium supplements significantly decreased bone loss from the lumbar spine and distal radius, but had no effect on bone loss from the femoral neck. Monitoring of serum calcium and renal function is required in patients on calcitriol, because of the risk of hypercalcaemia and renal impairment. Nevertheless, calcitriol may be useful in the management of younger patients with corticosteroid-induced bone loss, in whom other treatments such as HRT and bisphosphonates may be inappropriate.[20]

Hormone Replacement Therapy

There are few studies examining the effect of HRT in women with corticosteroid-induced osteoporosis. Early studies showed an increase in spine bone density with HRT, but continuing bone loss in the control groups. A small RCT in 42 women receiving corticosteroids for rheumatoid arthritis showed an increase in spine bone density with HRT, but continuing bone loss with calcium alone.[20]

Bisphosphonates

Other antiresorptive agents such as bisphosphonates have a major role in the prevention and treatment of corticosteroid-induced osteoporosis. In a small randomised controlled study of patients starting corticosteroid therapy, oral pamidronate prevented the bone loss from the spine and metacarpal cortex seen in the control group. An RCT of intermittent intravenous pamidronate infusions in patients starting oral corticosteroids showed significant increases in spine and hip bone density, compared with bone loss in the control group.[20]

Small controlled studies have shown that intermittent cyclical etidronate prevents bone loss from the lumbar spine in patients starting oral steroid therapy, significantly increasing spine bone density in patients on long term steroids with evidence of reduced bone density. The largest of these studies was an RCT in 141 men and women who had recently started oral corticosteroids (basal mean prednisolone dose > 20 mg daily), which showed prevention of bone loss from the lumbar spine and femoral trochanter with cyclical etidronate over a 12 month period of time. There was also a significant reduction in vertebral fracture incidence among the 70 postmenopausal women receiving etidronate, although the study was inadequately powered to accurately assess the effect of treatment on fracture rate.[20]

A small controlled study in patients starting oral corticosteroids for sarcoidosis showed that alendronate 5 mg daily prevented bone loss from the forearm. Preliminary results from a larger RCT demonstrate significant increases in bone density in the spine and femoral trochanter in corticosteroid-treated patients taking alendronate 10 mg daily.

Calcitonin

In a controlled trial in patients starting oral corticosteroid therapy for polymyalgia rheumatica, intranasal calcitonin significantly decreased but did not prevent bone loss from the spine. Another study in patients starting corticosteroids for polymyalgia rheumatica or temporal arteritis showed no effect of calcitonin on bone loss from the spine or hip. In contrast, an RCT in patients on long term oral corticosteroids for asthma demonstrated a significant increase in spine bone density with intranasal calcitonin, relative to the control group.[20]

Anabolic Steroids

A small controlled trial in postmenopausal women on long-term corticosteroids showed an increase in forearm bone density with nandrolone, compared with bone loss in the control group.[20]

Fluoride Salts

In a controlled study in patients with established corticosteroid-induced osteoporosis, monofluorophosphate and calcium increased spine bone density more than calcium alone, although no effect was seen at the femoral shaft or neck. Another RCT in patients on long-term corticosteroids showed a greater increase in spine bone density with monofluorophosphate and calcium than with calcium alone. A recent study compared enteric coated sodium fluoride and cyclical etidronate and calcium in patients with corticosteroid-induced osteoporosis. This showed greater increases in spine bone density in the fluoride-treated patients than the control group. Although the increases in bone density with fluoride treatment are encouraging, they may not necessarily be accompanied by a reduction in fracture risk, as the early studies in postmenopausal osteoporosis showed marked improvement in bone density, but no decrease in fracture incidence.[20]

Bone Densitometry in Corticosteroid-induced Osteoporosis

Although long term corticosteroid therapy is recognised as an indication for bone density measurement, its precise role in patient management is unclear. The relationship between bone density and fracture incidence is less well established in corticosteroid-induced than postmenopausal osteoporosis, but patients on corticosteroids appear to fracture at a higher bone density than other postmenopausal women.[4] It has, therefore, been suggested that treatment to prevent further bone loss is started at a higher bone density in patients on oral corticosteroid therapy, perhaps when the BMD is more than 1.5 SD units below the mean value for young adults (T score < –1.5).[20] In patients on treatment for corticosteroid-induced osteoporosis, BMD measurements should be repeated after one year, then every one to three years depending on the results.[20]

Transplantation Osteoporosis

With increasing survival after organ transplantation, osteoporosis is now seen as a significant complication of renal, liver, cardiac, lung and bone marrow transplants. Patients with liver disease such as primary biliary cirrhosis have lower bone density and higher rates of bone loss than age-matched controls. Bone density decreases further after liver transplantation, resulting in atraumatic fractures in up to 65% of cases. In the longer term, bone density increases again, suggesting that osteoporosis may become less severe. In a series of 40 patients studied after cardiac transplantation, reduced bone density was present in 28% at the lumbar spine and in 20% at the hip, whereas vertebral fractures were found in 35%. Patients undergoing cardiac transplantation tend to have low spine bone density before surgery, which may be due to immobility, poor nutrition and the use of loop diuretics. After cardiac transplantation, the spine bone density falls to values up to 50% lower than normal at six months, probably due to treatment with corticosteroids and cyclosporin A.

It may be worthwhile performing BMD measurements prior to organ transplantation, to identify patients requiring treatment to prevent bone loss. We have recently reported that most patients developing vertebral fractures after liver transplantation have a lumbar spine BMD T score < –2.0 before surgery. This observational study also suggests that such fractures may be prevented by the use of three-monthly intravenous infusions of pamidronate, started before transplantation is performed.[21] In view of the rapid bone loss occurring after transplantation, BMD measurements should probably be repeated 6–12 months after surgery, to assess bone loss and monitor the effect of any therapeutic intervention. Controlled trials are now required to establish the optimal method of preventing and treating osteoporosis after organ transplantation.

Male Hypogonadism

Hypogonadism is a well established cause of osteoporosis in men, occurring in up to 20% of men with vertebral fractures and 50% of elderly men with hip fractures. The diagnosis of hypogonadism may not always be clinically apparent in men with osteoporosis, so routine measurement of serum testosterone and gonadotrophins is probably worthwhile, as treatment may reverse the bone loss. Causes of hypogonadal osteoporosis in men include Klinefelter's syndrome, idiopathic hypogonadotrophic hypogonadism, hyperprolactinaemia, haemochromatosis and primary testicular failure.[19] Studies show an increased bone resorption and decreased mineralisation, which has been attributed to androgen or oestrogen deficiency, low plasma 1,25-dihydroxyvitamin D concentrations, malabsorption of calcium and reduced circulating calcitonin levels. These abnormalities may be reversed by treatment with testosterone replacement, which leads to an increase in BMD in the forearm and lumbar spine, particularly in patients with open epiphyses (Fig. 5.8). Serial BMD measurements may be useful in the management

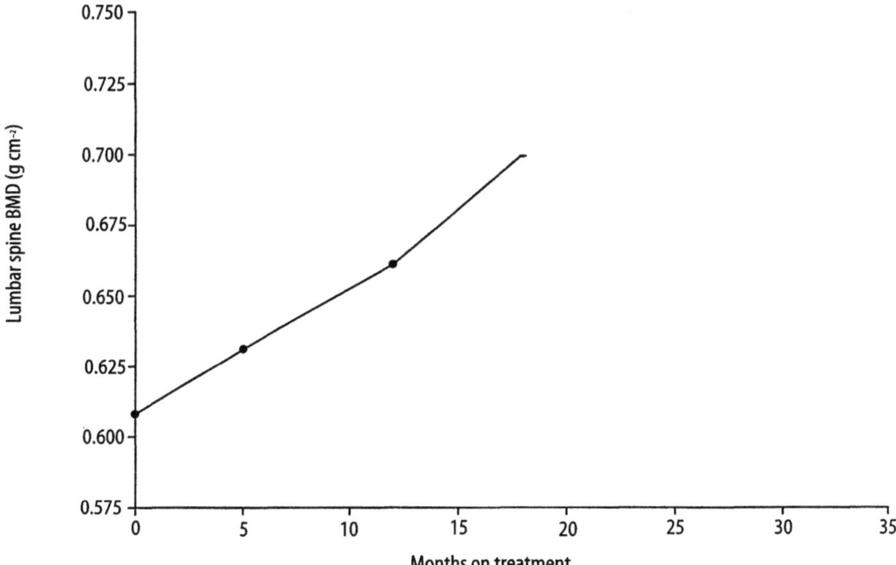

Figure 5.8 The effects of testosterone replacement therapy on lumbar spine BMD in a 36-year-old hypogonadal man.

of hypogonadal men on testosterone replacement therapy, to identify those who require additional treatment for osteoporosis.

Hyperthyroidism

The association between hyperthyroidism and osteoporosis is now well established, since the effects of severe hyperthyroidism on bone were first described by Von Recklinghausen in 1891. Hyperthyroidism is associated with an increase in bone formation and resorption, although resorption usually exceeds formation, such that bone is lost from the skeleton. Studies show a reduction in bone density with hyperthyroidism, which is more marked in women after the menopause. Hyperthyroidism may sometimes present with osteoporotic fractures, but the diagnosis is not always apparent, as elderly osteoporotic patients may have no other clinical features of hyperthyroidism. Exogenous administration of thyroxine may also reduce bone density, which is related to duration of treatment, rather than dose or serum thyroid hormone levels. Treatment of hyperthyroidism leads to an increase in bone density and partial reversal of the osteoporosis, particularly in younger patients.[19] As in other patients with underlying secondary causes of osteoporosis, serial BMD measurements may be useful to identify those who require additional treatment for osteoporosis.

Primary Hyperparathyroidism

Hyperparathyroidism increases bone remodelling and therefore magnifies the imbalance between bone formation and resorption seen after the menopause, leading to a greater rate of bone loss. The reduction in bone density in primary hyperparathyroidism is more marked in postmenopausal women than in younger women or men. Primary hyperparathyroidism may be associated with an increased risk of vertebral crush fractures, occurring in up to 20% of cases, although this has not been a universal finding. In patients with asymptomatic primary hyperparathyroidism, BMD measurements are useful in identifying patients who would benefit from surgery, as osteoporosis may be an indication for neck exploration. Parathyroidectomy significantly increases bone density, leading to a partial correction of osteoporosis.[19]

Amenorrhoea

Young women with a history of amenorrhoea have a lower than expected bone density, which is related to the duration of amenorrhoea and the severity of oestrogen deficiency, rather than the nature of the underlying disease. Rapid bone loss from the lumbar spine has also been reported in women with anovulatory cycles or cycles with short luteal phases. Together with the observations of the effects of hyperprolactinaemia, anorexia nervosa and amenorrhoea in athletes, it would appear that amenorrhoea is an important cause of bone loss and osteoporosis in young women.[19] Treatment of the underlying condition generally leads to an improvement in BMD, but oestrogen replacement may be necessary in the meanwhile, to protect the skeleton from the adverse effects of oestrogen deficiency.

Hyperprolactinaemia

Hyperprolactinaemia is found in up to 30% of young women with secondary amenorrhoea, and is associated with a reduction in forearm and vertebral bone density. The reduction in bone mass is most severe in those with the lowest circulating oestradiol concentration, suggesting that bone loss is due to oestrogen deficiency. Treatment of hyperprolactinaemia with either bromocriptine or surgery increases bone density, but only partially corrects the osteoporosis. It is therefore important that hyperprolactinaemia is diagnosed and treated early, to prevent further bone loss and decrease the subsequent risk of osteoporotic fractures.[19]

Anorexia Nervosa

Anorexia nervosa is associated with a reduced bone density in the forearm, spine and femur. Spine bone density may be as much as 30% below the expected value, particularly where the anorexia nervosa has developed during adolescence. Factors implicated in the pathogenesis of osteoporosis in this condition include poor nutrition, decreased body weight, early onset and long duration of amenorrhoea, reduced physical activity and hypercortisolism. Successful treatment of the anorexia nervosa is associated with an increase in bone density, although this is likely to lead to only a partial correction of the deficit in bone mass. Follow up of women with anorexia nervosa suggests that although treatment prevents further bone loss, the increased risk of fracture may persist.[19]

Amenorrhoeic Athletes

Although athletes tend to have a higher bone mass than more sedentary individuals, female athletes who become amenorrhoeic have a lower than expected bone density, developing stress fractures as a result. Amenorrhoea occurs in up to 50% of competitive runners and ballet dancers, probably due to hypothalamic–pituitary dysfunction secondary to low body weight. The bone loss in amenorrhoeic athletes is probably due to low circulating oestrogen levels. Amenorrhoeic athletes may also have a reduced peak bone mass, as many start training before the cessation of linear bone growth and have a delayed menarche. The reduction in bone density observed in amenorrhoeic athletes may be partly reversible, as decreased training leads to weight gain, increase in circulating oestrogens, resumption of menses and improvement in bone mass.[19]

Alcoholism

Alcoholism has long been recognised as a cause of osteoporosis, and more recent studies show reductions in bone mass of as much as 40% in the lumbar spine and 10% in appendicular cortical sites. There may be radiological evidence of osteoporosis with vertebral crush fractures in 50% of alcoholics. Alcoholism is associated with a decreased bone formation, which may be due to a direct effect of ethanol on osteoblast function. Acute alcohol intoxication causes transient hypoparathyroidism, hypocalcaemia and hypercalciuria. The transient suppression of parathyroid hormone after alcohol ingestion may be followed by a rebound increase above the normal range, which may then stimulate bone resorption. Other possible causes of bone loss in alcoholism include poor diet, malabsorption of calcium due to vitamin D deficiency, alcohol-induced loss of calcium in the urine, alcohol related liver disease and pseudo-Cushing's syndrome. Although alcohol-induced hypogonadism has been implicated in the pathogenesis of bone loss in alcoholic men, a recent study shows normal testosterone levels. The diagnosis of alcoholism may be overlooked, and should be particularly considered in osteoporotic subjects who are male, have a raised mean corpuscular volume (MCV), abnormal liver function tests or rib fractures on chest radiograph.[19]

Gastric Surgery

Although gastrectomy has long been considered a cause of osteomalacia, the precise role of gastric surgery in the pathogenesis of osteoporosis is unclear. Osteoporosis is encountered more frequently than would be expected by chance in men and women following gastric surgery. Possible factors in the pathogenesis of bone loss after gastric surgery include decreased absorption of vitamin D, the reduced food intake which commonly follows gastric surgery, and malabsorption of calcium due to marginal vitamin D deficiency, the absence of gastric acid and intestinal hurry.

Bowel Disease and Malabsorption

Osteoporosis is a well recognised complication of inflammatory bowel disease,[22] occurring in up 30% of patients with Crohn's disease. The reduction in bone density may be due to a number of factors, including corticosteroid therapy, short bowel syndrome, malabsorption, low body weight, hypogonadism and the release of inflammatory cytokines. Patients with extensive Crohn's disease and previous bowel resections are at high risk of vitamin D deficiency, hypomagnesaemia and secondary hyperparathyroidism. It is, therefore, worthwhile measuring serum magnesium, 25-hydroxyvitamin D and intact parathyroid hormone in such patients, as correction of any underlying biochemical abnormalities with vitamin D or its active metabolites and mineral supplements, may decrease bone loss and prevent the development of osteomalacia. Other treatments for osteoporosis in patients with Crohn's disease include HRT and bisphosphonates. Intravenous infusions of a bisphosphonate may prove more effective than oral treatment, but this requires confirmation in a clinical trial.

Although coeliac disease is a well-recognised cause of osteomalacia, it may also be associated with the development of osteoporosis. Underlying causes include malabsorption, vitamin D deficiency, secondary hyperparathyroidism and low body weight. The diagnosis of coeliac disease should be considered in patients with otherwise unexplained osteoporosis, but particularly those with low body weight. Investigations such as antiendomyseal antibodies and jejunal biopsy may be useful in such patients. Introduction of a gluten-free diet should lead to an improvement in bone density, but calcium and vitamin D supplements may be required if there is evidence of vitamin D deficiency and secondary hyperparathyroidism. Bone density may be used to assess the need for additional treatment for osteoporosis.

Other causes of malabsorption such as pancreatitis and cystic fibrosis may also increase the risk of developing osteoporosis, because of decreased absorption of calcium and vitamin D.

Anticonvulsant Therapy

Bone density in epileptic patients on anticonvulsant drugs is 70–90% of the expected value, whereas up to 8% of osteoporotic men with crush fractures are on anticonvulsant therapy. This suggests that anticonvulsant treatment is a genuine risk factor for the development of osteoporosis, rather than that fractures result simply from the trauma of convulsions. The adverse effect of anticonvulsant treatment on bone density has been reported with phenytoin, phenobarbitone, carbamazepine and sodium valproate. Some anticonvulsant drugs increase the hepatic microsomal metabolism of vitamin D, leading to low plasma 25-hydroxyvitamin D levels. This together with evidence of a direct effect on bowel mucosa, may account for the observed decrease in calcium absorption. Anticonvulsant treatment during bone growth and consolidation may also potentially reduce the peak bone mass, and therefore lead to osteoporotic fractures in early adult life.[19]

Immobilisation

Physical activity and weightbearing exercise are essential for the maintenance of skeletal mass, and declining physical activity probably contributes to age-related bone loss. Immobilisation leads to rapid bone loss of about 1% per week, which continues for about six months, when bone loss slows down and the bone mass reaches a new steady state. Bone loss in immobilisation is due to a stimulation of bone resorption and a decrease in bone formation. Immobilisation leads to more rapid bone loss in weightbearing bones, suggesting that bone loss is due to local mechanical factors, rather than changes in systemic factors. Therapeutic agents have been given to prevent further bone loss in immobilisation, but the results have been disappointing. Where practical, remobilisation should be encouraged, as this appears to increase trabecular bone mass by 0.25% per week, and may at least in part correct the osteoporosis.[19]

Joint Disease

Periarticular osteoporosis is common in rheumatoid arthritis (RA), as active synovitis leads to the release of cytokines which stimulate bone resorption.[22] There is also evidence of more generalised osteoporosis in RA, with an increased risk of vertebral and femoral neck fractures. Osteoporosis in RA may be related to disease activity, relative immobility and oral corticosteroid therapy. BMD measurements of the spine and hip are useful in assessing the need for osteoporosis treatment, whereas bone density measurements of the hand may be helpful in quantifying periarticular bone loss in RA.

There is also an association between systemic lupus erythematosis (SLE) and osteoporosis, which has been reported in up to 25% of patients. Possible causes include corticosteroid therapy and disease activity, but the interaction of these factors and bone loss is complex. BMD measurements may therefore be used to assess the risk of fractures and the need for treatment to prevent bone loss. Although HRT may have a beneficial effect on osteoporosis in postmenopausal women with systemic lupus erythematosus (SLE), it needs to be monitored carefully, as it may aggravate the underlying condition.

Ankylosing spondylitis is associated with ligamentous calcification around the spine, but studies show an overall reduction in spine and hip bone density and an increased risk of vertebral fractures.[22] The pathogenesis of osteoporosis in this condition includes relative immobility and disease activity.

Osteoporosis of Pregnancy

Although the onset of osteoporosis during pregnancy is a rare phenomenon, it presents an important clinical problem. The incidence and aetiology remain poorly defined and it is uncertain whether the association is coincidental or causal. Vertebral collapse with severe back pain and loss of height are the commonest features of the condition. These symptoms usually develop during the third trimester of pregnancy or in the postpartum period.[11] Transient osteoporosis of the hip during pregnancy has also been described, which may even result in femoral fracture. The pathogenesis is still unknown, but histological findings suggest that it is not due to increased resorption. In a small series of cases, plasma concentrations of 1,25-dihydroxyvitamin D were low. This suggests a transient failure of the usual changes in calcium regulating hormones, which normally prepare the maternal skeleton for the demands of pregnancy and lactation. We have observed marked increases in bone density after delivery in untreated women with osteoporosis of pregnancy, whereas others have suggested that the problem does not recur in subsequent pregnancy.[19]

References

1. Ross PD, Davis JW, Epstein RS et al. (1991) Pre-existing fractures and bone mass predict vertebral fracture incidence in women. Ann Intern Med 114:919–923.
2. Peel N (1993) Eastell R. Measurement of bone mass and turnover. Baillieres Clin Rheumat – osteoporosis 7:479–498.
3. WHO Study Group (1994)Assessment of fracture risk and its application to screening for postmenopausal osteoporosis. Report. World Health Organization, Geneva.
4. Peel NF, Moore DJ, Barrington NA et al. (1995) Risk of vertebral fracture and relationship to bone mineral density in steroid treated rheumatoid arthritis. Ann Rheum Dis 54:801–806.
5. Melton LJ, Chrischilles EA, Cooper C et al. Perspective: how many women have osteoporosis? J Bone Miner Res 7:1005–1010.
6. Francis RM (1998) Cyclical etidronate in the management of osteoporosis in men. Rev Contemp Pharmacother 9:261–266.
7. Eastell R, Boyle IT, Compston J et al. (1998) Management of male osteoporosis: report of the UK Consensus Group. Q J Med 91:71–92.
8. Anderson FH, Francis RM, Selby PL et al. (1998) Sex hormones and osteoporosis in men. Calcif Tissue Int 62:185–188.
9. Scane AC, Francis RM, Sutcliffe AM et al. (1999) Case–control study of the pathogenesis and sequelae of symptomatic vertebral fractures in men. Osteoporosis Int 9:91–97.

10. Baillie SP, Davison CE, Johnson FJ et al. (1992) Pathogenesis of vertebral crush fractures in men. Age Ageing 21:139–141.
11. Francis RM, Peacock M, Marshall DH et al. (1989) Spinal osteoporosis in men. Bone Miner 5:347–357.
12. Delaet CED, Van Hout BA, Burger H et al. (1997) Bone density and risk of hip fracture in men and women: cross-sectional analysis. Br Med J 315:221–225.
13. Anderson FH, Francis RM, Bishop JC et al. (1997) Effect of intermittent cyclical disodium etidronate therapy on bone mineral density in men with vertebral fractures. Age Ageing 26:359–365.
14. Scane AC, Francis RM, Johnson FJ et al. (1992) The effects of testosterone treatment in eugonadal men with osteoporosis. In: Ring EFJ. ed. Current research in osteoporosis and bone mineral measurement II: 1992. British Institute of Radiology, London, p. 54.
15. Anderson FH, Francis RM, Peaston RT et al. (1997) Androgen supplementation in eugonadal men with osteoporosis – effects of six months' treatment on markers of bone formation and resorption. J Bone Miner Res 12:472–478.
16. Reid IR, Wattie DJ, Evans MC et al. (1996) Testosterone therapy in glucocorticoid-treated men. Arch Intern Med 156:1173–1177.
17. Ringe JD, Dorst A, Kipshoven C et al. (1998) Avoidance of vertebral fractures in men with idiopathic osteoporosis by a three year therapy with calcium and low-dose intermittent monofluorophosphate. Osteoporosis Int 8:47–52.
18. Caplan GA, Scane AC, Francis RM (1994) Pathogenesis of vertebral crush fractures in women. J R Soc Med 87:200–202.
19. Francis RM, Sutcliffe AM, Scane AC (1998) Pathogenesis of osteoporosis. In: Stevenson JC, Lindsay R (eds) Osteoporosis. Chapman Hall, London, pp. 29–51.
20. Eastell R, Reid DM, Compston J et al. (1998) UK Consensus Group on management of glucocorticoid-induced osteoporosis: an update. Journal Intern Med 244:271–292.
21. Reeves HL, Francis RM, Manas DM et al. (1998) Intravenous bisphosphonate prevents symptomatic osteoporotic vertebral collapse in patients after liver transplantation. Liver Transplant Surg 4:404–409.
22. Boyle IT (1998) Secondary osteoporosis. Bailliere's Clin Rheumatol – Osteoporosis 7:515–534.

6 The Use of Bone Mineral Density Measurements in the Context of Osteoporosis Services

J.N. Fordham

Introduction

The purpose of this chapter is to explain the pivotal role that BMD measurement has in the management of patients with osteoporosis. This relates not only to the management of patients in the community under the care of their general practitioner, but also patients referred from within the hospital setting from specialties such as orthopaedics, endocrinology and gynaecology. It is obviously important to encourage good working relationships with public health physicians working in Health Authorities or with relevant physicians within commissioning groups. This is particularly so since the use of bone densitometry in the management of osteoporosis had become an emotive topic in the UK following the publication of the Effective, Health Care Bulletin report in 1992.[1] This is no longer the case following the Advisory Group on Osteoporosis report (AGO)[2] with its recommendation that the Department of Health should develop guidelines on the prevention and treatment of osteoporosis. Subsequently The Royal College of Physicians (RCP) produced a report which reviewed all available literature relating, among others, to the various techniques available for measuring bone density.[3] This recommended that the basis for the diagnosis of osteoporosis should be the use of such techniques rather than alternative options such as quantitative ultrasound or computed tomography. The latter techniques, however, can be used as independent assessments of fracture risk. The general thrust of the RCP Report was that a preventative strategy for osteoporosis be directed towards selective case findings rather than adopting population-based strategies designed to reduce the risk of fracture in the general population e.g. by advocating increased levels of physical activity, reduced smoking habit, and increased dietary calcium, etc. It is considered that the evidence for the effectiveness of such interventions on fracture risk coupled with the compounding effect of poor compliance, with such strategies was such that the writing group could not endorse such an approach. Official support for the use of bone densitometry followed the recommendations in the AGO Report and the subsequent instructions issued in the NHS Executive Letter (1996)[4] 1110 which gave responsibility to local Health Authorities to "purchase bone densitometry measurements by means of dual X-ray absorptiometry for particular clinical indications."

More recently a Health Service Circular[5] brought together a number of initiatives including: the RCP Guidelines; the Committee on the Medical Aspects of Food and Nutrition Policy report on nutrition and bone health[6] and a quick reference Guide for Primary Care Teams. This has been followed with Local Health Action Sheets which include, within the targets reduction in the rate of accidents. Although not explicitly including the goal to reduce the risk of osteoporosis, and hence lessen the morbidity and mortality associated with fractures, this does give sufficient leeway for local commissioners of health to include preventative and secondary strategies designed to reduce the impact of accidents where osteoporosis has a rôle. The effectiveness of such initiatives will ultimately depend to a large extent on the enthusiasm of local lead clinicians working with local health authorities and primary care groups. The Report on Osteoporosis in the European Community[7] also confirmed that bone density measurements provide the best assessment of fracture risk with selected case finding preferred above the option of population-based screening. It was noted that access to densitometry varied considerably from the best (Austria 32 units per million) to the worst (UK and Ireland 4–5 units per million population).

The style of the service in Teesside has evolved over a number of years and is described in some detail as a potential model for others to adapt to their own needs. Underpinning the service is the identification of patients with osteoporosis and osteopenia in accordance with the World Health Organisation criteria. On a purely pragmatic level, given these definitions of osteoporosis and osteopenia, BMD measurement is necessary in order to enable treatment decisions to be consistently applied. The debate about the particular technology used for measurement of bone mass is likely to continue. However, at the moment the "gold standard" method of investigation in the UK is dual-energy X-ray absorptiometry (DXA). The current techniques available are usually hospital-based and by their nature are large and cumbersome fixed machines although with the evolution of X-ray technology and miniaturisation, it is already possible to foresee services which will not be hospital- based but which will provide services at the GP practice setting. By improving accessibility, and most importantly, reducing costs, this would enable increased numbers of patients to be identified at risk. Later in the chapter, a potential way for re-providing such a service based on a small mobile, peripheral scanner is described.

Rationale

The evidence that bone mineral density (BMD) measurements are predictive of fractures is presented elsewhere. There is little debate that at present BMD measurement is the most useful, single measurement in predicting those patients at increased risk of fracture. Studies in vitro have shown that 60–80% of bone strength is determined by bone density.[8] However, it is important to note that the relative predictive importance of BMD measurements may vary through life. Thus, individual patients may have lifestyle or medical conditions associated with osteoporosis which may be more important in predicting fracture than bone density itself. This is particularly so in the elderly where the propensity to fall is of much more importance as a fracture risk than low BMD. It is also of note that, by definition, the incidence of osteoporosis in the elderly inexorably rises, thus at 80 years approximately 80% of patients will have osteoporosis at either appendicular or axial site.[9] Given this, the relative importance of BMD measurements in managing elderly patients declines. This contrasts with younger women in whom bone density measurements in the early postmenopausal years provides a useful index of the risk of fractures later in life. The studies by Wasnich et al.[10,11] and Ross et al.[12] all indicate that fracture incidence is related to BMD. This association is true at whatever site the bone density measurements are carried out and using different bone densitometry devices. The analysis of the gradient of risk using bone mineral measurements shows an association between bone density and fracture which is stronger than that between cholesterol or hypertension and the risk of ischaemic heart disease. Typically there is a doubling of risk of fracture for each standard deviation fall in BMD measurement.

Population screening leading to identifying patients at risk of osteoporosis is not recommended (RCP Report). Rather, a case finding strategy is recommended in those patients who have had a fragility fracture or who have strong risk factors for osteoporosis. The use of additional non-bone density risk factors that add additional information to fracture risk should be incorporated in the overall assessment of patients. However, the method for incorporating such additional information independent of bone density measurement, is in its infancy. The use of bone densitometry measurements on a case finding basis obviously conserves more resources than would the undirected use of such equipment.

The correct identification of patients at risk of fractures enables "targeting" of patients with antiresorptive agents. There is evidence that compliance with hormone replacement therapy improves if patients have had bone density measurements carried out. However, the study by Rubin and Cummings[13] noted that detrimental psychological affects on patients should not be disregarded, e.g. those patients identified as showing below normal density showed undue anxiety and inappropriate inhibition of lifestyle because of fear of fracture. Abnormal bone density results increased concern among women; 55% reported increased concern about their increased potential for fractures. Those women with below normal results (38%) became increasingly fearful of falling. Women of 65 years or over were more likely to limit their daily activity than women with normal results. Nevertheless the majority of patients in this study (92%) indicated that they were satisfied with bone densitometry as a procedure and would encourage other women of their age to undergo this test. A further study of perimenopausal women showed that disclosing the results of a BMD scan directly to women improves their knowledge of their bone density without any adverse psychological consequences.[14] There were no reported differences in anxiety levels between the randomised groups studied. It was concluded that, in this group of women, knowledge of their BMD results did not result in increased anxiety. Another study[15] showed that although increased usage of hormone replacement therapy (HRT) occurred after bone densitometry, 40% of women with low bone density were not using HRT 8 months after bone density measurement. Similarly, it is to be expected that those patients in whom lifestyle factors are of importance in the aetiology of osteoporosis, may be more amenable to suggested changes in lifestyle if their bone density measurements are low. The evidence for such an effect is at present tenuous but suggestive. Certainly the measurement of bone density enables the patient and doctor to make informed decisions about medication and changing lifestyle.

Those patients with osteoporosis associated with underlying medical conditions may be screened to assess the severity of the osteoporosis which, by correction of the underlying condition and supplementary treatment, may result in improvement in bone density and reduced risk of fracture.

Other secondary benefits of BMD measurement include effects on public awareness and conceptions about osteoporosis. Often a nihilistic view about the effectiveness of detection and management of osteoporosis is expressed by the general public (and for that matter some medical practitioners). Similarly the general level of understanding of osteoporosis may be limited to those of higher social class. Greater access to BMD measurement may increase public awareness with resultant increased expectations by patients for their "bone health care."

The use of bone densitometry to assess response to interventions is discussed later in this chapter.

Table 6.1 summarises the rationale for the use of BMD measurements.

Table 6.1. Rationale for the use of bone mineral density (BMD) measurements

- Predict fracture risk
- Enable targeting of patients for treatment
- Increase patient compliance
- Increase general public awareness of osteoporosis
- Enable objective monitoring of efficacy of interventions

Provision of Osteoporosis Services

The chief purpose of an osteoporosis service is to identify patients at increased risk of fractures and to provide appropriate targeted medical support to those identified at risk. In the hospital setting the consultant responsible for the provision of the service will often provide more detailed investigations and specialised treatments. Similarly access to education support groups may be via the specialist in charge. A hospital-based service may also provide, through its staff, health promotion advice to the local population and ideally should work closely with public health physicians in raising public awareness of osteoporosis by promoting lifestyle changes to reduce the impact of osteoporosis.

Access to Bone Densitometry

The RCP recommendations for case finding are indicated in Table 6.2. These are in essence a refinement of those published in the AGO Report but include in

Table 6.2. Selection criteria for patients for bone densitometry

Radiographic evidence of osteopenia and/or vertebral deformity

Loss of height, thoracic kyphosis (after radiographic confirmation of vertebral deformity)

Previous fragility fracture

Prolonged corticosteroid therapy (prednisolone greater than 7.5 mg daily for six months or more)

Premature menopause (age less than 45 years)

Prolonged secondary amenorrhoea (greater than 1 year)

Primary hypogonadism

Chronic disorders associated with osteoporosis

Maternal history of hip fracture

Low body mass index (less than 19 kg m^{-2})

BONE DENSITOMETRY (DXA SCAN) REQUEST FORM

INDICATIONS FOR SCAN

Measurement of BMD by DXA scanning <u>should only be undertaken when the result of the scan will influence patient management.</u> If a decision to treat with HRT has already been made on other clinical grounds, a DXA scan is not indicated, even in case of premature menopause.

REPEAT SCANS

A repeat scan to monitor those patients already on treatment for osteoporosis or those with a previous 'low normal' result is indicated at 2-5year intervals.

BONE HEALTH QUESTIONNAIRE

Patients will be asked to complete a questionnaire when attending for a scan and given appropriate advice supported by leaflets etc.

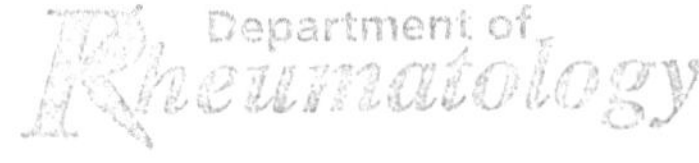

PATIENT DETAILS	REFERRING DOCTOR
Name:	GP/Hosp:...........................
Address:...........................	Name:...........................
....	Address/Hosp./Dept:...........................
Tel.No.:...............D.O.B.:......../........../............	....
	Tel. No.:...........................
D number:...............NHS/PP:...............	Fundholding : YES [ ] NO [ ]
	FHSA GP Code: [ ] [ ] [ ]
	Date of Referral:........../........../............

PLEASE RETURN COMPLETED FORM TO: BONE DENSITOMETRY SERVICE, RHEUMATOLOGY DEPT., SOUTH CLEVELAND HOSPITAL, MARTON ROAD, MIDDLESBROUGH, TS4 4BW. FAX NUMBER:(O1642) 854661

Please tick appropriate boxes

1. **THE RESULT OF A DXA SCAN WILL INFLUENCE MY DECISION TO**
   start treatment, stop treatment, continue/change treatment

2. **THE PATIENT IS IN THE FOLLOWING GROUP(S)**

AT RISK GROUP	CONFIRMATION OF DIAGNOSIS	PREVIOUS ABNORMAL DXA RESULT
long term steroid (>7.5mg prednisolone/day)	vertebral deformity	low normal
chronic renal failure	low trauma fracture	low
chronic liver disease	osteopenic X-ray	date of last scan....../....../.....
rheumatoid disease		
alcohol abuse		
malabsorption/malnutrition		
thyrotoxicosis		
hypogonadism (males)		
premature menopause		

ADDITIONAL INFORMATION / OTHER REASON FOR SCAN please specify :-

3. **CURRENT DRUG TREATMENT**

	Duration of treatment ? Years Months	CLINICAL DETAILS
HRT	....	height (cms):- ....
Bisphosphonate	....	weight (kg):- ....
Vit D	....	
Calcium	....	
Corticosteroid	....	
Other(s) please specify:-	....	

FAILURE TO COMPLETE SECTIONS 1 & 2 WILL RESULT IN THE DEPT.CONTACTING THE REFERRING DOCTOR BEFORE SENDING FOR THE PATIENT.

Figure 6.1 Example of bone density request form.

Table 6.3. Reasons for referral for bone densitometry

	Females (%)	Males (%)
Early menopause	18.5	--
? Use hrt	12.4	--
Fracture	11.6	20.5
Family history	12.2	1.3
Back pain	8.2	9.0
Steroid use	7.7	11.5
Patient concern	11.4	12.8
X-ray appointments	3.5	10.3
Medical conditions	7.0	17.9
Other	7.5	16.7

addition, maternal history of hip fracture, low body mass index, and primary hypogonadism.

Access to the service is best provided by the use of a validated referral proforma, an example of which is provided in Fig. 6.1. In essence it is important that those patients referred for bone densitometry fall within the criteria listed in Table 6.2. Furthermore the result of the investigation should, in some way, alter the management of the patient. It is important in this regard that, for example, women who take HRT or who would be willing to use HRT for its non-bone benefit should not be routinely scanned unless the patient is considering cessation of such treatment in which case knowledge of bone density may influence the patient's decision whether to continue treatment or not. The design of our own referral proforma correctly constrained referrals to the most appropriate groups of patients as indicated by the AGO report. The analysis of the major reasons for referral to our own service in the early 1990's is shown in Table 6.3. Patients with an early menopause with possible consideration of the use of HRT, history of fracture, and family history of osteoporosis were the major categories of referral. Overall these accounted for 54.7% of the total reasons for referral. Many patients had more than one reason for being referred, in our own experience 61.2% of patients were referred with a single risk factor, 32.8% had two risk factors and 6% had three or more risk factors. Patient concern regarding possible osteoporosis, but without any obvious underlying clinical risk factor, accounted for 11.4% of all female referrals. The most common reason for male patients being referred was a history of fracture (20.5%). Medical conditions associated with osteoporosis was the second major cause for referral

On receipt of the bone density referral request (Fig. 6.2) patients referred to bone densitometry are sent an appointment for the bone densitometry clinic where each patient is given a bone health questionnaire (Fig. 6.3). Those items relating to bone health are discussed in detail with a bone counsellor and appropriate written advice provided. The BMD measurements are carried out at the lumbar spine and femoral neck and the results of these measurements are reviewed by a consultant member of staff and interpreted in conjunction with the referral proforma and the completed bone health questionnaire. The report is issued to the referring general practitioner or consultant and those patients with osteoporosis (i.e. T-score < –2.5) are routinely given an outpatient appointment for the bone clinic where further investigations are undertaken and treatment

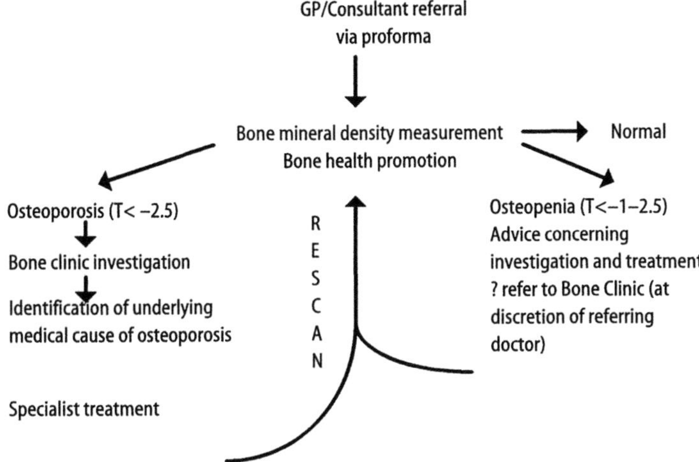

Figure 6.2 Service outline.

planned. Those with osteopenia (T-score $= \le -1$–2.5) are usually referred back to the general practitioner with advice to consider a repeat measurement in 2 years and to consider investigation and/or referral to the bone clinic. All patients who attend the bone densitometry clinic are advised to discuss their results with the referring doctor in the following week. Their reports are sent out to the referring doctor within 24 h of bone densitometry measurement.

Table 6.4 summarises the functional components of an osteoporosis service.

The design of the service is such that "inappropriate" involvement of senior medical staff for those patients with normal BMD is avoided. The referral proforma should guide general practitioners and hospital colleagues to make only appropriate referrals. This service style enables targeting of those patients with the highest risk of osteoporosis and enables them to be identified and managed most efficiently. The provision of health promotion at the time of maximum patient interest, i.e. the time of attendance for bone densitometry seems appropriate. Hand-in-glove with the development of bone densitometry services should be additional services including a nurse led education group for patients with osteoporosis, and a telephone helpline open to patients and doctors managing patients. Patients with osteoporosis can be put in touch with the National Osteoporosis Society or local groups (Table 6.5).

The most appropriate scanning site, i.e. the lumbar spine, femoral neck or peripheral site, e.g. wrist or heel, is dependent partly on the age of the patient and the clinical context. In general most patients referred to the service have both lumbar spine and femoral neck measurements carried out. However, patients over the age of 65 years are likely to have significant degenerative disc disease and therefore this site is unreliable for diagnostic purposes (Table 6.6).

Although peripheral scanning techniques do offer certain advantages in terms of cost, and size of the devices, measurement time and precision etc., the predictive relationship between peripheral bone density measurement, e.g. of the heel or wrist and hip and vertebral fracture is less strong than measurement at the potential fracture site itself. Therefore, the BMD threshold for therapeutic intervention on the basis of the peripheral measurement may have to be "set" at a

<u>Bone Density Questionnaire</u>

DATE-

GP-
REFERRED BY-
GP / Cons / Other
DISTRICT CODE-
ETHNIC ORIGIN-

D.O.B.   AGE-   SKINFOLD-
D.Number-   HEIGHT-
     WEIGHT-

****

PRE/PERI/POST   HYSTERECTOMY-Y/N
AGE AT MENOPAUSE-   YR-*19*______   OOPHORECTOMY-Y/N
FLUSHES / SWEATS-Y/N   No. PREGNANCIES-
DURATION-   No. CHILDREN-
MENARCHE-

     ORAL CONTRACEPTIVE-Y/N
HRT-Y/N   CURRENT / PAST
PAST/PRESENT   DURATION-

****

SMOKER Y/N   A DAY FOR-
PAST SMOKER Y/N   A DAY FOR-   STOPPED FOR-

****

REGULAR EXERCISE-Y/N
WEIGHT BEARING   TIMES PER WEEK-   MIN PER TIME-
NON WEIGHT BEARING   TIMES PER WEEK-   MIN PER TIME-
ACTIVE / SEDENTARY
ALCOHOL UNITS/WEEK-

****

PAST HISTORY FRACTURE-Y/N   WHICH BONES?-
FAMILY HISTORY FRACTURES/HEIGHT LOSS/DOWAGERS-

****

MILK/PINTS PER WEEK-   WHOLE / SEMI / SKIM
CHEESE/WEEK-   CUPS COFFEE-
YOGHURT/WEEK-   CUPS TEA-

****

CURRENT STEROIDS-Y/N   PAST STEROIDS-Y/N
DOSE-   DURATION-   DURATIONS-

CURRENT ANTICONVULSANTS-Y/N   PAST ANTICONVUL.-Y/N
DOSE-   DURATION-   DURATION-

SERIOUS ILLNESS/SURGERY-

OTHER ANTIRESORPTIVE THERAPY-   DURATION-
LMP-

Figure 6.3 Bone health questionnaire.

Table 6.4. Functional components of an osteoporosis service

1. Diagnostic and interpretative facility
2. Advisory service to patients, general practitioners and referring consultants
3. Specialist investigational services
4. Specialist medical treatment
5. Bone health promotion to general public and doctors
6. Educational service to patients with osteoporosis
7. Audit activities

Table 6.5. Osteoporosis dervice – personnel/facilities

1. Bone densitometer – bone densitometrist/bone counsellor
2. Bone clinic lead consultant with bone laboratory back-up support
3. Osteoporosis education group led by osteoporosis nurse
4. Specialist personnel – physiotherapist, occupation therapist, nutritionist
5. Consultant led advisory links with orthopaedic services, GPs, Accident And Emergency Department
6. Links with the National Osteoporosis Society/local group of NOS

Table 6.6. Most appropriate scanning sites at different ages

< 65 years – BMD lumbar spine. + BMD hip
> 65 years – BMD hip + BMD peripheral site e.g. os calcis

From Baran et al.[8]

different value from that at the lumbar spine or femoral neck (see below). In those patients over 65, where prevention of hip fracture is the main intention, the primary scan site should be the hip. The lumbar spinal values may still be useful for monitoring purposes provided that artefacts are not present. All too often this is not the case and use of peripheral sites may become more important, firstly because they are less likely to be affected in this manner and, secondly, in the elderly there is greater equivalence of bone density between peripheral sites and the axial skeleton than in younger patients.

In measuring the response to treatment, the site selected should be based on the precision of the measurement (ratio of SD to the mean as a percentage) and the response rate of these sites to the clinical intervention. In general the lumbar spine offers the most responsive site in those less than 65 years. In those over 65 years the most appropriate site to measure response to treatment is usually the hip. Peripheral sites may also be used provided they are rich in cancellous bone since these are less affected by artefact than the lumbar spine. In the later age group such peripheral sites may, therefore, provide important additional information (see Table 6.6).

Bone Densitometry Rescanning

Repeat bone densitometry measurements are often used to monitor either the response to therapy or the natural history of bone loss in patients who may have normal bone mass but who may be anticipated to fall, e.g. patients starting corticosteroid therapy. Although this approach is intuitively sensible, and it would plainly be desirable to measure the rate of bone loss both to assess the natural rate of bone loss and conversely to measure the increments in bone mass in response to treatment, the use of such equipment in this context is fraught with difficulties. This is partly due to variations in bone loss between patients, which may be considerable, and the fact that age related bone loss is normally only in the order of 1% a year so that changes in bone density can usually only be reliably detected over long periods. It has been suggested that the main use of repeat bone density measurements might be to improve compliance. It is not clear how much the measurement of bone density itself aids compliance beyond the effect of a review appointment and with it the opportunity to discuss medication. Other factors which need to be considered when interpreting sequel bone density measurements include the regression to the mean phenomenon. Also, since it is not known what proportion of patients fail to respond to treatments, be they HRT or bisphosphonates, it is possible that, even if a patient is losing bone while continuing on treatment, the loss might have been greater without such treatment. An additional area of difficulty relates to the question of consistency of the bone densitometry equipment used for monitoring purposes. Although there may only be small differences using similar machines at different geographical sites these differences may outweigh any effect of drug treatment. Similarly software upgrades may affect the reliability of measurements. This means that, for consistent results, patients should have the measurements repeated on the same machine.

Because of all of these difficulties, the reporting of serial BMD measurements should be cautious and over-interpretation of changes in bone density measurement should be avoided.

Table 6.7. Interval between measurements required for reliable bone loss detection over time

Technique precision error (CV%)[a]	Estimated bone loss (%)	Difference in measurements (%)[b]	Approximate follow-up measurement (years)[c]
1	1	2.77	2.77
1	3	2.77	0.92
2	1	5.54	5.54
2	3	5.54	1.85
3	1	8.32	8.32
3	3	8.32	2.77
4	1	11.08	11.08
4	3	11.08	3.7
5	1	13.30	13.30
5	3	13.30	4.43
6	1	16.63	16.63
6	3	16.63	5.54

[a]This table assumes that accuracy is invariable.
[b]Two scans (measurements) would have to differ by more than this amount to be confident that a real change had occurred with 95% confidence that the detected losses are real.
[c]Time frame for a reliable bone mass measurement follow-up.
Source: Agency for Health Care Policy and Research, US Department of Health and Human Services, Public Health Service. Health Technology assessment, No. 6: bone densitometry: patients with asymptomatic primary hyperparathyroidism. AHCPR Pub. no. 96-0004. December 1995. Rockville, MD.

The rescan interval period depends on the precision of the measurement and the rate of bone loss at the site scanned (Table 6.7).

Precision measurements typically at the lumbar spine and at the femoral neck are 1.25–2%, and 2–3%, respectively. In order to detect a difference either due to treatment, or the natural history of the underlying condition, a change of at least 2.8 at times the precision error is necessary. Thus changes of at least 3.5–5.6% would be necessary to pick up a "real" change in bone mass at the lumbar spine and larger changes would be necessary at the hip. Precision measurements at peripheral sites such as the forearm may be lower than at the axial sites. However, at the forearm the response to treatment or the rate of bone loss may be less than at the lumbar spine because of the relative excess of cortical bone at the former site. A peripheral site with a high cancellous bone content may be preferable. However, the use of peripheral sites in this context has been less well studied than "central" sites such as the hip and spine.

In practice the usual minimum rescan interval period at the lumbar spine and hip is 2 years although in certain circumstances earlier scans may be indicated. For example, those patients receiving high dose corticosteroids with normal bone density should have bone density measurements carried out at 6 months since the maximum rate of loss of BMD in patients receiving steroids occurs in the induction period. In addition there is evidence from drug trials that patients with very low bone density may respond to a greater extent than those with less severely depressed bone density. Therefore, early monitoring, e.g. at 6 months to 1 year, may give an early indication of the response of bone to the intervention. In general, perimenopausal women should have the lumbar spine as the primary monitoring site, although it is often routine to measure BMD changes at the hip as well. At this age, artefactual compounding factors at the lumbar spine are usually less than in those over 65 years. In the older age group the femoral neck can be used in this context and there is also evidence that the os calcis may now be used as a monitoring site.[8]

The precision of each measurement site used at any osteoporosis centre should obviously be subject to close scrutiny with periodic repeat measurements carried out. It needs to be borne in mind that precision measurements are usually under-taken using normal volunteers but should ideally be carried out using patients since this more closely mirrors clinical practice

As discussed repeat measurements may be routinely carried out at 2-year intervals but, where clinically relevant, interim measurements may be carried out on an individual basis to give an early indication of response to treatment and may be used in conjunction with other tests such as bone marker studies. Although lateral scanning has been suggested for monitoring in patients with artefacts which preclude PA scanning, in practice the poor precision of such measurements may preclude this method where older non fan beam technology is used.

Interpretation of Bone Densitometry Results

In the service described above, the interpretation of bone densitometry results is the responsibility of the consultant in charge of the osteoporosis service. In order to provide a meaningful report, the reason for the referral should be clear and to that end the referral proforma illustrated in the appendix indicates the reason for the original referral. With this information, and aided by the results of the bone health questionnaire (see appendix), it is possible for the reporting physician to provide an informed report which preferably should have narrative comments included as needed. Provided the referral proforma and the bone health questionnaire are available, there is no particular need for each patient to be interviewed by the reporting physician. In this way the osteoporosis service based at a hospital can be most efficiently used such that only those patients who have World Health Organisation defined osteoporosis are routinely reviewed in a bone clinic. Ideally the reporting physician should develop practical expertise and receive training in the interpretation of bone density measurements (see below). Depending on the size of the population served, the expertise in the interpretation of bone densitometry results should be focused on one or two individuals in a department. It is not acceptable to provide the hard copy print-outs of bone density measurement to the patients or to the referring physician without an accompanying interpretative report.

Although bone densitometry is the single most useful indicator for risk of fractures, other risk factors identified in the bone health questionnaire could be considered by the reporting clinician. There are many factors which determine risk of fracture independent of bone densitometry. The most important of which emanate from the study of osteoporosis fractures.[16] These include history of prior fracture after the age of 40 years, history of fracture of the hip, wrist or vertebra in a first degree relative and being in the lowest quartile in weight (less than 57.8 kg) and current cigarette smoking. It should be noted, however, that although these risk factors are validated in the USA their applicability in Europe remains to be tested. It has been suggested in a collaborative report led by the National Osteoporosis Foundation[17] that nomograms are used to collate all relevant information including age, BMD, risk factors, probabilities for fractures, etc., in order to come to an informed decision about treatment recommendations. The applicability of this approach will depend on the acceptability of the nomograms to reporting physicians and ultimate validation of such an approach in terms of effectiveness in reducing fracture. At present the application of this approach remains untested.

Effect of Artefacts on Bone Densitometry Measurements

Considerable care should be taken in the interpretation of bone density measurements particularly at the lumbar spine because of the risk of misclassifying patients. Most artefacts result in an increase in bone mass, particularly at the lumbar spine. The potential causes of increased bone density measurements of the lumbar spine are shown in Table 6.8. The scan of the lumbar spine takes in not only the vertebral body, but also the spinous processes of the vertebrae and their arches. It is generally well appreciated that degenerative changes in the facetal joints as well as degenerative changes in the discs and osteophytes may give rise to high bone density. It is important when reviewing bone densitometry scans that differences in BMD measurements which are greater than 10% between adjacent vertebrae are carefully interpreted. If necessary a disclaimer should be issued and the reporting site altered from the usual reporting site (the second to the fourth lumbar vertebra fourth to an alternative e.g. L2–3 Studies of the impact of degenerative changes on bone density including the effect of osteophytes,

Table 6.8. Factor affecting bone density measurements

Intrinsic abnormalities of the vertebrae and discs	OA facetal joints
	Degenerative disc disease/osteophytes/Schmorl's nodes
	Diffuse idiopathic skeletal hyperostosis
	Scheurman's disease
	Epiphseal dysplasia
Infiltrative processes	Metastatic disease
	Osteopetrosis
	Fluorosis
Structural	Scoliosis
	Kyphosis
Others	Myodil
	Overlying barium
	Positional
	Weight gain/fat effects
	Computer software upgrades

scoliosis and overlying vascular calcification have shown in general that over the age of 65 years these factors impinge significantly on the reliability of the DXA measurements. Thus, bone densitometry measurements at the lumbar spine should be interpreted with great caution after this age. Readers are referred to Wahner and Fogelman's text book for a review of this and allied topics.[18]

Where a single vertebra has significantly elevated BMD compared to its adjacent vertebra then a plain radiograph of the lumbar spine may be necessary (see examples). In an attempt to obviate the problems of AP scanning of the spine several bone densitometers have a lateral scan view option. Fan-beam based scanners also provide a similar more detailed facility with almost radiographic quality images. The potential advantage of lateral scanning in terms of localised measurement of true vertebral bone density and the ability to measure a true volumetric density have been outweighed to some extent by the poor precision of lateral scanning although this criticism does not apply to fan beam scanners.

The reporting physician should carefully check the BMD measurements of each vertebra as well as the area measurements, looking for any variation from the normal increase in bone mineral content, vertebral area, and BMD moving down the lumbar vertebrae. In the presence of a vertebral fracture there is characteristically a reduction in height and increase in BMD of the affected vertebra.

Other sources of errors should be considered, particularly when interpreting sequential scans, for example the effect of changes in body fat over time. Errors can also occur because of excess fatty deposition in the vertebral bone marrow.[19]

Differences in the normal ranges used by different manufacturers and the use of local "normal" ranges compiled using non-standard recruitment may give rise to very large differences in classification of patients.[20] There is a need for a UK normal range which can be used by all centres in order to have a consistent standard across the UK.[21]

Other complicating factors include the effect of misalignment or inconsistency in the positioning of patients, this particularly applies to femoral neck scanning. Computer software upgrades may give rise to changes in the reference range with potential for misclassification.

Examples of Difficulties in Interpretation of BMD Measurements

1. Patient F.D. A 75-year-old man, referred with a dorsal kyphosis. Note that the lumbar spine scan shows increased BMD of L1 and L2 compared with L3 with reduced height (3 cms for L1 and L2 compared with L3 and L4). A radiograph was suggested by the reporting physician and this showed sclerotic changes at L1 and L2. The patient's prostatic specific antigen was 331 establishing the diagnosis of carcinoma of the prostate (Fig. 6.4a).

2. Patient E.H. This 74-year-old woman was first referred in March 1991 with a history of numerous dorsal vertebral fractures. Note that the lumbar spine scan shows increased BMD of L2, L3 and L4 compared with L1. The chronological summary sheet shows progressive increases in BMD of the lumbar spine since the patient's first scan at the age of 67 years. Most of this increase was due to degenerative changes in the lumbar spine rather than any increase due to the antiresorptive agents used (cyclical etidronate and subsequently nasal calcitonin). Femoral neck BMD values over this same period of time

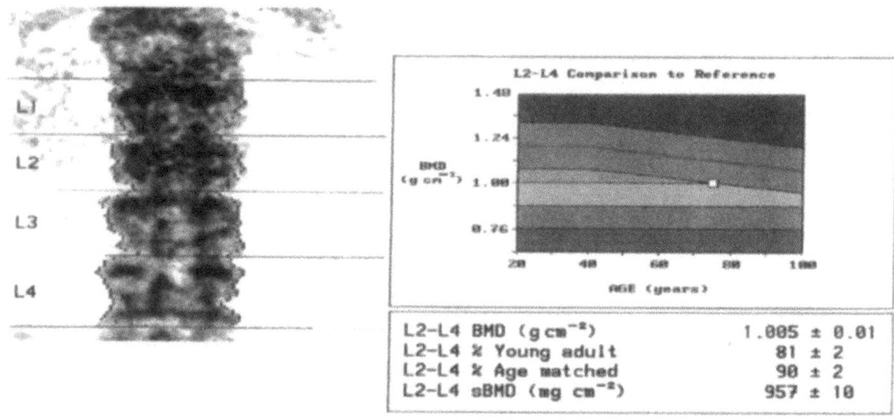

Region	BMD (g cm⁻²)	Young adult %	T	Age matched %	Z
L1	1.159	100	0.0	111	1.0
L2	1.160	94	−0.7	103	0.3
L3	0.987	80	−2.1	88	−1.1
L4	0.910	73	−2.7	81	−1.8
L1 – L2	1.159	97	−0.3	107	0.6
L1 – L3	1.094	90	−1.0	100	0.0
L1 – L4	1.039	85	−1.5	94	−0.5
L2 – L3	1.065	86	−1.5	95	−0.5
L2 – L4	1.005	81	−2.0	90	−1.0
L3 – L4	0.946	76	−2.4	84	−1.5

a

Figure 6.4 Bone density scans illustrating artefacts 1–11.

showed a fall for the first three readings on cyclical etidronate and then a period of consolidation following the use of nasal calcitonin (Fig. 6.4b).

3. Patient E.G. A 53-year-old woman referred because of a premature menopause. The bone mineral density measurement of L3 showed markedly increased bone mineral density at 1.851 gm cm^{-2} compared with 1.162 at L2. An isotope bone scan was carried out, this showed an increase in uptake. radiograph had shown increased density of the vertebral body of L3 (? early Paget's disease) (Fig. 6.4c).

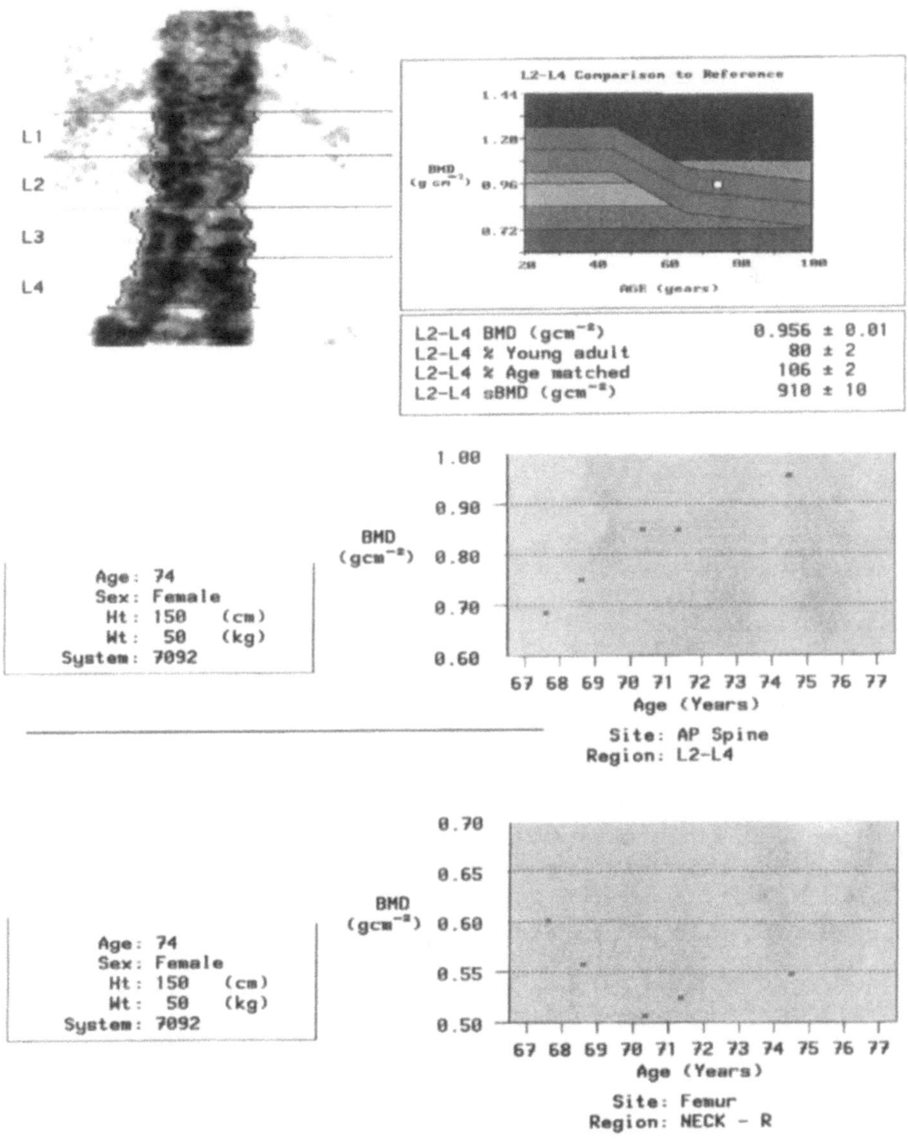

b

Figure 6.4 *continued.*

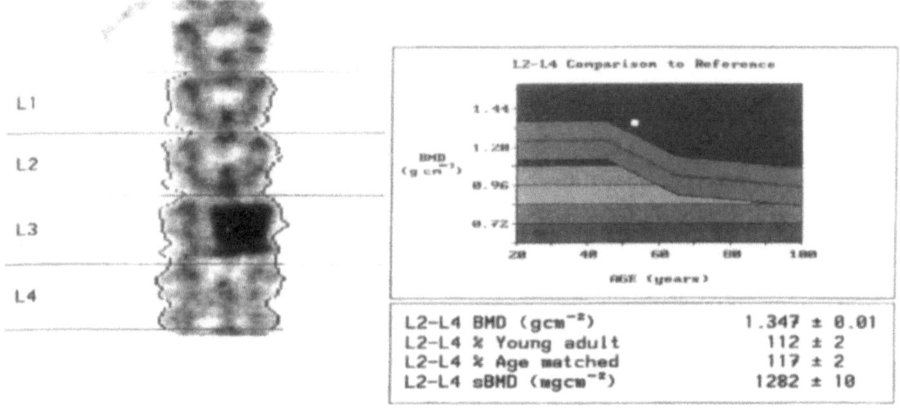

L2–L4 BMD (gcm⁻²)	1.347 ± 0.01
L2–L4 % Young adult	112 ± 2
L2–L4 % Age matched	117 ± 2
L2–L4 sBMD (mgcm⁻²)	1282 ± 10

Region	BMD (g cm⁻²)	Young adult %	T	Age matched %	Z
L1	1.207	107	0.6	112	1.1
L2	1.162	97	−0.3	101	0.1
L3	1.851	154	5.4	161	5.9
L4	0.977	81	−1.9	85	−1.4
L1 – L2	1.184	103	0.3	108	0.7
L1 – L3	1.443	123	2.3	129	2.7
L1 – L4	1.317	112	1.1	117	1.6
L2 – L3	1.541	128	2.8	134	3.3
L2 – L4	1.347	112	1.2	117	1.7
L3 – L4	1.424	119	1.9	124	2.3

c

Figure 6.4 *continued.*

4. Patient O.B. A 66-year-old woman referred for bone density measurement because of a premature menopause (aged 42 years). The scan of the lumbar spine suggests facetal osteoarthritis and associated scoliosis. The average value of L2–L4 (T-score = 0.01) is reassuring yet the bone density measurement of the femoral neck fell outwith the normal range with a T-score of –2.46 (Fig. 6.4**d**).

5. Patient M.S. A 53-year-old woman referred originally because of a premature menopause. She had been commenced on HRT and had been on such treatment for five years. Note that the chronological chart shows an increase in BMD of the lumbar spine amounting to 8.6% change, since baseline measurement. However, the femoral neck values were unchanged over this time. The scan of the lumbar spine itself suggested normal anatomy of the vertebrae. In this situation a plain radiograph of the spine should be requested and use of a further monitoring site considered, e.g. os calcis. In this case the radiograph of the spine was normal, the patient appeared to have a response to HRT limited to the spine (Fig. 6.4**e**).

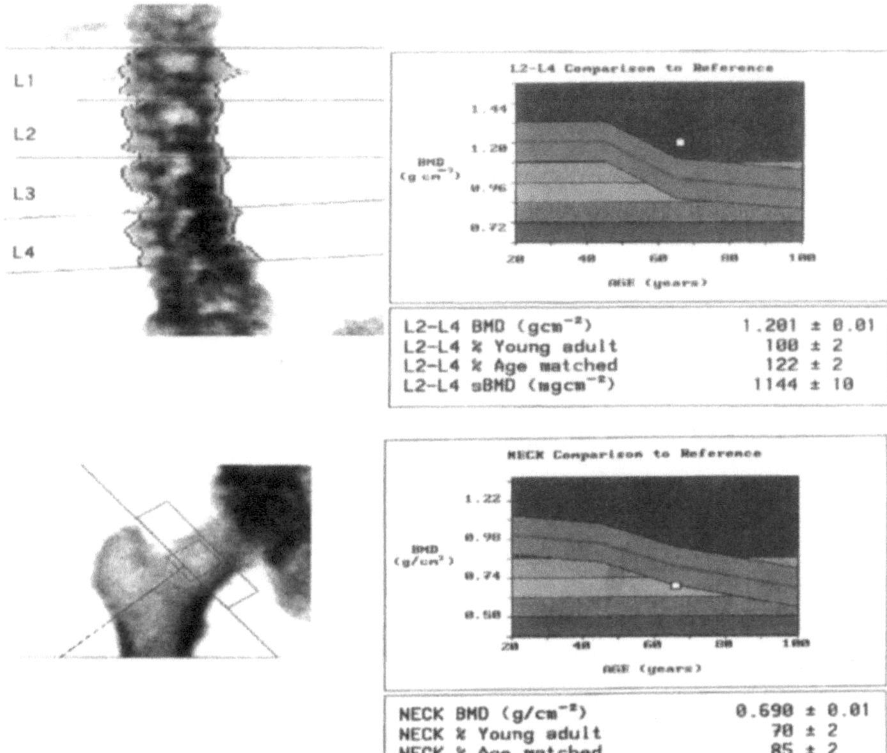

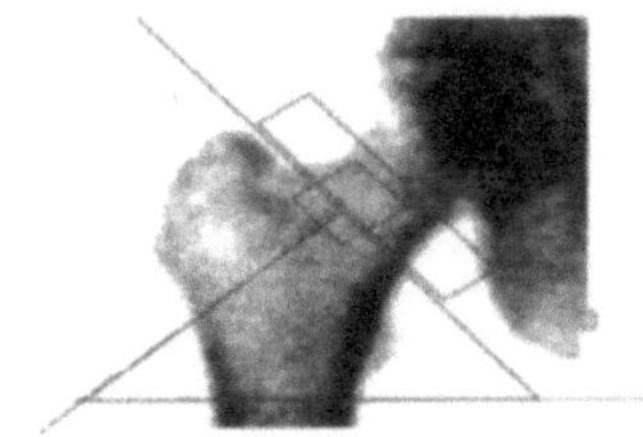

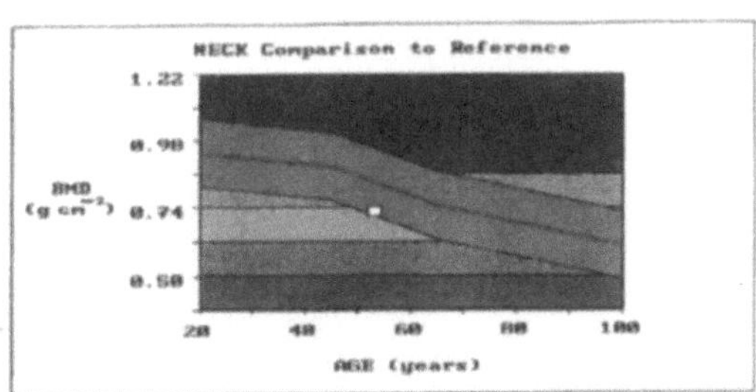

d

Region	BMD (g cm⁻²)	Young adult %	T	Age matched %	Z
NECK	0.728	74	−2.1	88	−0.9
WARDS	0.625	69	−2.2	88	−0.6
TROCH	0.592	75	−1.8	85	−0.9
SHAFT	0.881	−	−	−	−
TOTAL	0.758	76	−2.0	87	−1.0

e (part I)

Figure 6.4 *continued.*

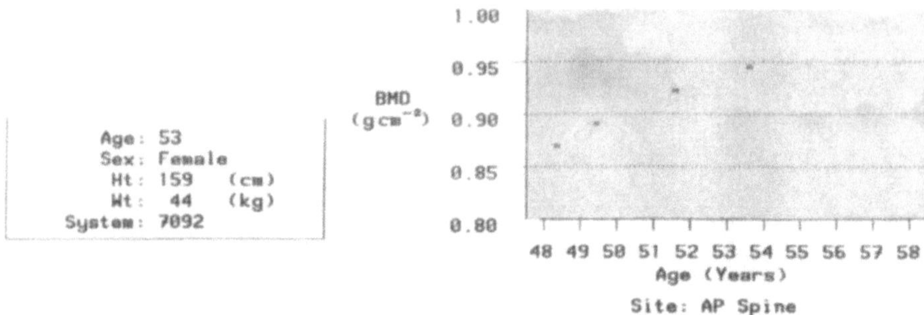

Scan Date	Age	BMD (g cm⁻²)	Change (%)	Change /SD
23.12.92	48.3	0.870	- - -	- - - -
26.01.94	49.4	0.891	2.4	2.1
20.03.96	51.6	0.923	6.1	5.3
20.03.98	53.6	0.945	8.6	7.5

e (part II)

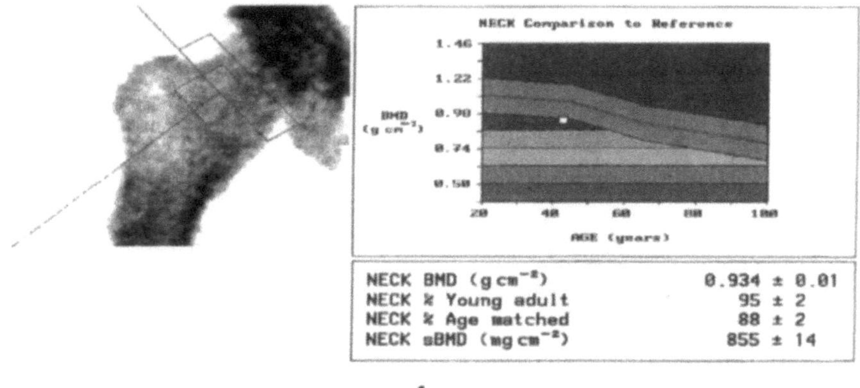

f

Figure 6.4 *continued.*

6. Patient S.B. A 54-year-old woman referred with a two and a half year history of amenorrhoea. The hip values are impossible to interpret because of the abnormally wide femoral neck. The patient was noted to have multiple osteochondromata when her radiograph were reviewed (Fig. 6.4f).

7. Patient F.W. An 81-year-old woman referred because of back pain. Measurements of the hip show normal bone mineral density values for her age although they are depressed in comparison with the young adult mean (T-score = –1.84 at the femoral neck). The appearances of the scan suggest osteoarthritis of the hip confirmed on radiograph therefore the bone density of the femoral neck is not reliable (Fig. 6.4g).

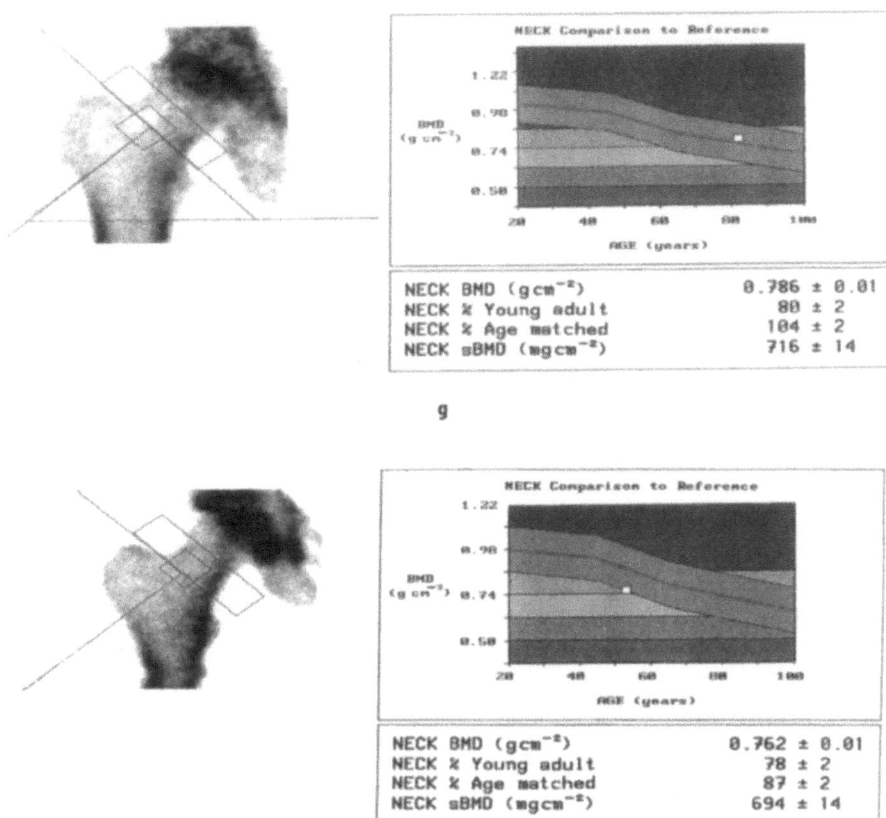

g

h

Figure 6.4 *continued.*

8. Patient E.C. A woman aged 47 with Down syndrome referred because of an early menopause and low trauma fracture. The appearance of the right hip is due to dysplasia. Caution must be used in interpreting such a result in view of the abnormal anatomy (Fig. 6.4h).

9. Patient R.W. A 65-year-old woman referred because of fracture of the neck of femur. As can be seen there is an area of increased bone density abutting the disc space of L3, L4 with increase in BMD at 1.36 gm cm^{-2} and 1.397 gm cm^{-2}, respectively. Radiograph of the lumbar spine (Fig. 6.5) showed degenerative changes at L3, L4. (Fig. 6.4i).

10. Patient M.H. A 70-year-old woman referred with low trauma fractures. Lumbar spinal DXA measurements are uninterpretable due to the scoliotic deformity of the lumbar spine (Fig. 6.4j).

11. Patient C.M. A 46 year-old-lady referred because of use of long term steroids for possible primary biliary cirrhosis. Her BMD values at the lumbar spine and femoral neck were very low. Subsequent investigation included a bone biopsy which showed evidence of severe osteomalacia. The aetiology of her condition was on the basis of renal tubular acidosis (Fig. 6.4k).

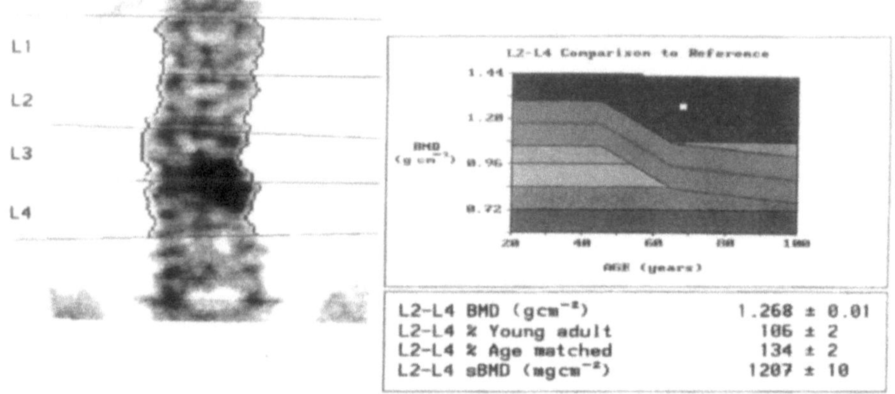

Region	BMD (g cm⁻²)	Young %	adult T	Age %	matched Z
L 1	0.889	79	−2.0	101	0.1
L2	1.042	87	−1.3	110	0.8
L3	1.360	113	1.3	144	3.4
L4	1.397	116	1.6	148	3.8
L1 – L2	0.965	84	−1.5	108	0.6
L1 – L3	1.091	93	−0.7	119	1.5
L1 – L4	1.173	99	−0.1	127	2.1
L2 – L3	1.196	100	0.0	126	2.1
L2 – L4	1.268	106	0.6	134	2.7
L3 – L4	1.380	115	1.5	146	3.6

i

Figure 6.4 *continued.*

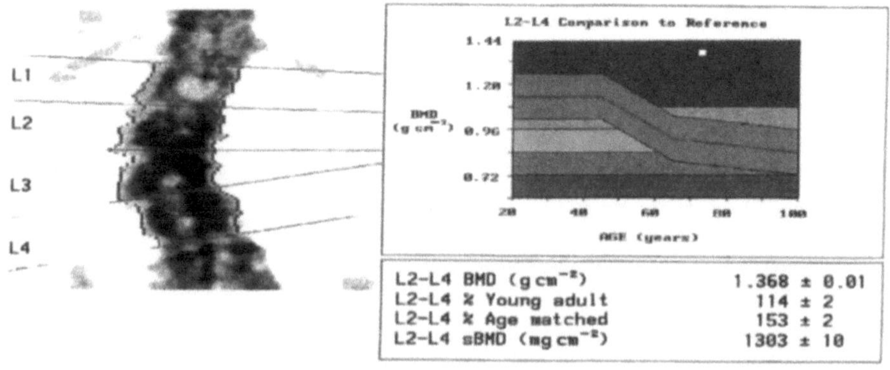

j

Figure 6.4 *continued.*

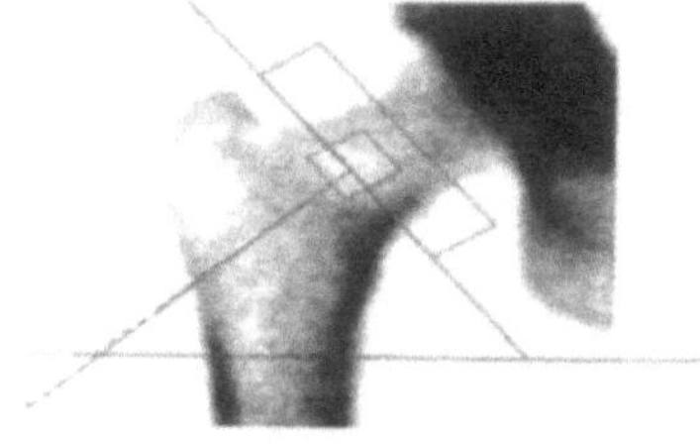

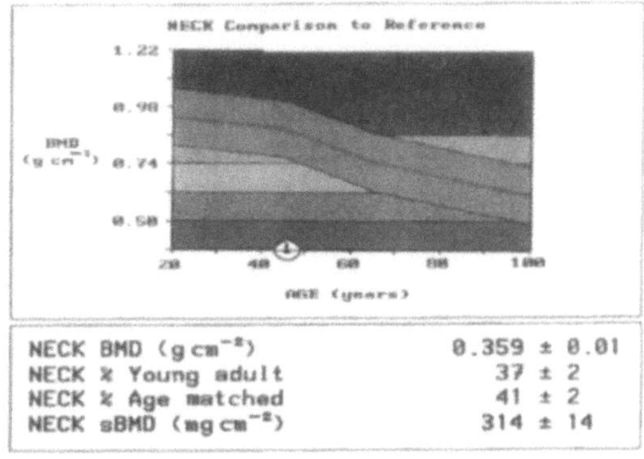

Region	BMD (g cm⁻²)	Young %	adult T	Age %	matched Z
NECK	0.359	37	−5.2	41	−4.3
WARDS	0.219	24	−5.3	28	−4.3
TROCH	0.351	44	−4.0	49	−3.4
SHAFT	0.546	–	–	–	–
TOTAL	0.464	46	−4.5	51	−3.8

k

Figure 6.4 *continued.*

Audit

Underpinning the use of BMD measurements in any osteoporosis service is the premise that identification of patients with low bone mass, and therefore the targeting of such patients with appropriate treatments, will ultimately reduce the incidence of fragility fractures in the community. At present there is no evidence that this is the case. Although the evidence for efficacy of HRT and bisphosphonates in terms of reducing fractures is increasingly compelling, because of the relatively few numbers of patients taking such agents and the delay in the effect of such agents in reducing fractures, it is unlikely that population surveys of incident fractures will show a downturn in the foreseeable future. Therefore, audit activity related to bone densitometry services may be directed more towards process rather than outcome measures. The Advisory Group on Osteoporosis[2] and the RCP report indicated appropriate patient groups to be considered for bone densitometry. These standards should be used in the audit of local bone densitometry services. Similarly the National Osteoporosis Society produced guidance on the local provision for osteoporosis services[22] and setting standards for access to services and the appropriate selection of patients for bone densitometry as well as other standards relating to the interpretation of results

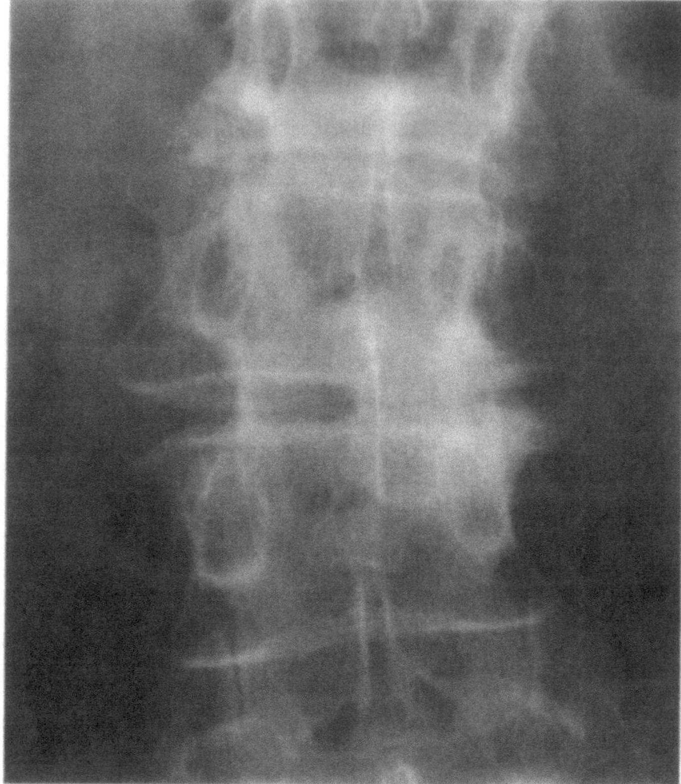

Figure 6.5 Radiograph of lumbar spine.

and the delivery of the results to the referring physician. There are also other requirements for any osteoporosis service, e.g. the provision of a local lead clinician leading a multi-professional team, the provision of a bone clinic and adequate laboratory support to such a clinic.

An example of a study to evaluate clinicians' and patients' awareness, use of, and satisfaction with, a local service is described below.

The purpose was to determine whether patient management changed as a consequence of BMD measurement and to obtain the views both hospital-based doctors and GP on how the service might be provided in the future. The results of this study were also used to influence local purchasers in their discussions about the future need for bone densitometry services. The approach was purely pragmatic on the basis of evaluating an, as yet unproven service, which had already been initiated by the local lead physician.

The study consisted of a survey of all doctors potentially using the service and a prospective survey of all patients undergoing bone densitometry over a 6 month period.[23] This was followed by a subsequent survey of the referring doctors of all those patients who had been seen in the 6-month trial period.

The review of doctors' perspective of the service showed a high awareness of the use of bone densitometry and the need to access the service by locally agreed guidelines. Table 6.9 shows the doctors' indications for referrals. Doctors were

Table 6.9. Usual indications and indications with resources constraints in the NHS for use of the bone densitometry sevice

Indication	Indications from GPs		Indications from consultant	
	Usual ($n = 131$)	With constraints ($n = 179$)[c]	Usual ($n = 24$)	With constraints ($n = 46$)[c]
1. Because patients ask for it	73(56%)	31(17%)	4(17%)	7(15%)
2. Population based screening of asymptomatic women	99(7%)	29(16%)	0	6(13%)
3. Selective testing of high risk patients (premature menopause, on steroids, family history)	119(91%)	165(92%)	19(79%)	40(87%)
4. To help decide whether to prescribe HRT to women	64(49%)	67(37%)	8(33%)	20(43%)
5. To monitor patients' response to treatment for osteoporosis	45(34%)	103(58%)	6(25%)	31(67%)
6. Diagnostic use in patients with symptoms suggestive of osteoporosis (back pain, height loss)	100(76%)	142(79%)	17(71%)	36(78%)
7. Other	4(3%)	4(2%)	0	1(2%)

[a]Only asked of those doctors who reported having used the bone densitometry service; [b]asked of all doctors; [c]one missing value.

asked what their usual indications for bone densitometry referral were and whether these would change in the event of resource constraints being applied. There were significant differences between GPs and consultants, for example more GPs than consultants referred patients because the patients had asked for the tests (73 out of 131 versus 4 out of 24; chi square 10.82, $p = < 0.0001$). Surprisingly, some doctors thought it would be appropriate for population-based screening despite the then recently published Effective Healthcare bulletin advising to the contrary.

From the patients' perspective 309 patients underwent bone densitometry measurement (mean age 57 years, 298 were women.) Subanalysis showed that almost three quarters of patients were aware of the facility for bone densitometry measurements before they had been referred and 86 of the patients had themselves suggested to their doctor that they be referred for bone densitometry. Patients' understanding of the results did not always correlate with the actual bone measurements. Overall the general level of satisfaction with the service was high. The level of apprehension engendered by the test was low. The study showed that the test result influenced the management of 72% of respondents although the form of management did not always necessitate a change in medication. In general the study confirmed a high level of awareness of the service and a high demand for it. There was also a high level of satisfaction of the service both from the patients and the referring physicians. Whether the service provided the most appropriate cost-effective yield remains an unresolved question. As a result of the study an osteoporosis education group was set up led by an osteoporosis nurse in order to improve patients' understanding of their condition.

Apart from detailed audit of services as exemplified, ideally an annual report should be published by each centre including information about the proportion of patients in the normal, osteopenic, and osteoporotic ranges.

Population Needs

It is clear that an osteoporosis service cannot operate in the absence of the technology needed to measure bone mass. Since dual energy absorptiometry is acknowledged as the gold standard diagnostic tool and since BMD is the single most useful indicator of risk of fracture the central role of DXA in the management of patients with osteoporosis is self-evident.

Based on the specific clinical indications for bone densitometry, indicative figures were derived by the Advisory Group on Osteoporosis. This suggested a total of 600 scans per 100,000 population. Based on this and a suggested cost of £25 per scan, this would yield a total cost of £15,000 for an average district of 300,000.

Our own experience of operating an open access bone densitometry service for eight years would suggest that the estimate of 600 scans per 300,000 population is an underestimate. Despite adherence to a constraining proforma the number of scans per 300,000 population averages 918 per year. This figure does, however, reflect the cumulative effect of rescanning patients over a number of years. The National Osteoporosis Society have carried out a national survey of the use of DXA and the findings suggest a need for 934 scans per 100,000 (Table 6.10). This average figure does not allow for patients who have repeat scans to monitor treatment effects.

The current higher price, as opposed to the cost, for DXA scanning charged by Health Trusts is an inhibition to the more widespread use of bone densitometry in the identification of patients with osteoporosis. The advent of cheaper

Table 6.10. Clinical indication/numbers of scans per 100 000 population

Target high risk group	Reason for referral	Nos of scans per 100,000 population[a]
Men and women with:		
Previous low trauma fracture	Assess bone density to decide need for treatment	147
Radiographic evidence of osteopenia	As above	194
Corticosteroid use (>7.5 mg prednisolone daily for 3 months or more)	As above	215
Family history of osteoporosis (especially maternal hip fracture)	As above	107
Ohter clinical risk factors: height loss, kyphosis, low BMI (<19 kg m^{-2})	As above	107
Possible secondary osteoporosis, primary hyperparathyroidism, poorly controlled thyrotoxicosis, malabsorption, rhumatoid arthritis liver disease, alcoholism		54
Women with:		
Oestrogen deficiency (menopause or hysterectomy <45 years, secondary. amenorrhoea >6 months not due to pregnancy, primary hypogonadism)	If HRT contraindicated and in those who are uncertain about or do not wish to take HRT	78
Total scans		902

[a]Based on national survey of DXA provision and epidemiological needs assessment (in press).

equipment may lower the threshold for referrals and thus more patients at potential risk may be identified. Assuming that treatment decisions result in reduced fractures, and that compliance is effected by bone density measurements, then the potential for reducing the incidence of osteoporotic fractures may be realised. Although the arguments against total population screening are overwhelming, particularly since HRT is increasingly used for its cardiovascular benefits as well as the effects on bone mass associated with its use, there are still potentially much larger numbers of patients currently not being referred by general practitioners. This is perhaps because of apprehensions about the long-term management of patients with osteoporosis, and the cost effects of treatment on GP budgets, as well as underdeveloped bone health counselling in general practice. The absence of funding for bone health in general practice is also a large inhibition to the development of such services. Despite this, assuming that the price of scans does drop with the potential advent of portable scanners, it is probable that increasing numbers of patients will have their bone density measured in the future.

The derivation of the costs for a typical bone densitometry service are indicated in Table 6.11.

Table 6.11. Costs of providing a bone densitometry service

	£	£
Direct costs per scan		
Access into system/referral		
File made up/appointment sent		
10 minutes radiographer	2.10	
15 minutes A & C	1.62	
		3.72
Patient care while in Department		
Questionnaire		
Weigh/measure and scan x 2		
40 minutes radiographer		8.43
Patient follow-up		
Analysis of scan		
Consultant reporting		
5 minutes radiographer	1.05	
10 minutes consultant	5.29	
		6.34
		18.49
Additional daily costs		
System back-up		
Re-filing/sorting		
Filing/indexing/card set-up		
Response to queries/telephone calls		
2 hours 55 minutes radiographer	36.86	
30 minutes A & C	3.25	
Cost per day	40.11	
Cost per scan (average 6 scans)		6.68
Summary of cost per scan		
Direct costs	18.49	
Daily costs	6.68	
Other costs	16.70	
Cost per scan	41.87	

The cost effectiveness of DXA scanning will be dependent on the costs of treatment. In general the more expensive the treatment, the more cost effective the use of bone densitometry. Cost utility analysis may further refine the appropriate use of this test in those patients where multiple risk factors are present.

Future Developments

As discussed, a major inhibition to the more widespread provision of osteoporosis services is not merely the relative dearth of bone densitometry equipment itself in the UK, but also that the site of the services provided is usually hospital-based. This is because such equipment is large and fixed rather than small and portable. The clinically important sites of osteoporotic fracture are the spine and femoral neck. The techniques developed have reflected this. The clinical usefulness of axial sites is dependent on their high precision and accuracy and the effect of menopausal bone loss is maximal at axial sites. The effects of antiresorptive agents on bone are also best documented at central sites. The applicability of such techniques is limited by the fixed nature of the densitometers and slow scan times and the fact that the lumbar spinal measurements are particularly prone to artefacts. Because of these difficulties, attention has turned increasingly to the use of peripheral sites, particularly the forearm and the heel which offer reasonable precision and accuracy. The competing merits of pDXA against ultrasound-based techniques continues to intensify. In the United States there has been a large increase in the number of peripheral DXA machines sold and similarly ultrasound-based devices. The types of peripheral scanning devices are indicated in Table 6.12.

The potential advantages of ultrasound techniques include short scan time, and ease of portability. They are generally cheaper than DXA-based techniques and do not carry the risk of ionising radiation. In the United States, three machines have been approved by the FDA (1998), two being os calcis scanners and one tibial. Although ultrasound techniques do not measure bone density, they do provide predictive risk of fractures. The American study of osteoporosis fractures[16] showed that there was a doubling in relative risk of hip fractures independent of BMD measurements for every standard deviation decline in ultrasound attenuation, the EPIDOS Study gave similar results.[24] A prospective study in younger women has also shown that a low stiffness index was associated with greater risk of hip and spine fractures.[25] The case for the use of ultrasound techniques for measuring response to treatment has not been fully made even though the FDA has approved two systems which measure bone stiffness at the calcaneal and tibial sites. The difficulties relating to the assessment of bone density response to treatment at peripheral sites are the relevance of changes in bone

Table 6.12. Peripheral scanning techniques

Peripheral quantitative computed tomography	QCT
Peripheral dual energy X-ray absorptiometry	pDXA
Quantitative ultrasonic attenuation	QUS
Single X-ray absorptiometry	SXA
Radio absorptiometry	RA

density at sites distant to those of clinical relevance. Central DXA is likely to remain the most appropriate technique for assessing response to treatment, not least because the lumbar spine reflects early changes in bone loss at the menopause and conversely shows prompt response to antiresorptives. Secondly, the response of antiresorptive agents at peripheral sites are less than at the lumbar spine. Studies of the effect of alendronate, HRT and placebo in post-menopausal women[26] show that forearm BMD measurements did not change or even decreased after treatment whereas spine and hip BMD measurements increased. After treatment with 5 mg of alendronate, bone density increased by 3.5% at the lumbar spine, HRT increased bone density by 4.5% at the spine. Bone density measurements of the forearm, however, continued to fall despite alendronate therapy and only increased slightly as a result of HRT. Changes in peripheral skeleton bone density therefore may be minimal and delayed compared with the central sites. Notwithstanding, therefore the increased precision of the newer ultrasound-based techniques, their applicability in monitoring responses to treatment remains dubious.

Ultrasound and DXA measurements at the os calcis would appear to be the most appropriate of the peripheral scanning techniques for future development. The site has a high proportion of trabecular bone and its weight-bearing site reflects physical activity. Evidence from Nelson's study[27] showed a similar prevalence of osteopososis attending a bone clinic, whether pDXA or central DXA, was used to classify patients. Although the fracture predictive capabilities are not as good as with central sites, it is likely that the advantages of using peripheral sites will mean that they are increasingly used for selective case finding.

The advantages and disadvantages of peripheral scanning are summarised in Table 6.13.

Thus the predictive value of these sites for the important clinically relevant fractures is less than for axial DXA and rates of bone loss at peripheral sites do not mirror the menopausal bone loss rate at the spine. The advantages of their greater applicability including low cost, ease of use, small size and portability as well as scan speed has never-the-less meant that such devices are increasingly promoted as potentially offering advantages over fixed axial scanners. A working party of the NOS Scientific Advisory Group have produced a position statement relating to the use of forearm bone densitometry partly addressing the question of appropriate thresholds to define fracture risk in relation to T-scores at axial sites.[28] This exercise is necessary because lumbar spine and femoral neck measurement remain the standard sites for the assessment of fracture risk. Correlation between peripheral sites such as the distal or ultra-distal forearm and the femoral neck or lumbar spine varies between 0.53 and 0.67. The threshold for intervention can therefore be adjusted by studying sensitivity and specificity data and using receiver operator characteristic analysis to compute an optimal threshold for patient classification. These exercises have been carried out at the forearm and at the heel.

In a study from the author's own practice (in press), the clinical usefulness of peripheral heel bone density measurements was tested against the lumbar spine and femoral neck sites. Sensitivity and specificity of bone density measurements at the os calcis were compared at these sites. Patients classified as osteoporotic at either the lumbar spine or femoral neck according to WHO T-scores were analysed: sensitivity and specificity; positive (PPV) and negative predictive (NPV) values, and likelihood ratios were calculated at different cut-offs for the os calcis

Table 6.13. Advantages and disadvantages of peripheral scanning

Advantages	Disadvantages
Inexpensive	Measurement sites may not be clinically relevant
Short scan times	Peripheral sites do not reflect response to treatments as great as at central sites
Portability	Ultrasound techniques involve many different measurements (direct and deduced) – lack of conformity
Reduced or little x-ray exposure	Correlation between peripheral and central measurements variable
Good fracture risk prediction	T-scores cannot be used in ultrasound techniques
Applicable to trabecular sites	

Table 6.14. Sensitivity specificity, positive (PPV) and negative (NPV) predictive values, likelihood ratio at various cut-offs of os calcis score

Cut-off for OC - T-score N = 443	Sensitivity %	Specificity %	PPV	NPV	LR
−0.5	91.9	51.1	0.517	0.917	1.88
−0.6	88.2	54.3	0.524	0.890	1.93
−0.7	87.6	58.2	0.544	0.891	2.09
−0.8	85.1	63.8	0.873	0.882	2.35
−0.9	82.0	67.4	0.589	0.868	2.51
−1.0	79.5	72.3	9.621	0.861	2.87
−1.1	76.4	74.8	0.634	0.847	3.03
−1.2	72.7	78.7	0.662	0.835	3.42
−1.3	**69.6**	**82.6**	**0.696**	**0.836**	**4.00**
−1.4	63.4	85.1	0.708	0.803	4.25
−1.5	60.9	86.5	0.721	0.795	4.52
−1.6	57.1	89.0	0.748	0.784	5.20
−1.7	53.4	90.4	0.761	0.773	5.58
−1.8	47.2	91.1	0.752	0.751	5.32
−1.9	46.0	92.6	0.779	0.750	6.17
−2.0	41.0	94.0	0.795	0.736	6.80
−2.1	36.6	95.4	0.819	0.725	7.95
−2.2	34.2	96.8	0.859	0.720	10.70
−2.3	29.2	97.2	0.855	0.706	10.29
−2.4	27.3	97.9	0.880	0.702	12.84
−2.5	23.6	98.2	0.884	0.693	13.31

Logistic regression analysis suggested that the optimum T-score was −1.3.

(Table 6.14). Logistic regression analysis shows that at T-score of −1.3 optimal assignation of patients will occur with a sensitivity of 69.6%, and specificity of 82.6%. Applying such a T-score at the heel would result in the predicted prevalence of osteoporosis at either the lumbar spine or femoral neck for women aged 50–60 years of 27.0%, and 60–70 years of 45.0%. The receiver operator characteristics (ROC) for the os calcis and related to osteoporosis at the spine or femoral neck are shown in Fig. 6.6. The area under the curve was 0.836 (standard error 0.02).

Obviously the choice of which cut-off point to adopt in peripheral bone density measurement depends on the number of false negatives and false positives which are judged acceptable. A low sensitivity will miss too many true cases whereas a low specificity will identify too many false positives. However, using this cut-off point would, we contend, enable consistent management of patients. It is important, however, to note that individual T-scores should not be slavishly interpreted to the exclusion of other clinically important information, for example prevalent fractures and other risk factors.

A change from axial to peripheral bone densitometry devices would depend on the support of primary care groups and health authorities to negotiate appropriate contracting arrangements. There is a risk that an unplanned, unsupervised dissemination of cheaper bone densitometry and ultrasound devices into the community and general practice may result in "uneven" management of patients.

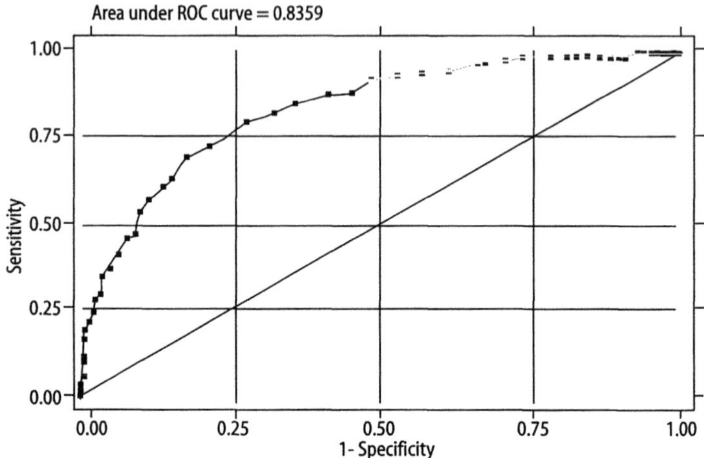

Figure 6.6 ROC analysis of T-score for os calcis in 443 women related to T-score of –2.5 or lower at lumbar spine or femoral neck.

It is crucial therefore that there is consistency of interpretation of bone density results and hence the appropriate medical management of patients. It is important that any expansion and dissemination of bone densitometry services is guided by a lead clinician in the locality in conjunction with any local interest groups including members representing local GPs and other service users. It is also important that the foreseen development and use of peripheral scanners remains within the NHS purview and does not, as has happened to some extent with ultrasound techniques, fall within a commercial umbrella.

The increased use of bone densitometry brings with it the need for maintenance of the quality standards relating to the interpretation of the reports. It is also inevitable that larger numbers of patients will be identified at risk and, assuming this to be the case, there will be increased requirement for specialist bone clinic services and the back-up in terms of laboratory facilities that such clinics require.

Assuming the above changes, the future use of the hospital-based scanners will be open to review. It is probable that in the future hospital scanners will be used primarily for monitoring purposes since measurements of the lumbar spine are of established use in this regard. However, should the early evidence suggesting that the os calcis is also an appropriate monitoring site be proven, then decreasing use of axial hospital scanners may occur.

In the expected scenario outlined above, it is evident that GPs will require continuing education in the field of osteoporosis as will hospital specialists not immediately involved in osteoporosis management. The implications in terms of medical training requirements need to be considered thoroughly. There will also be increased training requirements for nurses likely to become involved in the bone health/drug advisory role in conjunction with GPs. To that end the NOS courses for hospital and practice nurses specialising in osteoporosis will become increasingly relevant.

In the event of the predicted technological advances the "threshold" for the measurement of bone density will drop. The likelihood is that peripheral scanners could be used in fracture clinics and in accident and emergency centres at the time of presentation of patients with fractures such that the assessment of patients with fractures routinely include measurement of bone density. Other clinical contexts in which routine peripheral scanning can be envisaged include menopause clinics and well-women clinics. The use of peripheral scanners in school children may identify those children at increased risk of osteoporosis particularly girls who may benefit from life style advice to increase peak bone mass and hence reduce the risk of fractures in later life.

Other important issues which will need to be addressed include the probable burgeoning cost of drug treatment and, at the moment, the apprehensions of many general practitioners relating to the potential costs of long-term treatment of patients identified as osteoporotic.

Many questions remain to be answered of relevance to the above, not least the usefulness of "single peripheral bone density measurements" as opposed to axial and hip measurements in the diagnosis and management of patients with potential osteoporosis. The evidence at the moment would suggest that it is possible that a single peripheral measurement at a site of high trabecular bone content, may ultimately prove to be as appropriate as measurement at the lumbar spine and hip in identifying those for drug targeting and life style advice. This suggestion needs to be systematically tested by measurement at peripheral skeletal sites and by direct comparison between these sites and the lumbar spine and hip sites.

The ultimate usefulness of such change in practice will only be proven by evidence of reduced fragility fracture rates in local populations. Thus it is necessary to continue to collect and analyse local fracture incidence rates as these services are developed.

References

1. Freemantle N (1992). Screening for osteoporosis to prevent fracture. In: effective health care no. 1. School of Public Health. Leeds.
2. Department of Health (1994) Advisory Group on Osteoporosis report. Department of Health, London.
3. Royal College of Physicians (1999) Osteoporosis: clinical guidelines for prevention and treatment. Royal College of Physicians, London.
4. NHS Executive (1996) Letter. 1110.
5. Department of Health (1998) Health Service Circular. Strategy to prevent fractures caused by osteoporosis 124. Department of Health, London.
6. Department of Health (1998) Nutrition and bone health with particular reference to calcium and vitamin D. Department of Health, London.
7. Compston JE, Papadopolos SE, Blanchard F on behalf of a Working Party from European Member States (1998). Report on osteoporosis in the European Community: Current status and recommendations for the future. Osteoporosis. Int 8:531–534.
8. Baran DT, Faulkner KG, Genant HK et al. (1997) Diagnosis and management of osteoporosis: guidelines for the use of bone densitometry. Calcif. Tissue Int 61:433–440.
9. World Health Organisation(1994) Assessment of fracture risk and its application to screening for postmenopausal osteoporosis. WHO Technical Report Series. WHO, Geneva
10. Wasnich RD, Ross PD, Davis JN et al. (1985) Prediction of postmenopausal fracture risk with use of bone mineral measurements Am J Obstet Gynaecol 153:745–751.
11. Wasnich RD, Ross PD, Davis JW et al. (1989) A comparison of single and multi-site BMC measurements for assessment of spine fracture probability J Nucl Med 30:1166–1171.
12. Ross PD, Wasnich RD, Heilbrum LK et al. (1987) Definition of a spine fracture threshold based upon prospective fracture risk Bone 8:271–278.
13. Rubin S, Cummings S (1992) Results of bone densitometry affect women's decisions about taking measures to prevent fractures Ann Intern Med 116:990–995.

14. Cambell MK Torgerson DJ, Thomas RE et al. (1998) Direct exposure of bone density results to patients: effect on knowledge of osteoporosis risk and anxiety level Osteoporosis Int 8:584–590.

15. Ryan PJ, Harrison R, Blake G et al. (1992) Compliance with hormone replacement therapy (HRT) after screening for post menopausal osteoporosis Br J Obstet Gynaecol 99:325–328.

16. Cummings SR, Nevitt MC, Browner WS et al. for the Study of Osteoporotic Fractures Research Group (1995) Risk Factors for Hip Fractures in White Women N Eng J Med 332:767–773.

17. National Oskeoporosis Foundation (1998) Ostoporosis: review of the evidence for prevention, diagnosis and treatment and cost effectiveness analysis. Osteoporosis Int 8:Suppl 4.

18. Wahner HW, Fogelman J (1994) The evaluation of osteoporosis: dual energy X-ray absorptiometry in clinical practice. Martin Dunitz, London..

19. De Bisschop E, Luypaert R, Louis D et al. (1993) Fat fraction of lumbar bone marrow using in vivo proton nuclear magnetic resonance spectroscopy. Bone 14:133–136.

20. Simmons A, O'Doherty MJ, Barrington SF et al. (1995) A survey of dual energy X-ray absorptiometry (DXA). Normal reference ranges used within the UK and their effect on patient classification Nuc Med Commun 16:1041–1053.

21. Truscott JG, Simpson DS, Fordham JN (1997) A suggested methodology for the construction of national bone densitometry reference ranges: 1372. Caucasian women from four UK sites. Br J Radial 70:1245–1251.

22. National Osteoporosis Society (1995) Provision for a local osteoporosis service. Essential requirements for a hospital based clinical service in the health district. National Osteoporosis Society.

23. Madhok R, Kirby P, Fordham J et al. (1996) Bone densitometry at a district hospital: evaluation of service by doctors and patients Qual Health Care 5:36–43.

24. Hans D, Pargent-Molina P, Schott AM et al. (1996) Ultrasonographic heel measurements to predict hip fractures in elderly women: the EPIDOS Study Lancet 348:511–514.

25. Thompson PW, Taylor J, Oliver R et al. (1998) Quantitative ultrasound of the heel predicts wrist and osteoporosis related fractures in women aged 45–75 J Clin Densitometry 3:219–25.

26 Hosking D, Clair ED, Chilvers D et al. (1998) Prevention of bone loss with alendronate in post-menopausal women under 60 years of age N Engl J Med 338:445.

27. Nelson DA, Molloy R, Kleerekoper M (1998) Prevelance of osteoporosis in women referred for bone density testing: utility of multiple skeletal site J Clin Densitometry 1:5–13.

28. National Osteoporosis Society (1999) The use of forearm X-ray absorptiometry: A position statement. National Osteoporosis Society.

7 Developing Clinical Practice Guidelines (CPGs) for Bone Mineral Density Measurement and Osteoporosis Management

R.A. Hughes

Clinical Practice Guidelines: An Introduction

Definition

Clinical Practice Guidelines (CPGs) can be reduced to their driest form by defining them as "systematically developed statements to assist the practitioner and the patient in making decisions about appropriate health care for specific clinical circumstances".[1] Introduced with such excitement it is not surprising that CPGs have tended to become viewed as cumbersome and a hindrance rather than an essential aid to clinical practice.

Alternatively, on a more positive and optimistic note, CPGs can be viewed as a means of improving the standard of care that patients receive whilst reducing health costs by standardising treatment and eliminating unnecessary procedures.[2] CPGs presented as practice algorithms, with straightforward messages, written in simple English in a clear and unequivocal form, are likely to be of help to the busy clinician. Instead of having to assess the whole of the current literature on a certain subject, perhaps not central to their own specialty, doctors can use good CPGs to facilitate the practice of high quality evidence-based medicine; a CPG can act as a backbone around which local clinical management strategies can be based, allowing some uniformity of approach to a particular clinical problem. CPGs can be of particular use in general practice where doctors are regularly expected to deal with diverse clinical problems, with multiple investigation and treatment options available to them, and with limited specialist experience in any particular field. Surveys have shown that GPs are of the opinion that well-constructed CPGs will improve patient care.[3] Unfortunately, too many CPGs of a poor standard have been produced, providing the clinician with yet more unwelcome paperwork which ends up being ignored and subsequently forgotten.

One aim of CPGs may be to define optimal care. Unfortunately optimal care is a nebulous concept and must be approached with caution. In the development of CPGs remember that:

Science cannot define optimal care with certainty;

The process of analysing evidence and opinion is imperfect; unintended bias may cloud the analysis and the production of evidence-based CPGs runs the risk of a lack of objectivity;

Patients are not uniform and there are no absolutes in medicine

It is appropriate to consider development of specific CPGs for bone density measurement and osteoporosis management in the context of the considerable experience of CPG development in general. An analysis of the various steps that lead to the production and implementation of a generic CPG can lead to an understanding of the reasons why even the best intended CPGs have not always resulted in changes in clinical practice. To design CPGs with the appreciation and understanding that its primary purpose is to bring about a change in clinical behaviour can avoid a huge amount of wasted effort.

Pitfalls of CPG Development

A great deal of time and effort can be expended on the process of development of CPGs only to find that the end product fails to influence clinical practice. Before putting pen to paper the potential author should consider some of the ways to avoid such an ignominious destiny.

It is essential to understand that new CPGs must not suggest to the intended user any attempt to restrict free practice of medicine. Badly presented CPGs can be misinterpreted as a crude effort, perhaps motivated by the forces of management, to ration rather than to rationalise available resources.

New CPGs will not succeed if the authors have no clear understanding of the environment of practice of the intended user.[3] No CPG can, or indeed should, be developed in the isolated environment of the provider. An understanding of the environment and psyche of the intended audience can be gained by site visits and by involving the potential audience, or selected members, in the early stages of development. Time spent seeking suitable candidates for a development committee, although often frustrating, can be time well spent. Most CPGs will be developed by the secondary or tertiary care provider or academic from a hospital base with the express purpose of changing the clinical behaviour of the primary care physician. Therefore, the development of most new CPGs will require an understanding of the environment of general practice and an involvement of GPs at an early stage in the development process.[4]

Successful CPGs require the investment of time and effort both in the preparation and the dissemination and implementation. A motivated champion prepared to invest that time is essential for the development of a successful CPG. He or she must be prepared to develop both the CPG and the implementation strategies to accompany that CPG. The strategy for implementation becomes as important as the development and content of the CPG.[2,5] Publication can sometimes be viewed as the end of the process of development of a new CPG but this is a false belief. The methods of dissemination and implementation are vitally important if a CPG is to change clinical behaviour. Even the very best and most appropriate CPG will fail to influence clinical practice if they are merely disseminated rather than implemented. A lot has been written about the development of CPGs but very little work appears to have been done to focus on effective strategies of implementation.[5,6]

An appropriate emphasis must be placed on the anticipated modes of communication between CPG producer and intended user with, where possible, provision of incentives to encourage use. Appropriate auditing of adherence to guidelines will determine both effectiveness and usefulness of a CPG. It is a change in clinical behaviour that will signal the successful implementation of a CPG.

The following points should be considered before starting to develop new CPGs.

1. CPGs must be produced to fulfil an existing need rather than for their own sake.
2. CPGs must allow for flexibility and adaptation to local needs.
3. CPGs should be based on best available evidence – preferably from randomised controlled trials.
4. CPGs must not threaten by overtly restrictive statements and should be sensitive to the possible perception of loss of autonomy and guide rather than demand.
5. CPGs should be developed with input from the potential users at the earliest stages.
6. Local CPGs must take the local environment into account.
7. CPGs must be written in clear simple English – preferably producing unequivocal algorithms that are easy to follow – and should be produced in a professional style.
8. Don't entirely re-invent the wheel. Use previous CPGs and experience of their development to avoid pitfalls.
9. A predetermined implementation strategy is essential.

It is the view of this author that the considerable effort required in the production of effective CPGs can prove worthwhile. It is to be hoped that some of the suggestions and hints given in this chapter will ease the pain of the process for the development team and lead to a successful outcome – change in clinical practice. If the barriers to successful implementation of CPGs are to be broken down the emphasis needs to be placed on better communications between developer and audience, perhaps aided by the generation of a set of acceptable principles for CPG development and a clear focus on generation from a strong evidence base.[7]

Clinical Practice Guidelines: General Hints on Preparation

Need

It is estimated that the American Medical Association has been involved in the production of over 1600 sets of CPGs to date and there are even Guidelines prepared for guideline development! Not all CPGs will have been developed in response to a clearly defined need. CPGs should only be produced where there is clear evidence of that need.

CPGs are best provided for conditions that are prevalent, that have costly implications for investigation and treatment, for diseases that are currently managed inappropriately and where clinical practice variation could result in disparate outcomes and varying costs. The management of osteoporosis in general and the use of BMD measurement in particular would appear to be an appropriate area of need for the use of CPG.

In an individual unit the decision as to whether the development of CPGs is considered appropriate must lie with the local service providers. In the case of bone mineral density (BMD) measurement, the local clinical expert in the field of osteoporosis together with the providers of BMD measurement services, local management and the users of that service will decide on the need for CPGs. An analysis of the potential uses of new CPGs can help to determine need.

Undoubtedly, one of the functions of a CPG in BMD measurement is to provide a logical mechanism whereby limited resources can be used rationally to target the groups at high future or present risk of osteoporotic fracture. However, to fuel a perception that any health service resource is being rationed will be unpopular and can be politically hazardous. In the assessment of need for CPGs consider that, despite the limited resource for BMD measurement in the NHS, CPGs should not be used primarily as a means of restricting access to and, therefore, cost of BMD measurement. Rather, if sensible CPGs are developed that adhere to the principle of improved patient outcome, the use of limited resources will be seen to be rationalised rather than rationed. In an environment of unlimited resources, any approach to BMD measurement other than widespread screening, especially in postmenopausal women, can be criticised. However, in the case of BMD a strong argument can be made for the restriction of BMD to high-risk groups on health economic grounds, especially as, in real life, there is always likely to be a restriction of available scanning facilities. Difficulties do arise in the definition of who is at high risk and this problem will be discussed later in the chapter. CPGs for BMD measurement do allow the primary care physician and the hospital doctor to decide on which patients will best benefit from BMD scanning rather than creating an environment where limited resources are allocated on a first-come first-served basis. If CPGs for BMD are used as one part of an overall strategy to define osteoporosis management, then factors other than measurement of BMD can assume important roles. Lifestyle advice, calcium supplementation and HRT prophylaxis can be seen as being of equal importance to all, and a focus can be placed on appropriate use of measurement of BMD measurement as part of the whole strategy.

Where CPGs are introduced coincident with the setting up of a new osteoporosis service, an initial estimation should be made of the anticipated demand on the BMD service to determine that the CPG being devised will not generate a work/demand overload. Conversely, where a scanning unit has spare capacity and relies for its survival on a continued demand for the service, CPGs can be used to help to generate appropriate business.

High quality CPGs can raise the service profile of a unit with local users and can be used as an 'advertisement' for that service and a public relations exercise.

CPGs have an educational potential.[7,8] CPGs for BMD measurement can be used to highlight the importance of osteoporosis to the non-specialist. Ignorance of the importance of osteoporosis is still widespread. This remains unacceptable with unequivocal evidence that effective identification and management strategies in osteoporosis can reduce subsequent fracture rates. In a field where physicians (and surgeons) in so many disparate disciplines, from general practice to more esoteric hospital specialties, will see patients who are at risk of osteoporosis, there is a need for the osteoporosis experts to lead from the front. Provision of appropriate CPGs, especially for BMD measurement, may help those without the time to keep up to date with the specialist literature on osteoporosis to include within their practice a rational approach to this potential problem. CPGs can act as an important prompt to include assessment of secondary management issues such as corticosteroid osteoporosis when the primary reason for consultation may be for a completely different condition.[9]

There is a need for CPGs in any condition where there may potentially be inappropriate variation in clinical practice. Use of CPGs is most logical where clear evidence of improved outcome exists to favour a certain set approach. Inappropriate use of a resource such as BMD measurement can be potentially wasteful, expensive and may lead to a denial of the service to some at high risk of osteoporotic fracture. Although it is clear that not all facets of osteoporosis management have a single best practice pathway there is now enough evidence to justify general statements of best practice to be based on evidence from well-conducted research studies. The need for CPGs in osteoporosis management extends beyond the need to define best practice. In lobbying for the development of an osteoporosis service and provision of BMD scanning facilities it is essential to engage the interest of the Director of Public Health and team at the District and Regional Health Authorities as well as relevant members of local primary care groups. CPGs can be the basis on which this dialogue is conducted. CPGs are usually viewed favourably by public health departments especially if presented as a move towards evidence-based practice. A good CPG may both define the need for a local BMD scanning service and demonstrate the mechanism by which an osteoporosis service will run.

Finally, the use of CPGs in medical litigation must be mentioned. The potential for legal action in situations such as corticosteroid-induced osteoporosis has become clear with the emergence of a large number of litigation cases brought by patients who claim never to have been warned of the risks of osteoporosis. CPGs that purport to represent accepted best practice in Osteoporosis may be considered to have potential for use in such cases.[9] In general, the attempted use of CPGs by lawyers in malpractice suits may become more common.[10] A successful action for medical negligence must prove that harm occurred to the patient as a consequence of a breach of the doctor's duty of care. The standard of care is usually judged by the Bolam test; "whether the doctor acted in accordance with a practice accepted as proper by a responsible body of medical men skilled in the particular art".[11] As the law stands at present, CPGs have little role to play in legal cases as their status as a reflection of a reasonable standard of care would be called into question. Not only do CPGs vary widely between different hospitals or health districts but CPGs are often oversimplifications of complex medical situations. As such CPGs represent a poor substitute for "expert medical opinions". This is especially the case with osteoporosis where CPG variation is common and best practice often remains uncertain in the absence of adequate evidence. The emergence of CPGs generated by national committees representing professional bodies such as the Royal Colleges may begin to change this situation as CPGs may start to be considered to represent consensus opinion. The 1998 consultation document on quality in the national health service has resulted in the setting up of the National Institute of Clinical Excellence (NICE) which will appraise evidence, develop and disseminate guidance and audit methods and co-ordinate CPG development. A body such as this may provide CPG with more potential for use in a legal capacity.

Medical belief in the legal relevance of CPGs remains uncertain, reflecting the actual situation. When questioned, hospital physicians (US internists) expressed the view that adherence to CPGs is not likely to reduce malpractice suits[12] and GPs were of the opinion that adoption of CPGs may provide a potential defence to litigation.[4] Whatever current or future potential CPGs have as tools to be used in medical negligence cases, they must attempt to provide a definition of accepted best clinical practice. CPGs do serve to highlight certain areas of medicolegal hazard for the practising clinician. It has become increasingly clear that a clinician who prescribes high dose corticosteroids without discussing the risks of steroid-induced osteoporosis runs a potential risk of litigation. Inappropriate management of osteoporosis in general is likely to move further into the legal limelight. At very least, guidelines serve to highlight the importance of having appropriate management strategies for osteoporosis.

Acceptance

Despite enthusiasm for CPGs from policy makers and those involved in health service management, CPGs are not universally viewed with such optimism. The launching of CPGs in a certain field can raise the hackles of those for whom they may represent perceived restriction of free clinical choice. Clinicians are worried about the imposition of "cookbook" medical practice.[4,7] Osteoporosis has an advantage over more established areas of clinical practice such as cardiology and respiratory medicine in countering this criticism. Osteoporosis is a relatively new field and medical school teaching in the subject is not yet written in tablets of stone. In this area CPGs may more easily be welcomed as representing new knowledge rather than attempting to dislodge old ideas or misconceptions. In addition, osteoporosis management is the potential province of the vast majority of practising doctors, whether in hospital or in the community and not merely confined to a single specialty. As such, most doctors will encounter patients at high risk of osteoporotic fracture and may welcome practical advice on management. Organisations such as the National Osteoporosis Society, in particular, have raised the awareness of the condition among both patients and doctors.[13] Guidance towards a standard approach to this new subject area may well be welcomed by those without an in depth knowledge of advances in the area. However, care must still be taken while there is still a belief that "clinical freedom, like other sorts of freedom, cannot be limited without being lost".

To change clinical practice CPGs must engage interest, maintain that interest and be perceived as being of benefit to the patients and doctors alike. The content and mode of implementation will play an important role but factors such as the working practice, environment and personality type of the audience must be appreciated in order to steer the development of the CPG. Acceptance of an attempt to alter clinical behaviour with a CPG, however well written and presented, is likely to be influenced by the personality types in the anticipated audience. Although CPGs cannot be tailored to the individual, a basic knowledge of behavioural psychology may be of help in designing them. These concepts apply equally to any situation involving acceptance and implementation of new ideas that lead to behavioural change.

People can be considered to be;
Innovators – venturesome
Early adopters – respectable

Early majority – deliberate

Late majority – sceptical

Laggards – traditional

The development of guidelines represents a challenge for it must attempt to alter clinical behaviour in people of different personality types. The innovator may need enthusiasm for a new technology such as bone density scanning to be curbed, whereas the laggard may need more positive incentives, financial or otherwise, to be convinced of the merits of a change to their traditional practice. More effort will need to be made to change the behaviour of the sceptical majority whereas any amount of effort with the laggards may meet with failure. The position is made more complicated by the coexistence of a number of different personality types within any single large GP practice. As the strains on health care providers increase so the need to seek and provide a suitable "reward" structure to encourage practice change in the context of new CPGs will become more important.

Acceptance of guidelines advocating the rational use of bone density measurement may run into some difficulty if bone density services have been set up for financial gain, whether under the auspices of the NHS or in the private sector. It is hard to see clinical practice changing in such a situation unless there is a financial disincentive introduced to discourage inappropriate use. Happily, a case can usually be made for BMD measurement in the majority of patients, many of whom may not necessarily demonstrate high risk factors for osteoporosis and BMD measurement will not be indicated. Because BMD measurement is quick and easy to perform with minimal radiation exposure, variance in practice is unlikely to be harmful clinically if the technique is overused.

Development

GPs have expressed the view that the majority of CPGs they have received concerning a wide variety of clinical topics have been of no use as they have been developed by academics with little reference to, or knowledge of, the day-to-day running of a general practice surgery. Such criticism has undoubtedly been of some relevance and great care must be taken to involve GPs in the development of CPGs especially if the aim of the CPG is to change GP behaviour. In a health world where primary care is becoming increasingly powerful one of the main barriers to effective development of new guidelines seems to be lack of GP involvement at an early stage. In an area of practice such as osteoporosis where GPs are likely to remain as central players, this involvement is especially vital. The development of CPGs aimed towards empowering the GP as the central figure at the centre of the osteoporosis service will be viewed positively by health authorities and policy managers. However, the GP may view new CPGs with disdain if it is presented as yet another imposition on the time, resources and energy of the GP practice, presented by hospital doctors or academics with little or no knowledge of general practice.

The validity of the new guidelines will be a function of the quality of factual evidence on which the contents are based. There now exist acceptable standards by which the quality of the evidence that influences CPG development and content can be judged. It is important to have some knowledge of these standards to be able to justify CPG content. There are several protocols for appraising published evidence[14] and one well-known and much quoted grading hierarchy is presented below.

I   Randomised controlled trials
II-1   Other clinical trials
II-2   Prospective cohort studies
II-3   Case–control (retrospective) studies
III   Observational studies
IV   Opinions

It could further be argued that a well-presented meta-analysis or formal systematic review might carry the most weight and be graded as I–+.

There is no gold standard for scoring methodological quality but for any single clinical decision appearing in a CPG a checklist or tabulated approach to weighting evidence is suggested. Increasingly CPGs are being developed and formulated when formal evidence is equivocal or even absent such as in the development of a new CPG that relates to male osteoporosis. The development team may even consider comment in the CPG relating to whether or not CPG content has an evidence base.

The conclusions or recommendations contained within guidelines may be graded further according to one of several different systems. One example puts a value judgement on recommendations depending on the strength of evidence. I – implementation implies watertight evidence and a need for action. D – development implies the need for implementation with on-going monitoring and usually involves some degree of experimental innovation or pilot study. Research implies the need for further study. Whether these grades need apply to new CPGs is debatable but the concept of some degree of weighting is still valid.

GPs tend to prefer guidelines that have valid scientific evidence at their core,[4] rather than those drawn up by panels of experts whose views may be swayed by personal experience or prejudice. In areas where clinical research evidence is inconclusive, such as BMD measurement, CPGs can still be drawn up using information from both sources. An alternative "explicit approach" to CPG has been used in areas of clinical uncertainty. Such CPGs include a clear exposition of the relative risks and benefits of adopting a certain clinical strategy and allow the user the final choice.

Implementation

There is a widely held belief, shown repeatedly in surveys, that CPGs do represent good educational tools in theory but prove useless in practice. The counter to this perception would appear to depend on the methods of implementation.

The key to eventual efficacy lies in the method of implementation.[5,6] Literature searches show that surprisingly little effort appears to have been made in researching effective implementation strategies for CPGs. One suspects that much well-intentioned effort has been expended in the development of new CPGs that, in reality, have had little effect on changing clinical practice because they have been inadequately implemented.

The problems inherent in this field have been examined in studies comparing the recommendation in CPGs and actual practice resulting from their dissemination. For example, American Cancer Society Guidelines for investigating for gastrointestinal (GI) cancer recommend primary care routine rectal examination, occult blood tests of stool samples and sigmoidoscopy. Follow up studies showed adherence rates for these procedures running at well under 50%.[15] Poor adherence to these guidelines resulted from lack of a sophisticated technique for their dissemination and implementation. Such attention to sales techniques can do much to draw attention to the importance of a particular CPG and to avoid a perception of irrelevance to the busy GP.

It is simple to see that there is a difference between straightforward dissemination of CPGs and implementation at different levels. Dissemination may involve direct mailing by post, publication in a journal, mailing guidelines to members of a specialist society, posting on the Internet or by presentation at a clinical meeting.[16] These "soft" methods tend not to change attitudes. "Harder" methods of implementation include audits, computer-generated reminders and embedded guidelines. This area warrants a little more discussion. One could borrow a definition of a "dissemination strategy" to describe an educational intervention that aims to influence targeted clinicians attitudes to, and awareness, knowledge and understanding of a set of guidelines. Implementation describes a strategy aimed towards improving targeted clinicians' compliance with guideline recommendations.

Before devising an implementation strategy for new CPGs, the following important factors should be considered:[17]

Source: Who is going to be seen as leading the implementation initiative. Are they knowledgeable? Are they respected?

Channel: Is this formal (media) or informal (face-to-face)?

Message: Content and format must convey the desired message and achieve the desired aim

Audience: Who are they and how will they best be influenced?

Setting: Where will the communication occur? Is this the most influential setting?

New guidelines will only achieve success if a strategy for each area of implementation is carefully thought through.

Channel and source can be considered together. The source must not only be plausible but must also have the necessary energy and enthusiasm. What emerges from the little research that is available regarding the channels of dissemination is the singular lack of success that results when the channel of dissemination has been limited to posting and publishing. Posted CPGs have fared better when accompanied by some form of follow-up package involving personal contact and further education. Face to face methods appear to have a more powerful impact.[16] With lectures and presentations, the dissemination of CPGs can be viewed as an educational experience. Knowledge gain is received better than the burden of yet more paperwork. The introduction of guidelines incorporated into a comprehensive care package as an embedded guideline has been used to try to achieve greater effect. For example, CPGs for infertility can be part of a package containing a structured infertility questionnaire and a semen analysis kit.[18] In the same way, BMD CPGs may accompany a general osteoporosis management package, hormone replacement therapy (HRT) education and advice on how to audit osteoporosis management and treatment to determine compliance with CPG recommendations.

The audience for new CPGs is often made up of GPs working in the setting of the GP surgery. Several factors within the GP surgery can influence whether or not the CPG will be implemented.

GPs work in practices and the currently held beliefs of colleagues who are considered as the thought leaders in that area of medicine within the practice will tend to shape attitudes. If the general attitude of the practice is against implementing or following guidelines then more junior individuals who would, under other circumstances, be keen advocates may remain silent. Whether to target the practice or the individual in the practice may vary. Doctors within the practice who are already involved with the development of other CPGs may be more likely to help with implementation.

Confidence and competence may also influence uptake. Where a CPG involves assessment and subsequent referral, as is the case with BMD measurement, confidence and competence may be of secondary importance compared with, say, CPGs that involve procedures requiring special skills. Unfortunately all the best theorising in the world may be defeated by the constraints of practice within the NHS. Pressures on time, finances, space or pressure from colleagues to prioritise different, perhaps more lucrative, areas of practice may constrain GPs from adopting new guidelines. These must offer a certain degree of local flexibility to allow adaptation to these constraints.

Having a broad concept of the psychosocial mechanisms of a "process of persuasion" may be of some help in designing an implementation strategy. When an individual receives a message the following processes occur on the path to a change in attitudes and behaviour;

- Attention
- Comprehension
- Yielding
- Retention
- Behaviour change

All the steps must be experienced before behaviour is altered.

The target audience must listen to the message and must be able to understand the form in which it is delivered. They must accept the message, remember it and finally act on it. The receiver must be taken through all these steps if the message is going to have any lasting effect. Not surprisingly, it is with the first two stages of CPG implementation that most effort seems to have been expended, perhaps because these areas are the easiest to achieve tangible results with well-constructed and well-presented guidelines. Maybe the conversion of CPGs into practice behaviour has proved so difficult because of the lack of attention to the rest of the pathways that leads to behaviour change. There has been very little guidance towards strategies to maximise yielding and retention of new information in the implementation of CPGs.

To reinforce behaviour change and to ensure adherence there is a necessity to design some form of follow-up strategy. A time course for the introduction of CPGs must include provision for secondary dissemination at an interval from the initial efforts and the use of computer generated reminders and embedded guidelines may help. It is also necessary to put some thought into mechanisms of audit.

Whether this should be carried out at source by monitoring adherence to referral criteria or in certain GP surgeries by examining change of practice will vary according to the parameters to be assessed.

Overall, the implementation presents the greatest challenge in the development of a new CPG.[5,6]

The general considerations relevant to the development of effective CPGs are summarised in Table 7.1.

Table 7.1. General considerations relevant to the development of effective CPGS

Development
Develop CPGs on scientifically valid, evidence-based data
Make them clear and not confusing
Offer interest and education within the CPGs
Implementation
Allow for paced introduction
Apply two or more methods of dissemination – concentrate on methods of communication
Make implementation as easy as possible
Allow for flexibility
Consider embedded CPG as part of a complete management package
Develop an audit and follow up assessment strategy

How to Develop CPGs for BMD Measurement and Osteoporosis Management

What existing CPGs are available to consult?

Basic advice on the clinical indications for BMD measurement have been given in a large number of research papers and editorials and summarised in documents such as the Advisory Group on Osteoporosis Report from the Department of Health of 1994.[19] The principles of CPGs in BMD measurement have been summarised as follows:

Selective case finding

Confirmation of diagnosis

Quantification of response to treatment

Quantification of bone loss

Although an outline of the areas of clinical applicability for BMD are relatively simple to define, the actual processes involved in the development of guidelines for BMD measurement will take a surprisingly long time to complete. Effort can be minimised if experience of previous development is shared across the UK. Building new CPGs for local use on the basis of knowledge gained from studying a published series of CPGs on BMD measurement allows the user to modify the consensus opinion whilst adapting to local needs. In addition, reference to other guidelines in use can increase the confidence of the development team when clinical evidence on which to base CPGs may be equivocal.

Government bodies are becoming increasingly interested in the concept of guideline-driven health care. Enthusiasm is building for the development stage of CPG production to take place at a national level, drawn up by appointed committees of experts, with implementation strategies varying at a local level. The results of nationally based efforts are in the process of publication.

The European Foundation for Osteoporosis (EFFO) has been set up as a non-profit-making organisation, with the aim of collaborating with patient, medical and research societies, health care professionals and the pharmaceutical industry to improve the management of osteoporosis. EFFO is attempting to establish pan-European protocols for osteoporosis management including BMD measurement. The conclusions of their consensus conferences have been published and further protocols are likely to follow.

The National Osteoporosis Society (NOS) is responsible for encouraging initiatives to develop acceptable national guidelines for osteoporosis management and use of diagnostic techniques for BMD measurement. Pharmaceutical companies are engaged in initiatives to set up National and Regional consensus bodies, part of whose brief is to help to develop widely acceptable CPGs for osteoporosis management. The Primary Care Rheumatology Society (PCRS) is an organisation with the aim of educating, informing and encouraging GPs interested in rheumatology and related clinical research. The PCRS has published consensus CPGs on diagnosis and treatment of osteoporosis. These CPGs are unusual in that they were drawn up with full and equal collaboration between GPs and a panel of hospital specialists under the auspices of the NOS. A number of publications exist that have attempted to define a template for CPG for BMD and osteoporosis. The position paper published in 1997[20] in Osteoporosis International is among the most helpful. Such documents should be read as part of the preparatory phase of development for a new local CPG and will give a broad and generally acceptable position regarding the most contentious issues.

New Clinical Guidelines on Osteoporosis Management have been produced by the Royal College of Physicians (RCP) together with the Royal College of Obstetrics and Gynaecology and the Royal College of Surgeons.[21] It is too soon to determine the impact that these will have but they may well serve as a template for the development of local CPGs in the future. The Royal College of Physicians Clinical Guidelines were published in 1999. Whilst providing a comprehensive set of evidence-based CPGs the full RCP document is useful in including the full evidence-base in the form of a literature review of randomised-controlled trials in osteoporosis. The weighty tome that comprises these CPGs will be a useful reference work but is, in itself, unlikely to change clinical practice without extensive investment in their implementation. The RCP report represents the best source of information for the prospective author of a new CPG.

Many CPGs have been developed at a local level. Although there are many of these documents available, there is no all-encompassing reference that details all published CPGs. This author holds 17 different CPGs relating to BMD measurement, many of which have been produced as part of a wider osteoporosis management initiative (Appendix 1).

What clinical areas should be covered by CPGs?

CPGs for BMD measurement could take one of several forms and each of the outlined methods has been attempted. Because there is so little information relating to implementation strategies and clinical effectiveness of CPGs in osteoporosis, the prospective author/s should consider their local needs and existing practice before deciding on the exact form for local development.

The following points need to be taken into consideration.

1. They should help the user to decide who requires BMD measurement according to risk factors for osteoporotic fracture.
2. The more important risk factors may require separate management strategies (i.e. steroid-induced osteoporosis).
3. They should offer help in the interpretation of BMD results.
4. They should guide towards further investigation of an osteoporotic patient.
5. They should help the user to formulate a treatment strategy on the basis of the BMD result.
6. They can act as a reference to guide for referral from primary care to a specialist unit.
7. They can act as an educational aid for all aspects of osteoporosis management.

Risk Factors

It is advisable to consider the age and sex of the patient when devising any CPG. Some authors have decided that it is necessary to include management of premenopausal women, postmenopausal women and men, whilst others simply list risk factors regardless of age or sex.

Most existing CPGs have adopted the conventional risk factor approach when determining for whom BMD measurement is advisable. The user is encouraged to systematically identify those with risk factors for the development of osteoporosis. It is envisaged that the first part of the guidelines will list those risk factors that might prompt the user to send a patient for BMD scanning (Table 7.2).

There will be a different emphasis placed locally on the relative importance of risk factors and whether or not there is an absolute need to measure BMD in all cases. However, a CPG that takes most, or all, of these risk factors into account will prove generally acceptable to all users and could be accompanied by clear instructions on modes of access to the BMD scanner or to the clinic.

CPGs for Separate Risk Factors?

A classic example of the need to consider risk factors separately is the issue of steroid-induced osteoporosis. Studies carried out in general practice and in hospitals have demonstrated that use of oral corticosteroids in doses greater than 7.5 mg prednisolone for more than six months is widespread. Such doses are clearly implicated as accelerators of bone loss, which can be minimised with appropriate anti-resorptive intervention. However, the identification of at risk individuals is still inadequate and should be the subject of a subsection of local guidelines. The definition of a suitable management strategy for these patients is still not clear cut but, currently, efforts are underway to help establish best practice[22]. In the same way, separate attention could be paid to formulating advice to deal with patients who suffer one or more low trauma fractures at the hip or wrist. Guidelines should help to alert the orthopaedic surgeon and the GP to the

Table 7.2. Risk factors for osteoporosis

Women

Premenopausal
History of:
  Thyrotoxicosis
  Amenorrhoea
  Eating disorders
  Multiple fractures
  Prolonged bed rest
  Excess alcohol
  Malabsorption or low dietary calcium
  Oral steroid use for longer than six months
  Co-existent chronic inflammatory disease (rheumatoid arthritis, chronic liver or renal disease)

Perimenopausal
Above plus:
  Menopause before age 45
  Family history of osteoporosis
  Risk factor and reluctant to take HRT

Postmenopausal
Above plus;
  Vertebral fracture
  Developing kyphosis
  Low trauma hip or wrist fracture

Men
Oral steroid use for longer than six months
Male family history
Excess alcohol
Hypogonadal
Prolonged non-weight bearing
Thyrotoxicosis
Low dietary calcium or malabsorption
Low trauma fracture

possibility that the identification of osteoporosis might form an appropriate part of the management of fractures postfixation.

Interpretation of BMD Data

There is a need to provide advice on the interpretation of the BMD scan data and the subsequent path towards treatment. Many problems have been precipitated, especially in general practice, when patients are sent for a BMD scan and the scan is returned with a very basic interpretation of the values but with no clear instructions relating to the next stage of management. Both doctor and patient may end up with a distorted view of the current risk of fracture. Incorrect management strategies and exaggerated pessimism may be the result for the patient. Authors of new guidelines should consider whether the same CPG that determines the risk factor approach to BMD measurement should also include advice on inter-

Table 7.3. A proposed scheme for BMD DXA scan interpretation

	T-score	Z-score
Normal	> 1	Low risk >0
Osteopenia	$-1.0 - -2.5$	Medium risk $0 - -1.0$
Osteoporosis	< -2.5	High risk < -1.0

pretation of BMD values and subsequent treatment. This serves as an educational exercise and empowers the primary care physician as the osteoporosis clinician without the necessity of seeking further specialist advice in uncomplicated cases. As with hypertension, it is this author's belief that the management of osteoporosis should be the province of the GP with reference to specialist advice only when the management is complex.

When considering the results of a dual-energy X-ray absorptiometry (DXA) scan it may be considered acceptable practice to use both T- and Z-scores in the prediction of fracture risk and in calculating the threshold below which to start antiresorptive treatment. Such an approach should avoid undue criticism and allow a clinical algorithm for treatment to be constructed (Table 7.3).

It may prove necessary to modify such a scheme in the future as correlation between DXA values and fracture rates is refined.

Further Investigation

One of the functions of the guidelines is to guide the user towards the need for further tests to exclude secondary causes of osteoporosis in patients with abnormally low BMD. The nature of these investigations and in whom they are to be used will differ in different local settings. As a general principle the CPG can be used to guide the user towards a basic screen suitable to exclude any serious disease likely to have caused low BMD. Such a list will probably include the following tests:

Full blood count

Erythrocyte sedimentation rate

Renal and liver function

Calcium, phosphate and alkaline phosphatase

Serum and urine electrophoresis

Thyroid function

Sex hormone profile

Some authorities also suggest measuring parathyroid hormone and vitamin D (25-OH) in the elderly or housebound.

The Treatment Strategy

Clinical guidelines should guide the user towards rational decisions on treatment. They should preserve the element of choice of treatment whilst giving an up to date exposition of treatment options according to the scan result. Reference to adverse effects and cost of treatments can be made if the CPGs are provided in a fuller educational form. In addition, they can give advice on non-pharmacological "lifestyle" advice such as reducing cigarette smoking and intake of alcohol, taking exercise and ensuring an adequate dietary intake of calcium and vitamin D.

Treatment options are usually linked with scan interpretation according to the use of the T- and Z-scores as discussed, with additional lifestyle advice for all groups, calcium and vitamin D supplementation for osteopenic patients and intervention with antiresorptive drugs for those with established osteoporosis.

Different CPGs may be necessary for different groups of at-risk patients. An easy split would be to consider premenopausal women, postmenopausal women and men as comprising discrete categories. The CPGs for pre-menopausal women and for men will be more difficult to develop as the evidence base for proposed treatment and investigation is less well-established.

Baseline Information on the Current Practice of the Audience

As part of the decision making process, attention should be given to collecting data on the current practice of the anticipated audience. This enables the development of guidelines to focus locally on weak areas and the baseline data facilitate subsequent practice audits that will be designed to assess behavioural change as a consequence of their successful implementation. Collection of baseline data can be very time consuming. The use of postal questionnaires has some advantages but still requires considerable time and is likely to result in poor response rates. Data collection by other methods usually depends on available resources to conduct interviews or scan clinical notes. It is sometimes possible to obtain sponsorship for such exercises, especially from pharmaceutical companies.

The author has had experience of collecting data in the following ways prior to the development and dissemination osteoporosis-related CPGs.

Hospital Practice: Audit Projects

Prevention of Steroid-Induced Osteoporosis

A study was conducted to audit all clinical notes from all medical outpatients seen over a three month period in a district general hospital. The aim was to identify all patients treated with > 7.5 mg prednisolone and to assess the prevalence of any osteoporosis prevention. The study was conducted by a D grade staff nurse employed full time for four months, funded by an educational grant from a pharmaceutical company. There was local presentation and publication.

Management of Osteoporosis in Orthopaedic Practice

Using a postal questionnaire, a study was conducted to define attitudes of orthopaedic surgeons toward their role in the identification of osteoporosis in-patients after treatment of hip or forearm fractures Results were presented at the British Orthopaedic meeting in Cardiff 1997.

Audit of Referral Patterns for BMD Measurement

With the help of the bone densitometry unit it was possible to determine the referral patterns of local general practices and compare them across the anticipated referral area: local reference only.

General Practice: Audit Projects

A Survey of Current Attitudes of GPs Towards Osteoporosis

This study was conducted as a postal questionnaire to gather basic information regarding BMD measurement, osteoporosis treatment and referral patterns: local reference only.

The net result of such data collection is to obtain a much clearer picture of the local practice of osteoporosis management. In the author's particular local area, a need was demonstrated for CPGs for steroid-induced osteoporosis in hospital and a CPG for the local orthopaedic surgeons to define best practice post-fracture.

Starting the Development Process

The first step is to convene a development committee. The membership of such a development committee need not follow a pre-defined format but should include representatives from the following groups, if suitable individuals can be identified:

Lead consultant in osteoporosis (rheumatologist/endocrinologist)
BMD measurement representative (medical physicist or radiologist)
Gynaecologist
Orthopaedic surgeon
Principal pharmacist (or a member of the local Drugs and Therapeutics Committee)
Physician – care of the elderly
Local NOS representative
Local community health care representative
A representative of the local primary care group
A representative from the local Public Health Department at the district health authority
A member of the local Hospital Audit Committee

As can be imagined, such a committee can become a leviathan, providing minimal hope of achieving a consensus of opinion. To avoid this fate, it is

Table 7.4. Suggested timetable for committee meetings

Meeting 1 – Time 0
    Introduce the committee; discuss aims, existing osteoporosis service locally with presentation of baseline data and need for CPGs. Full discussion. Determine timetable of development.

Meeting 2 – Time 1 month
    Present and discuss drafts (? for BMD measurement and interpretation, steroid-induced osteoporosis and algorithms of management). Allow time for full discussion and ensure documents have been precirculated.

Meeting 3 – Time 3 months
    This meeting should allow discussion of further amendments to draft documents having offered the opportunity for members to study the documents and give further feedback.

Meeting 4 – Time 4 months
    Present final guidelines. Discuss issues of publication, endorsement, dissemination and implementation. Seek guidance and involvement of Public Health team.

imperative to limit the membership to those who appear keen to cooperate and who express a common desire to facilitate the project.

The first meeting of such a committee can be used to discuss the current osteoporosis service, the proposed CPG and the anticipated timetable of development including the dates of future meetings of the committee (Table 7.4). At this stage it might be useful to discuss other issues such as sponsorship, printing and mode of publication and who to ask to write the foreword and endorse the finished product.

The subsequent meetings will be used to their maximum efficiency if preparatory work is conducted by either the lead in Osteoporosis or nominated members and the other members of the committee given the opportunity to read draft documents before the meeting. In a committee meeting of this size it is best to use the expertise of the committee to amend initial drafts and to suggest additions if there are areas of omission. Hopefully, the committee meetings will have encouraged the active involvement of all parties interested in osteoporosis management prior to the publication, allowing the presentation of as united a front as possible to the anticipated audience.

Publication Considerations

CPGs are more likely to have some initial impact if presented with clear graphics, an attractive typeface, a good layout and if they are printed using good quality paper. Lack of money may seem to preclude high quality printing but experience shows that sponsorship can be obtained to ease the burden. It is a good idea to seek professional help in the layout, perhaps from the local hospital department of Medical Illustration or from a local design and printing company if this is not available.

It can be of benefit to get a local celebrity or community representative to write a short forward expressing support for the CPG.

Guidelines for osteoporosis management have been published in several different forms. Some have been published as concise sheets, laminated and presented separately, or contained in a hinged folder. Such an approach is valid and, if presented in isolation, must be used as a component part of a wider implementation campaign. Some have been incorporated in a larger osteoporosis manual as a reference document; these can serve as a desktop reference manual but size is likely to preclude close study. One solution is to present as a large reference document with additional laminated summary sheets as enclosures. These laminated sheets may serve as day-to-day working documents for the desktop with the need for occasional reference to the larger document for explanation. It is likely that imaginative or innovative packaging will draw more attention to the contents.

It is important to decide on the number of copies for the first print run. Allow enough copies for postal dissemination to local GPs and hospital staff, together with copies to hand out at implementation meetings, for NOS, CHC and other groups and spares to meet specific requests for extra copies.

Implementation and Dissemination

The importance of this stage and its contribution to the ultimate success or failure of the whole project cannot be overemphasised.[23] There is no correct way to implement CPGs but experience has shown that there are many modes of implementation that result in CPGs finding a place, at best, as coffee mats. They are weak instruments for effecting change if used on their own. It is better that CPGs are to be aimed towards influencing practice at the level of primary care as part of a wider initiative to influence GPs as the main providers of health care. This view is likely to have a profound influence on the choice of implementation.

The following pointers should be considered in devising an implementation strategy for your CPG:

Implement with a **timed** strategy

Consider the employment of a **primary care facilitator**

Consider using **at least two different methods of dissemination**

Consider incorporation into the **practice computer system**

Use **audit** as a tool to encourage implementation

Use **educational meetings** to launch guidelines

Try to encourage use CPGs from within the health authority.

The need for a timed strategy implies that the implementation of guidelines must take place within the wider context of other local CPG development and implementation. Experience suggests that there is little point in trying to implement more than one or two in a single year. The involvement of a member of the audit department on the CPG committee may help to avoid a potential CPG overload on local GPs.

For guidelines to make a big impact on local practice the use of a primary care facilitator may be considered worthwhile. This facilitator can spend time within the local GP practices explaining the CPG and answering queries whilst exploring practical ways of implementation on the "shop floor". They would be expected to conduct subsequent audits of adherence to CPG pathways and behavioural change.

Postal dissemination will usually provide the mainstay of dissemination but the use of alternative additional methods of dissemination should be considered. Some hospitals now have web sites which could be used. If not, consider the use of a web site on the Internet or local network systems. Embedding the CPG within a more strategic overhaul of osteoporosis services may prove effective. The addition of referral criteria to the back of referral forms used to book DXA scans may act as a reminder to referring physicians. There is now a move towards developing software systems that can be incorporated within and accessed from GP desktop computers. One such system has been developed at Arrow Park Hospital on the Wirral in Cheshire, UK and is now used by a national network of hospitals to give GPs reference to information concerning practice pathways and specialist referral criteria at a local level.[24] The use of software to "flag" patients at risk of osteoporosis at the GP level would appear a potential tool for CPGs implementation.

It would appear that educational meetings provide a very good forum for the launch of osteoporosis CPG. Such meetings could utilise the various skills of members of the development committee to offer a day or half day designed to cover all issues of osteoporosis service, emphasising a unified CPG-led approach to the use of BMD measurement, prophylaxis and treatment of osteoporosis.

Audit and Quality Assurance

Audits of adherence to a new CPG can determine how much local practice has changed. The design of an audit will obviously depend on the nature and aims of the CPG.

Audit carried out in a hospital setting will be considerably easier to conduct than one set in general practice but it is the latter that will usually be the test of the effectiveness of CPGs. Some instruction on the design and method of accomplishment of CPG audit in general practice has been described.[25] Dr Peter Stott, a GP in Surrey gives a number of insights into the possibility of conducting osteoporosis audit in general practice. Audit centres around the practice computer files showing diagnosis of osteoporosis, use of high dose steroids, surgery including hysterectomy and fracture identification. Computer records also identify prescription of antiresorptive medication and calcium supplements. The following points are made.

- Doctors are generally too busy to collect audit data.
- Doctors are expensive data collectors.
- Dedicated staff such as nurses are good at collecting data and may be cost effective.
- One person should collect data.
- Funding and time need to be dedicated to this purpose.
- The data collector must be given a vested interest in the collection of data.
- A group leader experienced in audit may facilitate the process.

In simple terms audit should be separated into an audit of structure, process and outcome. Firstly, an audit of structure is possible by predicting the probable number of patients in a practice who should receive investigation and treatment for osteoporosis and determine the actual numbers receiving attention. Secondly, setting audit standards for the process will involve statements such as "all women who take steroids at a dose of 7.5 mg prednisolone or more for six months or more should be referred for BMD measurement." And comparison with recorded practice. The audit of outcome will involve a determination of factors such as treatment with statements like "all women who undergo premature menopause before the age of 45 should be offered HRT prophylaxis to protect their bone density."

Audit performed to a standard template and repeated over time can be used to identify effective CPGs and good implementation strategies that lead to behavioural change. By conducting both hospital and GP based audit the true value of a CPG can be assessed.

Conclusion

The development of new CPGs requires time, effort and dedication, and their true value remains debatable with respect to effecting a significant change in clinical practice. In the field of osteoporosis the need for some form of guidance towards the achievement of a standard of evidence-based practice is demonstrated by the wide variation of current management both in hospital and in general practice.

The worth of guidelines will be a function of the effort put into initial development, the imagination and enthusiasm expended in design, publication and implementation and the forging of close links with an anticipated audience. Feedback with audit studies, second wave implementation strategies and further educational meetings must follow initial publication and dissemination. New electronic methods such as e-mail and the Internet may be used to re-capture attention and allow the hospital-based CPGs to be conveyed directly into the GP surgery.

A CPG should be provided as a document written in clear concise English, and published using a professional layout with considerable efforts made to ensure accuracy with maximum of interest. There should be as much emphasis on implementation of the advice conveyed in the document as on the content.

The Health Services Research Unit at the University of Aberdeen have now set up a Clinical Guidelines Review Group to co-ordinate the development of evidence-based CPG and to help facilitate their implementation (Epoc @ abdn.ac.uk). The setting up of central advice agencies is likely to aid individual units in determining CPG strategy and will, hopefully, prevent duplication of work. Resources such as the Cochrane Database, providing fingertip access to evidence-based reviews should also help in the prospective preparation of local CPGs.

Do CPGs work ?[26] Experience would lean towards the view that good CPGs that are thoughtfully written and well implemented can change clinical practice for the better. There remains a strong suspicion that they are easier to write than to implement and that a large number are worth little more than the paper they are written on – beware.

Appendix 1

The following CPGs have come to the author's attention in the recent past. This list is by no means exhaustive but may act as a guide to past experience of CPG:

West Cumberland Health Care NHS Trust, West Cumberland Hospital, Whitehaven.

Osteoporosis 2000, PO Box 888, Sheffield S8 OHU.

North West Herts, St Albans and Hemel Hempstead NHS Trust, Waverley Road, St Albans AL3 5PN.

Derby Osteoporosis Service, Derbyshire Royal Infirmary, Derby DE12QY.

Bradford Bone Densitometry Service, St Luke's Hospital, Bradford BD5ONA.

Management of Osteoporosis in Wales, University of Wales College of Medicine, Heath Park, Cardiff CF4 4XN.

Osteoporosis Management Guidelines, Morecambe Bay Health Authority, Lancaster Moor Hospital, Lancaster LA1 3JR.

Somerset Osteoporosis Service, East Somerset NHS Trust, Yeovil District Hospital, Higher Kingston, Yeovil, Somerset BA21 4AT.

Guidelines for Bone Densitometry, South Kent Hospitals, William Harvey Hospital, Ashford, Kent TN24 0LZ.

Forest Healthcare Osteoporosis Unit, Chingford Hospital, Larkhall Road, Chingford, London E4 6NL.

Osteoporosis, Northumberland Health Authority.

Osteoporosis Treatment Guidelines, Royal Devon and Exeter Healthcare NHS Trust, Exeter EX2 4UE.

Guidelines for the management of Osteoporosis, Wessex Regional Health Authority.

Primary Care Osteoporosis Management Guidelines, Merton, Sutton and Wandsworth, St George's Hospital, London SW17 0QT.

Southampton Osteoporosis Unit, Southampton General Hospital, Southampton SO16 6YD.

Osteoporosis Guidelines, Havering Hospitals NHS Trust, Waterloo Road, Romford, Essex RM7 OBE.

South West Region Osteoporosis Initiative, Management Resource Pack.

Osteoporosis Management Guidelines, St Peter's Hospital, Chertsey, Surrey KT16 OPZ.

Osteoporosis, Worthing and Southlands NHS Trust Worthing BN11 2DH.

Appendix 2

The following information was produced on laminated sheets with double sided text for convenience of use

1 Side A The Osteoporosis Service at St Peter's Hospital

Referral Criteria
The clinical osteoporosis service at St Peter's Hospital will provide access to bone densitometry, the interpretation of DXA scans and clinical decisions regarding treatment and follow up. Referral to the Osteoporosis Clinic should be considered for any individuals who fulfil any of the following criteria;

- **Oestrogen deficiency –**
  premature menopause   < 45 years
  primary ovarian failure   oophorectomy or hysterectomy < 45 years
  prolonged amenorrhoea   6 months

- anorexia • hyperprolactinaemia • female athlete syndrome

- **Vertebral deformity, multiple low trauma fractures or osteopenia noted on X-rays**

- **Patients with conditions known to accelerate secondary osteoporosis** • Hyperthyroidism • Hyperparathyroidism • Malabsorption • Hypogonadism

- Long-term corticosteroid use (7.5 mg or more daily for > 3 months)

- Women at the time of the menopause considering HRT for bone conservation

- Monitoring antiosteoporotic therapy

- Men suspected of osteoporosis

1   Side B

Other factors that may increase fracture risk:

Family history of osteoporosis
Excess alcohol   Heavy smoking
Dietary calcium deficiency   History of prolonged bed rest (> 3 /12)

? Secondary Cause

In the case of established osteoporosis or multiple vertebral fractures on X-rays it is important to rule out secondary causes.

History and Examination

- FBC (Hb Total WBC Platelets)
- ESR
- LFT's (Alk Phos ALT)
- Serum and urine immuno-electrophoresis
- Calcium and phosphate
- Thyroid function tests (T4 and TSH)
- Serum testosterone (in men)
- Glucose

Referral Procedure

Please send referrals to the Consultant Rheumatologist at St Peters Hospital.

2   Side A   The Interpretation of DXA Scan Results

The scan data are plotted graphically. BMD is shown as a cross (+) allowing for a visual comparison between the BMD for the patient and BMD mean in an age- and sex-matched group. In the spine the value plotted is that for the average of L1–L4. In the hip the BMD for the femoral neck is plotted as this represents the most common fracture site.

BMD values are expressed in relation to reference data in terms of percentages or standard deviations (SD) from the mean: T-scores and Z-scores are given.

- T-score: this represents the number of SD between the patients BMD and the mean reference value for young sex-matched adults with peak BMD.

- Z-score: this represents the number of SD between the BMD and the mean value for a sex-and age-matched individual.

2 SD in either direction will be indicated by dark or light blue shading. An arbitrary fracture threshold line is plotted at 2 SD below the mean for a young sex-matched adult. If BMD falls below this line there is a theoretical increased risk of fracture. A reduction in BMD of 1 SD is associated with a 1.5–3.0-fold rise in fracture risk.

2   Side B

At St Peter's Hospital, DXA scans are interpreted in accordance with the WHO report which recommends osteoporosis to be defined in terms of BMD according to the T-score. Individuals will be placed within one of four diagnostic categories according to the T-score:

- Normal
  A value for BMD within 1 SD of the young adult reference mean.
  Lifestyle advice

- Osteopenia (low bone mass)
  A value for BMD more than 1 SD below the young adult mean but less than 2.5 SD below this value (defined as a T-score between –1 and –2.5)
  Treatment will be calcium and vitamin D. HRT or bisphosphonate prophylaxis may be considered. Lifestyle advice.
  Rescan at 2 years.

- Osteoporosis
  A value for BMD 2.5 SD or more below the young adult mean. (defined as a T-score below –2.5)
  Secondary causes will be excluded. Treatment will be HRT or bisphosphonates, calcium and vitamin D. Lifestyle advice.

- Severe osteoporosis (established osteoporosis)
  As above

There is no absolute threshold for BMD that will determine whether a patient will fracture or not.

References

1. University of Leeds (1994) Effective health care. Implementing clinical guidelines. Bulletin 8 Leeds.
2. Forrest D, Hoskins A, Hussey R (1996) Clinical guidelines and their Implementation. Post Grad Med J 72:19–22.
3. Newton J, Knight D, Woolhead G. (1996) General practitioners and clinical guidelines: a survey of knowledge, use and beliefs. Br J Gen Pract 46:513–517.
4. Siriwardena AN (1995) Clinical guidelines in primary care: a survey of general practitioner's attitudes and behaviour. Br J Gen Pract 45:643–6474.
5. Haines A, Feder G (1993) Guidance on guidelines [editorial], Br M J 305:785–786.
6. Delamothe T (1993) Wanted: guidelines that doctors will follow Br M J 307:218.
7. Woolf SH (1990) Practice Guidelines: A new reality in medicine. I: Recent developments. Arch Intern Med 150:181–1818.
8. Grimshaw JM, Russell IT (1994) Achieving health gain through clincial guidelines II: Ensuring guidelines change medical practice. Quality Health Care 3:45–52.
9. ACR (American College of Rheumatology) (1996) Taskforce on osteoporosis guidelines. Recommendations for the prevention and treatment of glucocorticoid – induced osteoporosis Arthritis Rheum 39:1791–1801.
10. Hyams L, Brandenburg JA, Lipsitz SR et al. (1995) Practice guidelines and malpractice litigation: a two-way street. Ann Intern Med 122:450–455.
11. *Bolam v Friern Barnet Hospital Management Committee.* All ER2 1957:118–122.
12. Tunis SR, Hayward RSA, Wilson MC et al. (1994) Internist attitudes about clinical practice guidelines. Ann Intern Med 120:956–963.
13. NOS Publications. National Osteoporosis Society Bath UK.
14. Woolf SH (1990) Assessing clinical effectiveness of preventive manoeuvres: analytical principles and systematic methods in reviewing evidence J Clin Epidemiol 43:891–905.
15. Mc Phee SJ, Bird JA, Jenkins CNH et al. (1989) Promoting cancer screening. a randomised, controlled trial of three interventions. Arch Intern Med 149:1866–1872.
16 Carter AO, Battista RN, Hodge MJ et al. (1995) Report on the activities and attitudes of organisations active in the clinical guidelines field. Can Med Assoc J 153:901–907.
17? Conroy M, Shannon W (1995) Clinical guidelines: their implementation in general practice Br J Gen Pract 45:371–375.
18. Emslie C, Grimshaw J, Templeton A (1993) Do Clinical guidelines improve general practice management and referral of infertile couples? Br M J 306:1728–1731.
19. Barlow DH (1994) Advisory group on osteoporosis. Department of Health, London.
20. Kanis JA, Delmas P et al. (1997) Guidelines for the diagnosis and management of Osteoporosis Osteoporosis Int 7:390–406.
21. Royal College of Physicians (1999) Osteoporosis. Clinical guidelines for treatment and prevention Lavenham Press, Suffolk (available from the RCP).
22. Eastell R on behalf of a UK Consensus Group meeting on Osteoporosis (1995) Management of cortico-steroid induced osteoporosis. J Intern Med 237:439–447.
23. Suarez-Almazor ME, Russell A (1998) The art versus the science of medicine. Are clinical practice guidelines the answer? Ann Rheum Dis 1998;57:67–69.
24. Buchan IE, Kennedy T (1995) Path finder: an interactive clinical information system. Int J Health Care Qual Assurance 8:32–35
25. Stott P (1994) Osteoporosis audit. Medicom UK Limited.
26. Grimshaw JM, Russell IT (1993) Effect of clinical guidelines on medical practice: a systematic review of rigorous evaluations Lancet 342:1317–1322.

8 Use of Bone Mineral Density Measurement in Orthopaedic Practice

S.M. Hay

Introduction

The consequences of osteoporosis produce a considerable burden on the health service resources both in the United Kingdom and throughout the Western world. Within the past two decades osteoporosis has been the subject of extensive research and major advances have occurred in our understanding of the disease, our ability to assess bone mass, and our ability to reduce fracture risk by the introduction of drugs which will slow the rate of age-related bone loss. Although the study of the mechanisms and the management of osteoporosis is not central to the training of orthopaedic surgeons, the effects of the disease process, which is manifest commonly as fragility fractures of the hip, the wrist and the vertebrae, represent a significant part of our trauma workload. (Fragility fractures, for the purpose of this chapter are those which occur as pathological fractures through bone which has been weakened by the process of osteoporosis. They are therefore low energy fractures, often diagnosed in the elderly, most commonly seen in the wrist, the spine and the hip.)

Osteoporosis may be defined conceptually as "A systemic skeletal disorder characterised by low bone mass and microarchitectural deterioration of bone tissue with a consequent increase in bone fragility and a consequent increase in fracture risk".[1] There has, however, been some controversy with this definition, some believing that the presence of a fracture is necessary to make the diagnosis. This has recently been resolved by the World Health Organisation[2] which has suggested that

Table 8.1. World health organisation classification of osteoporosis[2]

Definition	Criteria
Normal	A value for BMD that is no more than 1 SD below the young normal mean.
Low Bone Mass (Osteopenia)	BMC or BMD 1–2.5 SD below the young normal mean.
Osteoporosis	BMC or BMD more than 2.5 SD below the young normal mean.
Established osteoporosis	Osteoporosis (above) with one or more fragility fractures

BMD, bone mineral density: expressed in g cm^{-2} ie. an areal density. BMC, bone mineral content: expressed in g. SD, standard deviation.

the concept of reduced bone mass and the presence of a fracture should be combined into a stratified classification which includes four categories (Table 8.1).

The value of the WHO definition in particular is that it helps to provide clinical guidelines for the management of osteoporosis based on bone mineral density (BMD) measurements, which nowadays will usually be made using dual-energy X-ray absorptiometry (DXA).

Epidemiology of the Common Osteoporotic Fractures

Osteoporosis is a major health problem in the elderly population leading to more than 150,000 new fractures in the UK each year.[3] On average an individual's peak bone mass is achieved in their mid 30s, after which bone loss begins to occur, although the rate of this will vary between individuals. Bone mass is an important contribution to bone strength and consequently as mass diminishes so the risk of fracture necessarily increases. The incidence of fractures within the community is bimodal, the peaks occurring in youth and in the elderly.[4]

In younger people fracture episodes are generally precipitated by significant trauma and tend to affect the long bones. Young men are affected more often than young women probably reflecting a testosterone driven indulgence in more dangerous activities. After the age of 35 years the overall incidence of fractures in women increases dramatically and the female rates eventually double those of their male counterparts (Fig 8.1).[5] Indeed Donaldson[6] has confirmed that 90% of the fractures due to ageing occur in women and this in part reflects the gonadotrophic hormonal changes which accompany the menopause. An addi-

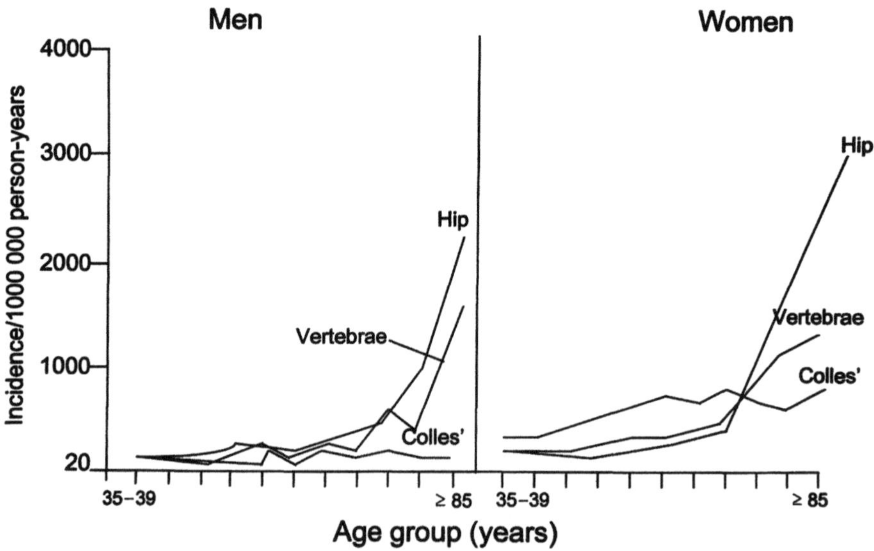

Figure 8.1 Age-specific incidence rates for hip, vertebral, and distal forearm fractures in men and women. Data derived from the population of Rochester, MN, USA. Reproduced with permission from Cooper and Melton.[5]

tional important influence on the increased incidence of fractures among the elderly is their increased tendency to fall. This is greater among women than men and a third or more of all elderly individuals may experience a fall annually. The causes of falls are often mutifactorial, but more than 50% are associated with a definite organic dysfunction and this increases with age. Indeed several organic mechanisms may be contributory including diminished postural control, changes in gait, muscle weakness, decreased reflexes, poor vision, postural hypotension, vestibular problems, confusion or dementia. Specific diseases or disease states including parkinsonism, hemiplegia, cardiac dysrthmias, arthritis and alcoholism will also facilitate falls in vulnerable people. The cause may also be iatrogenic such as the over-zealous use of sedatives and antihypertensives. In addition, the ordinary domestic environment may represent a dangerous assault course for the elderly and contributory factors include slippery surfaces, rugs, steps, kerbs etc.

The age- and sex-specific incidence of osteoporotic fractures is increasing in many countries and if the trends continue it will more than double over the next 15–20 years. Coupled with the fact that the proportion of elderly members within the community is rising due to increased life expectancy, one can begin to appreciate both the enormous health resource implications of this epidemic and the orthopaedic workload conferred.

The fractures most commonly associated with osteoporosis are those of the hip, the spine and the wrist although evidence is emerging that other sites including fractures of the proximal humerus, the clavicle, the toe and the rib are also significantly related to low bone mass.[7,8] However, although fragility fractures are common in an elderly populus, it should be remembered that not all fractures within this age group will be due to osteoporosis, and conversely some fractures even within a younger age group *will* be due to underlying osteoporosis.

The Hip

Estimates suggest that approximately 60,000 new fractures of the proximal femur occur within the UK annually[3] and the greatest total incidence occurs in the 70–80 year age group. The estimated lifetime risk of hip fracture in a 50-year-old white British woman is 14%.[9] These may be intracapsular [Fig. 8.2] or extracapsular [Fig. 8.3] occurring in a ratio of approximately 1:1.[10] Both fracture types are associated with low bone mass, and the relative proportion of extracapsular fractures has gradually increased.[10] The injury usually occurs with a fall from body height and reflects age-related bone fragility and an increased tendency to fall with increasing age, due to general system deterioration and poor neuromuscular co-ordination. Some of the factors which influence the tendency to fall have been discussed above. However, Bonjour et al.[11] have also pointed out the important influence of malnutrition, especially undernutrition, on both the pathogenesis and the consequences of hip fracture in the elderly. They comment that where deficient, the administration of vitamin D and calcium supplements can reduce both femoral bone loss and the incidence of hip fractures in institutionalised patients. In addition a deficiency in vitamin K will increase bone fragility and should be corrected. They have also suggested that reduced protein intake is associated with lower femoral neck BMD and that the administration of an

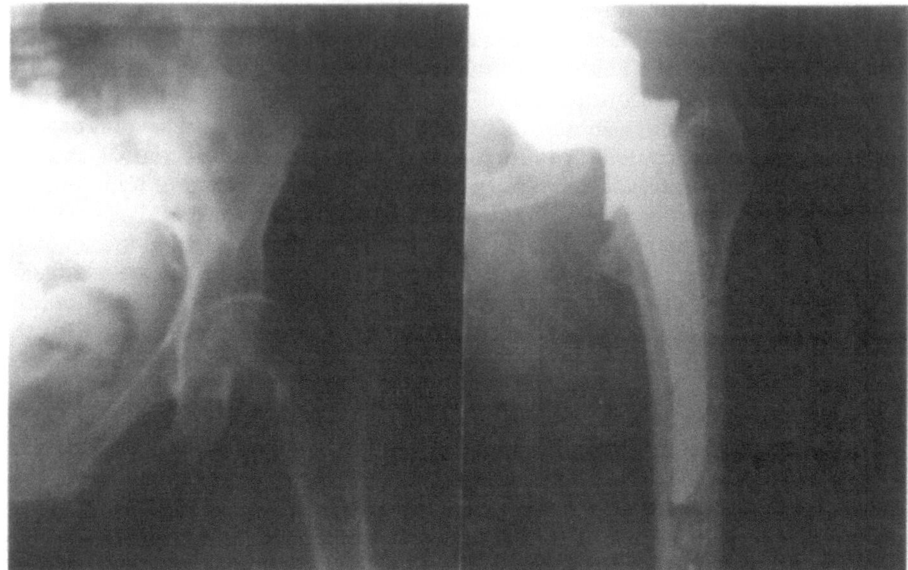

Figure 8.2 Intracapsular fracture of the proximal femur treated by cemented hemiarthroplasty.

appropriate protein diet can improve the outcome of hip fracture both in terms of complication rate and length of stay.

The relationship of the fracture line to the capsule is of particular importance to the orthopaedic surgeon as it reflects the surviving vascularity of the femoral head and will influence the type of surgical procedure undertaken. Displaced intracapsular fractures with an avascular femoral head will usually be treated by a replacement hemiarthroplasty [Fig. 8.2], whereas those which are undisplaced and the femoral head thought to be viable, will be fixed in situ. A proportion of these will inevitably develop avascular necrosis and require revision to total joint arthroplasty or hemiarthroplasty. Extracapsular fractures will normally be reduced and fixed with a dynamic screw and plate, which allows for fracture collapse (Fig. 8.3).

The prevalence of osteoporosis within the femoral neck is 5.1% in the 50–54 year age group but increases to over 60% at 85 years and correspondingly the incidence of hip fractures demonstrates an exponential increase with age. (In males alone the increase is from 0.4% to 29% within these respective age groups.)[12] Hip fractures are the most devastating of the three common osteoporotic fractures usually requiring expensive hospitalisation, surgery, intensive, often prolonged rehabilitation, and are commonly accompanied by significant mortality and morbidity. Various surveys indicate that 12–40% of all hip fracture patients die within six months of the injury and the mortality rate has been reported to be 12–20% higher than in similar populations of the same age and sex without fracture.[13] In addition, it has been reported that only one-third of the survivors are fully mobile 6 months after injury and only 32% of those over 65 years will regain their previous mobility. It is therefore understandable that a large number of patients will require long term institutional care even after intensive rehabilitation.

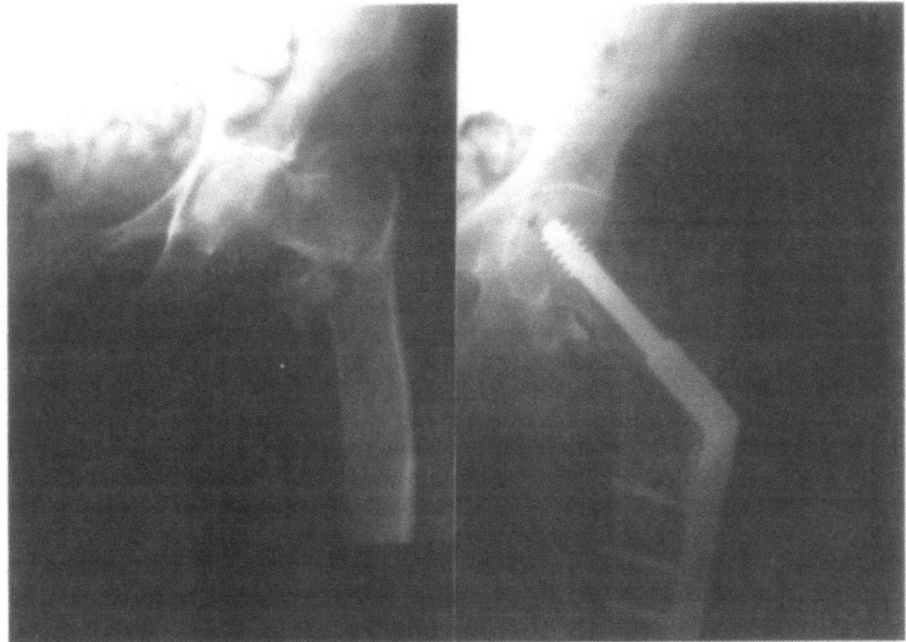

Figure 8.3 Extracapsular fracture of the proximal femur treated by a dynamic hip screw and plate.

The average length of hospital stay for hip fractures is 30 days (1992/93 data) and these fractures account for 20–30% of orthopaedic bed occupancy, which on a mixed trauma/elective orthopaedic ward will inevitably restrict elective admissions. Recently, approaches to this problem have been introduced in an attempt to offload the burden from the orthopaedic wards. Physicians specialising in the care of the elderly are becoming involved in the management of elderly fracture victims at a very early stage following admission, both to help with their preparation for theatre and also to take a lead role in the management of their rehabilitation once the immediate post operative rehabilitation is complete. In addition, the concept of patient management by the "hospital at home" has evolved in some areas whereby, if appropriate, the patient is discharged from hospital at a relatively early stage and rehabilitation is continued, with relevant support services, in the context of the patient's own home environment. One study using this approach suggested that 40% of patients with proximal femoral fractures were suitable for early discharge to such a scheme and this reduced direct hospital costs down from £5606 to £4884 per patient (ie. a saving of £722 per patient).[14]

In 1989 The Royal College of Physicians produced a working party report entitled "Fractured neck of femur – prevention and management".[15] This excellent report thoroughly examined the general management of this increasingly common problem, addressing aetiology, diagnosis, medical and nursing management both during and after admission, the importance of rehabilitation services and the important potential role of preventative measures. Through its laudable recommendations, the report emphasised an "ideal" management system for such patients, some of which has been discussed above. In 1995 the Audit Commission also produced a publication which assessed the overall management of this group of patients entitled "United they stand: co-ordinating care for elderly patients with hip fractures".[16] Once again this document emphasised a number of excellent recommendations, many of which coincided with those listed in the RCP report.

Constraints on such an "ideal" system may be of a practical nature, for example more urgent or deserving cases may inevitably result in delay in treatment of hip fracture patients, later than the recommended 24 h period after admission. However, unquestionably the biggest constraint to an ideal management system is a mixture of finance and resources, especially against a background of an increasingly elderly and vulnerable populus and an enormous nationwide increase in general trauma admissions. The importance of "resource implications" among hip fracture patients is emphasised by Hollingworth et al.[17] They comment on the future need for additional hospital beds to accommodate these patients and the importance of both a preventative strategy and improved community care. However, returning to the reports cited above, despite a lack of resources, it is encouraging that many of these recommendations have, where practical, been introduced and have consistently focused our attention on this important group of patients.

The Spine

The relationship between osteoporosis and vertebral fracture is well established, but the epidemiology of this fracture has been difficult to determine for two reasons. The first is that clinicians differ in their definition of spinal fracture, based on their interpretation of normal and abnormal thoracolumbar vertebral morphology. The second is that a large number of fractures occur without the diagnosis ever being made. Sometimes this is because the fracture has been entirely asymptomatic and sometimes because the patient did not bother approaching their doctor despite the development of pain. Unlike hip and wrist fractures, there is often no specific history of trauma and a fracture will occur spontaneously. The number of clinically diagnosed vertebral fractures is around 40,000 per annum in the UK,[14] but it is estimated that up to 66% may not seek medical attention, suggesting that the true incidence is considerably higher than hip fracture i.e. possibly 120,000.

Whether or not patients present for medical assessment and treatment, the morbidity following spinal fracture may be quite disabling, and includes persistent back pain, kyphosis and loss of height. Population studies suggest an exponential increase in vertebral fracture incidence with age and a 50 year old white British woman will have an estimated remaining lifetime risk of osteoporotic spinal fracture of 11%.[9]

Wasnich et al.[18] have examined the predictive relationship between spinal fractures and non spinal fractures. They have commented that subjects with prevalent non-spine fractures have a threefold increased risk of a vertebral fracture. Furthermore, in subjects with both non-spine and spine fractures the risk rises to sixfold and where also associated with women in the 50th percentile of bone mass or lower, the risk rises to eightfold.

The Distal Forearm

This is the third most common of the fragility fractures and in the UK represents approximately 50,000 new cases per annum[4] [Fig. 8.4]. A 50-year-old white

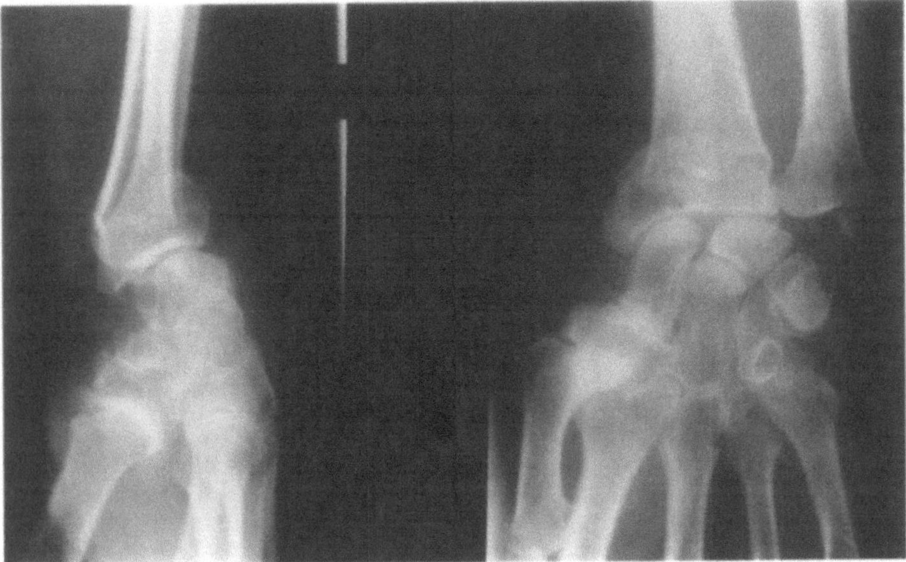

Figure 8.4 Fragility fracture of the distal radius (Colles' fracture)

British woman has a remaining lifetime risk of 13% for developing a distal radial fracture.[9] It is usually caused by a fall on an outstretched hand and as anyone will know who has worked in a hospital accident service during winter, has a marked seasonal influence. It is common in the middle aged and elderly and similar to hip fracture, the majority occur in women, half of which occur after the age of 65 years. Men show no increased risk of wrist fracture with age, the incidence remaining constant between 20 and 80 years. For women however, there is a marked increase in incidence in the five years after menopause but this peaks between the ages of 60 and 70 years, the incidence levelling or slightly declining thereafter, probably reflecting a slowing of bone loss[19] or a change in the pattern of falling. Although most patients with osteoporotic wrist fractures are managed as out-patients, usually requiring at least three out-patient attendances,[20] as the age of the patient increases so the need for hospitalisation following injury also increases, often on social grounds, because of a dependency on help while the arm is immobilised in plaster for 5–6 weeks. However, admission may also be necessary for fracture manipulation, remanipulation or wire fixation under anaesthetic. The injury is painful, may be complicated by neurological injury, and may be followed by algodystrophy in approximately 30% of cases.[21] Despite intensive physiotherapy some residual pain and functional deficit is common and this is therefore not always a benign injury.

Eastell et al.[22] have demonstrated a relationship between bone loss in the ultra distal radius and an increased risk of wrist fracture. In their series of patients with Colles' fractures, 90% had an ultradistal radial BMD of < 0.4 g cm^{-2}. This BMD level is referred to as the "fracture threshold". They found that the fracture risk increased with diminishing levels of bone density. Other studies have also demonstrated a decreased lumbar spine BMD in patients with Colles' fracture[23] suggesting an increased risk of vertebral fracture. A relationship has also been established between Colles' fractures and subsequent risk of hip fracture. In fact it has been reported that women over the age of 70 years who have a wrist fracture had double the expected risk of hip fracture, whereas those under the age of 60 years were at no increased risk.[24]

Financial Cost of Osteoporotic Fractures

Clearly osteoporosis has emerged as a major health problem in the Western world and one which will inevitably increase as the elderly population expands over the next 20–30 years. It has enormous health care resource implications related to both its prevention and its treatment and this has generated considerable interest in the past 10 years. The 1994 estimated cost of managing 150,000 new osteoporotic fractures in England and Wales was £742 million, most of which was attributable to the direct hospital costs of hip fractures.[25] More recently, in 1997 the National Osteoporosis Foundation of the USA has reported that previous financial analyses of osteoporosis have underestimated the costs associated with non hip fractures and this they address in their report on the 1995 figures.[26] During 1995, health care expenditures due to osteoporosis in the USA were estimated at $13.8 billion, of which $8.6 billion (62.4%) was spent on in-patient care, $3.9 billion (28.2%) on nursing home care and $1.3 billion (9.4%) on out-patient services; 75.1% of the total, representing some $10.3 billion was used for the treatment of white women, who are at particular risk of osteoporosis. Besides the economic costs of the disease, there are other costs to be considered, including the psychological effects on the patient, the residual disability experienced, the burden to friends and relatives and the resultant quality of life. Indeed patients with osteoporotic fractures have been shown by some studies to have a reduced quality of life which worsens as the severity of fractures increases. This is reflected by the significant disability incurred by hip fracture patients as demonstrated in Fig. 8.5.[27] Indeed most patients move down one level of dependency after this fracture.[28]

The report from the National Osteoporosis Foundation[26] of the USA emphasises that once an osteoporotic fracture has occurred considerable health care expenditure is incurred and concludes that preventive educational campaigns should be introduced at midlife or earlier in an effort to prevent or ameliorate the

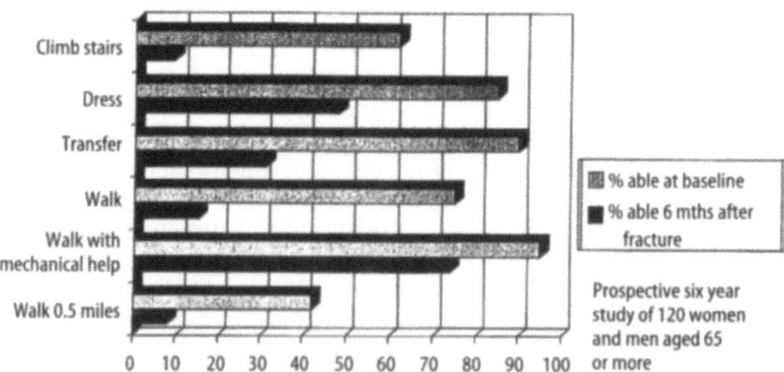

Figure 8.5 Disability following hip fracture. Reproduced with permission from Cooney and Marotolli 1993.[27]

complications of osteoporosis. Consequently a reduction in morbidity and costs could ultimately be realised.

Osteoporosis: Developing a Role for the Orthopaedic Surgeon

To date, the role of the orthopaedic surgeon in the management of osteoporosis has been quite literally to pick up the pieces. The role has focused on the restoration of function following fracture. Usually the surgeon will meet the patient at a stage when advanced bone loss has resulted in a fragility fracture, commonly of the hip or the wrist, but also at other sites, and this in turn will precipitate admission. The surgeon is usually presented with a patient who has poor bone quality and is often a poor anaesthetic risk due age-related multisystem disease, making operation very challenging for both surgeon and anaesthetist alike. A period of fluid resuscitation and drug manipulation is often required to optimise the patient's physiology for the rigours of surgery, which inevitably carries a risk of mortality either in the peroperative or perioperative phase (20% at six months). Against this, the surgeon is aware that an early operation will reduce the risk of the patient succumbing to the dangers of immobility and is likely to improve both the functional end result and the speed of discharge from hospital. This is obviously of considerable importance to the patient's well being but also has cost implications. The management of hip fractures has become a major burden on orthopaedic in-patient beds and if patients remain longer in hospital and acquire complications, so the efficiency of the service drops and the costs escalate. The orthopaedic surgeon therefore has a vested interest in trying to improve the general management of osteoporotic patients over and above the technicalities of surgery, in order to reduce the incidence of such fractures in the longer term.

Within the last ten years three published reports have focused on the management of Osteoporosis:

1. The Royal College of Physicians, "Fractured Neck of Femur – Prevention and Management".[15]
2. The Department of Health, "Osteoporosis – Advisory Group on Osteoporosis"[28]
3. The Audit Commission, "United They Stand – Co-ordinating Care for Elderly Patients with Hip Fracture".[16]

Each has examined the general management of osteoporosis and in particular the management of hip fractures. Each has suggested that the treatment of hip fracture victims has been unsatisfactory. The need for a more efficient, higher standard of preoperative, peroperative and postoperative care is emphasised. The important role of ortho-geriatric liaison is also made and clearly the orthopaedic surgeon is well placed to exercise a pivotal role in facilitating this.

Dual Energy X-Ray Absorptiometry

Bone mass relates to bone strength and is a determinant of hip fracture risk, which increases by 1.5–3 0 times for a 1 SD (standard deviation) reduction in mass.[3] Cummings et al.[29] demonstrate this well with changes in bone density of

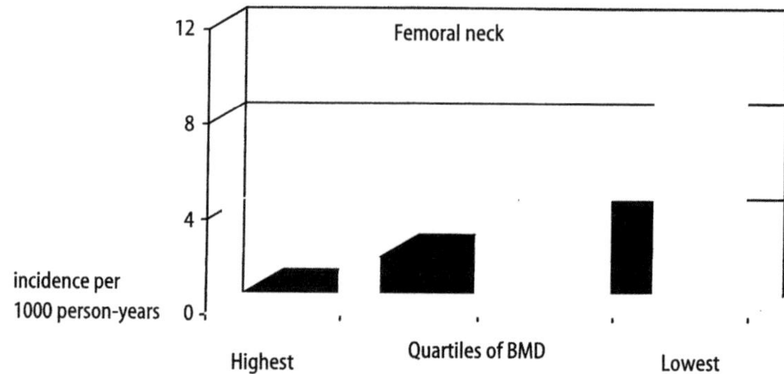

Figure 8.6 Change in hip fracture risk with declining bone density. Reproduced with permission from Cummings SR et al.[29]

the hip (Fig. 8.6). The internal architectural structure is also a determinant[1] as is the patient's risk of falling, which increases with age, although interestingly only approximately one fall in 70 among elderly patients actually results in a fracture. The rate of bone turnover and its plasticity are also relevant factors. Among the elderly, residual bone mass reflects both the peak mass gained in earlier life and the individual's rate of bone loss. The assessment of bone mass may be achieved by several techniques, but since the late 1980s the most popular, and the preferred technique at the 1993 Fourth International Symposium on Osteoporosis, is by DXA (Fig. 8.7).

This technique uses an X-ray tube to generate dual energy photon beams and produces a large photon flux. During scanning, the transmitted photons of two energies are detected separately. Although both energy beams are attenuated by

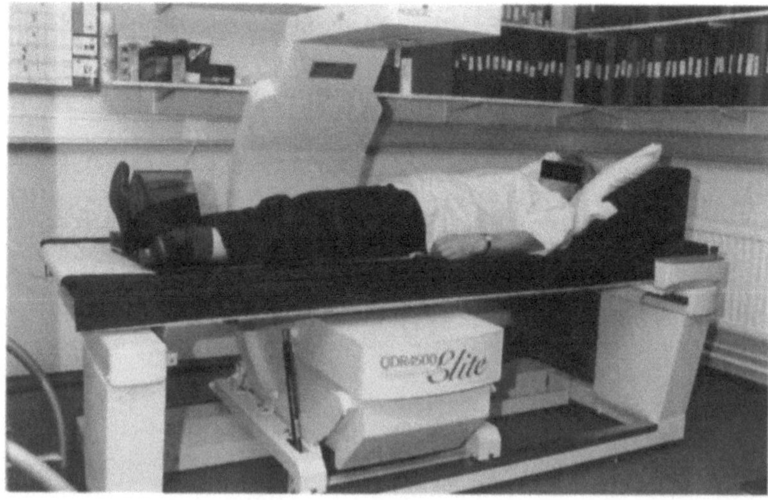

Figure 8.7 The DXA scanner.

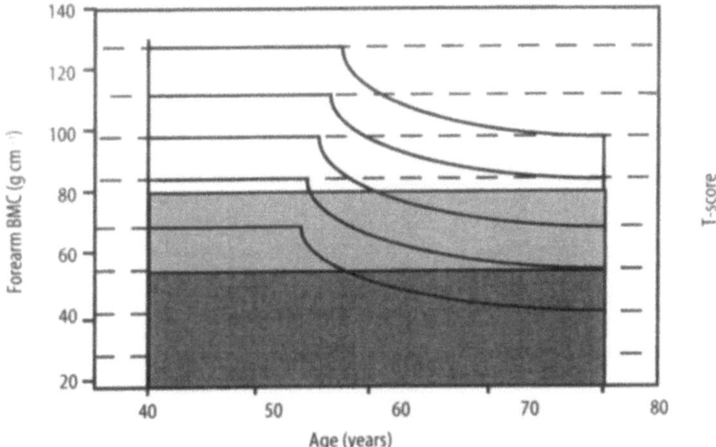

Figure 8.8 World Health Organisation definition of osteoporosis. Light grey represents women with osteopenia. Dark grey area represents women with osteoporosis. T-score is units of standard deviation, compared to the young normal mean. (Adapted from ref. 12)

both soft tissue and bone, the attenuation is greater in bone. Using mathematical formulae the attenuation within bone and the bone mineral content (BMC) can be established. The scan presents the data expressed either as BMC (in grams) or as BMD (in g cm^{-2}), which is expressed as an areal density. To coincide with the clinical treatment guidelines related to the WHO definition of osteoporosis, the result is expressed as a T-score which relates the bone mass to the young normal mean. The T-score value is expressed in standard deviations, therefore the more negative the score, the further from the young normal mean and hence the more porotic. By definition, in a normal distribution, 66% of patients will be within 1 SD either side of the mean and approximately 95% within 2 SD either side of the mean (Fig. 8.8). Density results can also be expressed as a Z-score which relates the bone mass to the same age and sex as the patient, but this is not part of the WHO definition.

DXA can be used to measure bone mass at any site including axial and appendicular sites; it is very reproducible and exposes the patient to very low levels of radiation (less than the daily background levels, or approximately equivalent to 1/15 the dose of a chest radiograph). Scanning occurs in a rectilinear fashion, using a fan beam and the procedure is fast, with some scan times being as quick as 30 s. Measurement of density levels at the hip, the spine and at the wrist[19] can each be used to predict future fracture risk, but the most commonly used sites are the proximal femur and the spine (Fig. 8.9). It is, however, important to point out that axial, spinal density measurements in elderly patients can cause some difficulty in interpretation because of the frequent co-existence of degenerative change within the lumbar facet joints and across the vertebral end plates. This may give the false impression of normal or even high bone density, especially when scanned in the coronal plane. Scanning in the sagittal plane with machines capable of recognising vertebral morphology has helped to reduce this problem.

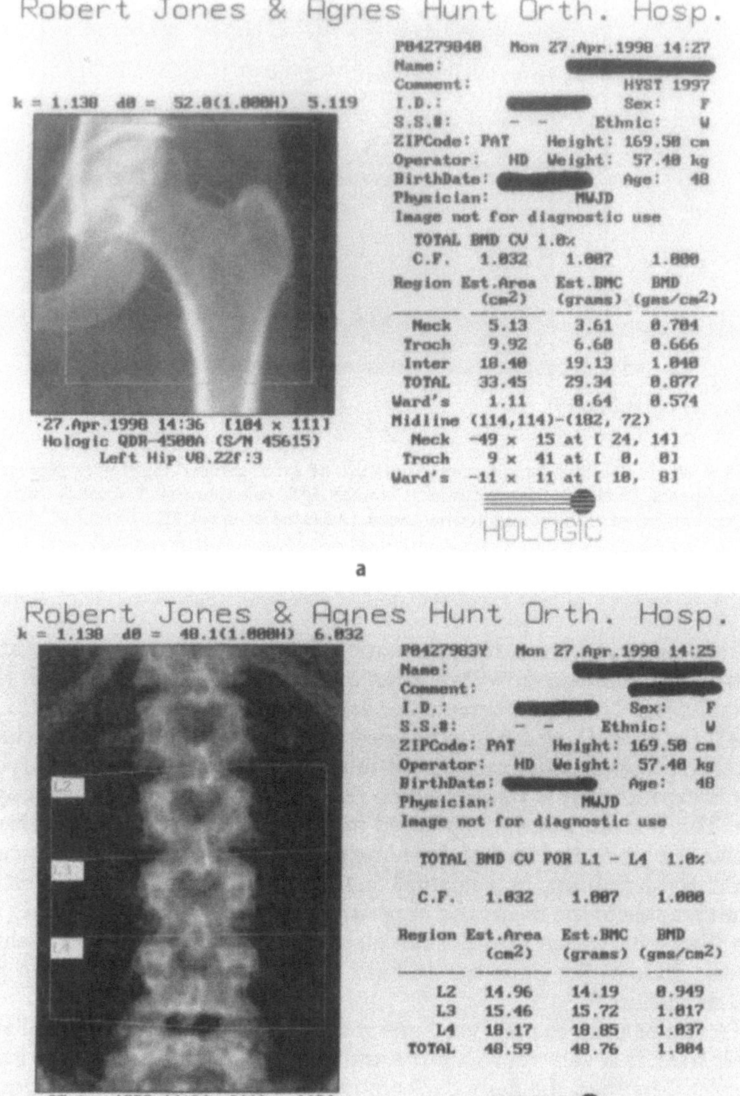

a

b

Figure 8.9 DXA scan results for the hip (**a**) and the lumbar spine (**b**).

Treatment of Osteoporosis

An individual's peak bone mass is achieved in their mid thirties and bone loss begins shortly after this at the femoral neck, although bone loss subsequently follows at other sites. The most dramatic loss occurs in women after the

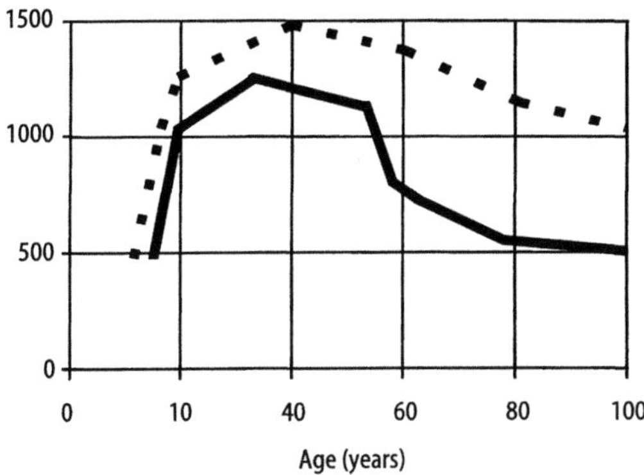

Figure 8.10 Changes in bone mass with age. Male ‑‑‑; Female ——. Reproduced with permission from Cooper and Melton.[5]

menopause as the protective effect of the gonadotrophic hormones is lost and by the age of 80 years women have lost over 30% of bone mass (Fig. 8.10)[5]

The drug treatments available for osteoporosis include those that decrease bone loss (antiresorptive agents) and those which increase bone mass (Table 8.2), although the only cost-effective management is by primary prevention. Realistically however, most patients present with established osteoporosis once a fracture has occurred. Although some clinicians advocate the use of densitometry for general screening for low bone mass in perimenopausal women, currently the case for this cannot be justified. Returning to the WHO stratified definition of osteoporosis (Table 8.1), osteopenia is defined as a T-score of between –1 and –2.5 SD below the young adult mean, osteoporosis as a T-score below –2.5 SD and established osteoporosis below –2.5 SD in the presence of a fracture. Osteopenia may constitute an indication for prophylactic treatment depending on the age of the woman and the relative risks and benefits of the proposed treatment. Both osteoporosis and established osteoporosis are usually regarded as indications for treatment. Given that both the diagnosis and the initiation of treatment is based on a score established by densitometry, how can this best be used to target the population? One approach is to select those patients for bone densitometry who have strong risk factors, for example those patients with premature menopause, those patients who already have a fragility fracture and those with radiological evidence strongly suspicious of osteopenia. (Table 8.3).

In practice the most common treatment used is the administration of hormone replacement therapy (HRT) which acts by reducing bone loss, therefore the

Table 8.2. Therapeutic agents in osteoporosis[12]

Anti-resorptive drugs	Bone formation	Others
Oestrogen ± progestogen Analogues	Fluoride	Vitamin D
Bisphosphonates	Parathormone	Anabolic steroids
Steroids		
Calcium		Ipriflavone
Calcitonin		

Table 8.3. Clinical indications for bone densitometry[3]

Presence of strong risk factors(secondary osteoporosis):
Premature menopause (<45 years)
Prolonged secondary amenorrhoea
Primary hypogonadism
Corticosteroid therapy (>7.5 mg day^{-1} for one year or more)
Anticonvulsants
Heparin
Anorexia nervosa
Malabsorption
Primary hyperparathyroidism
Organ transplantation
Chronic renal failure
Myelomatosis
Skeletal metastases
Hyperthyroidism
Prolonged immobilisation
Radiological evidence of osteopenia
Previous fragility fracture of the hip, the spine or wrist
Monitoring of therapy in patients with osteoporosis
Hormone replacement therapy
Newer drugs, for example, bisphosphonates, calcitonin, vitamin D metabolites, sodium fluoride.

earlier it is started, the more effective it will be in maintaining bone mass and reducing the fracture risk. However, to be most effective the treatment must be started in patients in their early postmenopausal years and continued over many years, since discontinuing will lead to bone loss and an increased fracture risk. This has some important practical implications in the epidemiology of the common fragility fractures as noted by Eastell.[19] The peak total incidence of hip fractures and vertebral fractures occurs with patients in their 70s–80s when considerable bone loss has already occurred, but the peak incidence of forearm fractures occurs a whole decade earlier, at which stage therapeutic intervention will be more effective in *preserving* bone stock, thereby reducing the risk of further fractures. Given that a wrist fracture is a risk factor for other fragility fractures, we should be particularly vigilant in targeting these patients for investigation by densitometry. However, investigation and treatment where indicated, should also be initiated for those with fractures of the spine, the hip and possibly also the proximal humerus, the rib and the clavicle.[7,8]

Once an antiresorptive drug such as HRT has been initiated, during the first 2 years of treatment bone resorption decreases rapidly towards premenopausal levels (Fig. 8.11).[30] This, therefore, is an effective treatment not only in preserving bone mass and also has the very beneficial effect of reducing the risk of cardiovascular disease (risk of myocardial infarction reduced by 50% or more). Despite these benefits, patient compliance with treatment is often poor because of (a) the side effect of breast tenderness, (b) the small increased risk of breast carcinoma with prolonged treatment, and (c) the unacceptable return of cyclical menstrual bleeding. It is likely that treatment compliance will improve now that HRT preparations are available which do not produce cyclical bleeding.

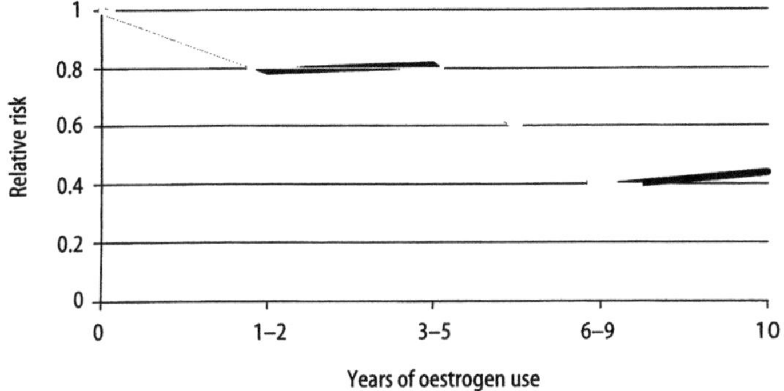

Figure 8.11 Reduction of fracture risk with HRT. Reproduced with permission from from Weiss et al.[30]

Besides HRT the other available drug treatment regimens include the use of calcium and vitamin D supplements which are of benefit where deficiencies exist, such as in cases of nutritional deficiency in the elderly and in cases of malabsorption eg. postgastrectomy. Another group of therapeutic agents are the bisphosphonates, which act by indirectly preventing resorption.

The bone mass in elderly patients reflects both the peak mass achieved in their mid-thirties and the subsequent rate of loss. Although genetic factors are important in determining peak mass, dietary calcium is one of three environmental factors namely physical activity, sex hormone status and calcium nutrition, which are also important determinants.[31] Indeed the protective effect of physical activity on bone mass is an extremely good reason for trying to mobilise patients as early as is feasible following a fragility fracture, quite apart from the protection conferred against the dangers of immobilisation (e.g. pressure sores, urinary tract infection, pneumonia, confusion and dependency).

Recently considerable interest has been shown in the use of external hip protectors which consist of elliptical plastic shields sewn into modified underpants. These are designed to deflect forces away from the hip following a fall, thereby reducing the risk of fracture. They have been shown to be effective in nursing-home residents,[32] but are not yet commonly prescribed in the UK.

Osteoporosis: Management Guidelines for the Orthopaedic Surgeon

Selecting Patients for Investigation

Although orthopaedic surgeons have an essential role in the surgical management of osteoporotic fractures, which represent a substantial proportion of their trauma practice, traditionally they have had little role in the investigation or treatment of this disorder. Indeed, despite the guidelines for the the management of osteoporosis-related fractures published by the UK Department of Health, these are by no means followed uniformly by orthopaedic surgeons.[33] Historically the responsibility for this has fallen to endocrinologists, geriatricians rheumatologists with a special interest, gynaecologists with a special interest or by specialist metabolic bone physicians. With the general recognition of the huge financial and resource implications of the disease and with the introduction of DXA within the last decade, this has sparked considerable clinical and research interest in osteoporosis, which now exists almost as a specialty in its own right. Consequently, most units around the UK which manage fracture patients, will have a local clinician with a special interest in osteoporosis to whom referral for investigation and treatment can be made. Indeed this has been a recommendation of the advisory committee to the National Osteoporosis Society (UK).[20] Currently the vast majority of patients with osteoporotic fractures are discharged by the surgeon once the fracture episode has been treated, without further investigation of their bone quality. This represents a lost opportunity to investigate and treat a large, important "at risk" group for osteoporosis. Clearly this is unacceptable since with treatment, this patient group will reduce their risk of future fracture and potentially lessen the future burden on both the fracture service and all the departments allied to the management of such patients. This is particularly pertinent when one considers that the elderly population is growing substantially and the incidence of osteoporosis is also increasing. The argument can also be extended to include the increased risk and complexity of surgery in those who have already had operations for fragility fractures. This point is illustrated well in Fig. 8.12 in which a 75-year-old patient sustained a femoral shaft fracture in weakened, porotic bone beneath a hemiarthroplasty stem, which had been inserted to treat an intracapsular hip fracture some three years previously. Poor quality bone makes such revision surgery difficult and unpredictable, and this patient's hemiarthroplasty was revised to a total hip replacement using both impaction and strut allografting in an attempt to replace bone stock.

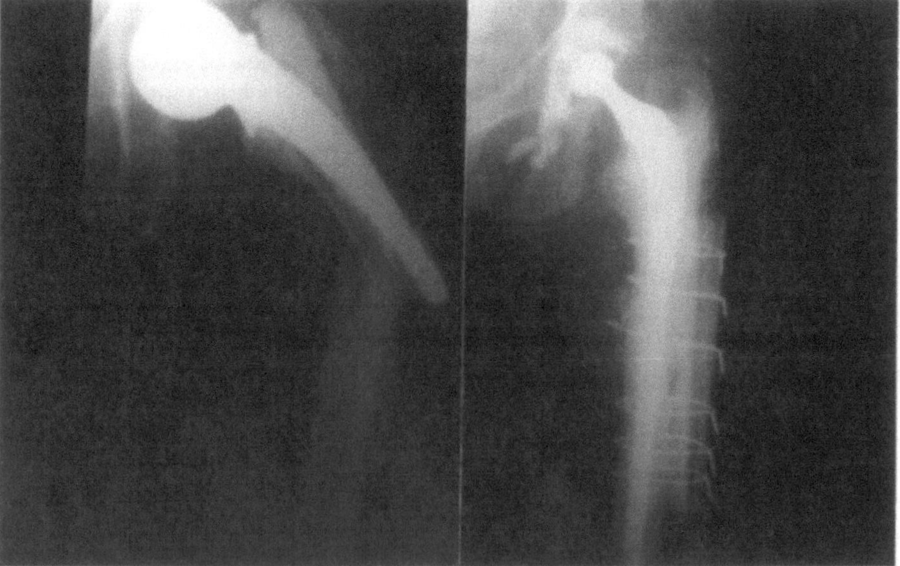

Figure 8.12 Complex, revision arthroplasty in weakened osteoporotic bone.

It would seem reasonable that the "at risk" patient group should be targeted within the fracture clinic, and where indicated this could set in motion an automatic process of investigation and referral to the appropriate "osteoporosis" specialist.

Fracture clinics within the UK are notoriously busy departments treating a large throughput of patients who are often disappointed at the length of time they have to wait and at the short period of time for which the doctor is able to consult with them. Under the circumstances it is unlikely that the orthopaedic surgeon will have the resources to personally take on the role of screening and investigating such patients, in the absence of a dramatic increase in staff. However, this is a void within the fracture service which should be filled. It may be appropriate that a dedicated specialist "osteoporosis" nurse be appointed to identify the "at risk" in-patients and out-patients who are suitable for investigation by way of a questionnaire, screening blood tests and DXA, on the assumption that such facilities are at their disposal locally.[20] The specialist nurse would work under the supervision of the local osteoporosis physician and help to provide close liaison between the fracture service and the local osteoporosis service. Where indicated, further investigation or treatment could then be initiated either via the osteoporosis physician or via the patient's general practitioner.

An Approach to Fracture Patient Management

The treatment guidelines for osteoporosis according to the WHO definition relate specifically to the patient's bone mass, therefore one of the important decisions to be made is whether or not the patient requires investigation by DXA. A simple

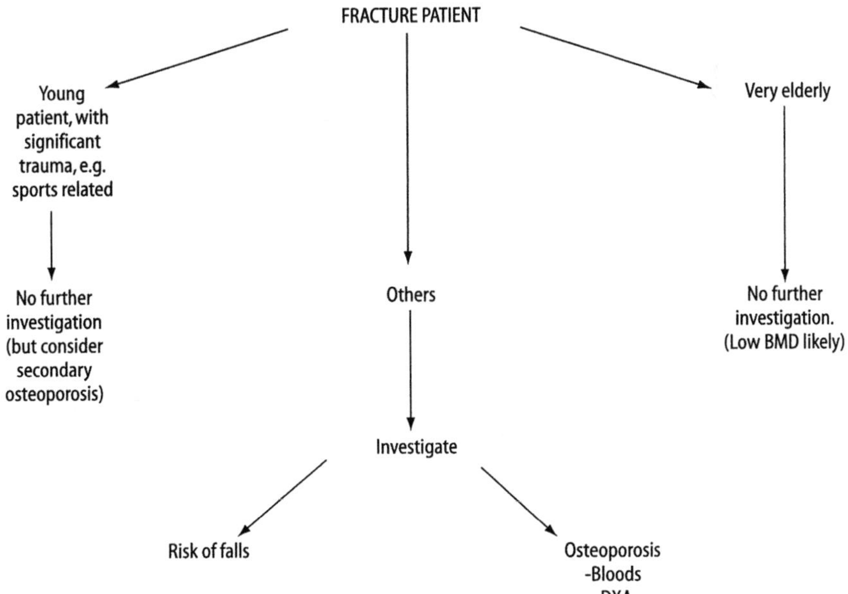

Figure 8.13 An algorithm for fracture patient management.

algorithm for use in a fracture service is shown in Fig. 8.13. This is designed to help to identify those patients in whom further investigation would be indicated.

Although osteoporosis is usually an idiopathic condition, secondary osteoporosis may be found in up to 30% of women and 54% of men who present to a metabolic bone clinic with symptomatic vertebral fractures. It is important always to be vigilant to uncover this by taking a careful history and examination and by performing the appropriate investigations when secondary osteoporosis is suspected. These investigations are listed in Table 8.4.[12]

Returning to the algorithm and setting aside the limitation of both cost and accessibility of facilities, a suggested management plan is as follows. It is reasonable to propose that two groups of patients probably do not require further investigation. These are first those young patients in who a fracture has been caused by an episode of significant trauma, for example as a result of a sports-related incident and whom may reasonably be assumed to have good bone stock. (It is however important to consider the possibility of secondary osteoporosis within this patient group. If suspected, the relevant investigations including blood tests and DXA would then be indicated.) Secondly, are those patients who are very old and in whom low BMD may be assumed (e.g. > 75 year olds). These may be treated empirically by calcium and Vitamin D supplements.[34]

In all other fracture patients further investigation may be undertaken, and will consist of DXA scanning and screening blood tests. In addition it will also be important to assess an individual's "risk of falls", taking into account both intrinsic factors (e.g. eyesight, neurological disease etc.) and extrinsic or environmental factors (e.g. loose carpets, poorly fitting footwear etc.). Simple intervention may help to reduce these risks. Patients should also be given general advice on lifestyle measures to decrease further bone loss including eating a balanced diet, maintaining regular exercise and moderating tobacco and alcohol consumption.[34]

The algorithm as suggested represents ideal circumstances but some departments whether for practical or financial purposes may wish to tailor investigation to the more common fragility fractures such as wrist, hip, spine and proximal humerus. However, where such an algorithm has been introduced it would be important to conduct an audit at regular intervals to ensure that the service was running efficiently. Applying the criteria in a "clinical management" algorithm such as that suggested here, one technique might be to critically review all the notes from randomly selected clinics to ensure that the appropriate referrals for investigation had consistently been made. Naturally as problems arise in the delivery of the service, these would be addressed and re-audited to ensure the satisfactory evolution of the service.

Table 8.4. Investigations for secondary osteoporosis[12]

Full blood count
Erythrocyte sedimentation rate
Urea and electrolytes
Thyroid function tests
Calcium, phosphate, alkaline phosphatase
Liver function tests
Testosterone, follicle stimulating hormone, luteinising hormone
Serum and urine electrophoresis
Prostate specific antigen

Clearly the availability of local facilities and the degree of interest within a department will influence both the establishment and the potency of such a service. Interest may develop as the accessibility of bone densitometry increases. For example, whereas most departments will use the standard, departmental DXA machines, smaller, portable devices for calcaneal densitometry are gradually becoming available. These may revolutionise the accessibility of densitometry and indeed may eventually establish densitometry as part of the routine fracture clinic investigation.

Osteoporosis in Males

Although the incidence of osteoporotic fractures among females is high, bone loss with advancing age does occur in males, but to a lesser extent (Fig. 8.10). In England and Wales during 1985, 7000 hip fractures in males over 65 years were caused by osteoporosis, and this number is rising. In fact 15% of all vertebral fractures and 20% of all hip fractures occur in males and the lifetime risk of fracture of the proximal femur, the spine and the forearm in a 50-year-old man are 6.0%, 5.0% and 2.5%, respectively.

Often there is an underlying cause (55% of men with vertebral fractures) such as corticosteroid therapy or hypogonadism and sometimes it reflects a low peak bone mass as occurs in delayed puberty. It may also relate to influential lifestyle factors such as cigarette smoking, alcohol, poor diet or inadequate exercise. Where suspected, a good history and examination is mandatory following which a bone density scan and routine screening blood tests are appropriate (Table 8.4). Once again, as for the investigation of females, the interpretation of results and the patient management thereafter should be undertaken by the osteoporosis physician, in liaison with the osteoporosis nurse.

Developing the Role for an Osteoporosis Specialist Nurse

Specifically, a role for an osteoporosis specialist nurse in this situation might be to trawl through the patient referral letters within the clinic in order to identify potential "at risk" patients. Such patients could then complete a simple lifestyle and health questionnaire whilst waiting, before seeing the doctor. This would help to focus attention on those patients for whom there might be a significant suspicion of osteoporosis. In addition such a nurse could liaise with the wards in order to identify those in-patients who had bypassed the fracture clinic sieve. Indeed the ward staff could provide invaluable assistance in this process. For example, the use of a short screening questionnaire introduced as part of the "Trauma admission care plan" would help to identify high risk individuals.

Despite the involvement of a specialist nurse, vigilance would however remain important among the medical staff within the fracture clinic to avoid missing the occasional patient who does not on the surface appear to be at risk of osteoporosis, but in whom the diagnosis would be made with investigation.

Having used the algorithm to identify those patients for further investigation, interpretation of results and decisions regarding treatment should be undertaken by the local osteoporosis specialist or the local metabolic bone clinic. Once again the specialist nurse would be in a strong position to liaise between the fracture clinic and the osteoporosis service to encourage efficiency in the continuity of management of such patients.

In the absence of DXA facilities or an appropriate osteoporosis specialist, management of these patients will obviously be more difficult and treatment decisions may necessarily be undertaken by the patient's GP.

The suggested guidelines outlined above represent the ideal scenario which could be achieved in a world of limitless financial and manpower resources. In reality however, this is not the case. In many parts of the country facilities for the investigation and treatment of osteoporosis are sparce and even where present, resources are often stretched. Realistically then, where such problems exist, as a priority we should aim to target those patients in whom the gains in terms of fracture protection, are likely to be the greatest. Consistent with the evidence we have, this group would seem to be the perimenopausal women with wrist fractures, in whom bone stock can theoretically be maintained by treatment. Once we have succeeded in helping this group, maybe then the therapeutic net could be cast a little further.

Estimated Potential Service Costs of Bone Densitometry

In 1995 Compston et al.[3] suggested several clinical indications for bone densitometry (Table 8.3) among which they include fragility fractures of the spine, the hip and the wrist. On the basis of these indications, it is suggested that the densitometry service demands in Britain would be relatively modest. Furthermore they have suggested that in an average health district of 300,000, facilities would be needed to scan 125 women per year with either premature menopause or other strong risk factors, who when counselled on treatment decide to defer their decision until after they have had densitometry. In addition, scans would be required for 200 men and women with vertebral deformities or radiological osteopenia; 40 men and women with established secondary osteoporosis and 160 patients who require BMD monitoring for treatment response. The predicted annual requirement of 175 scans per 100,000 population in 1994 was similar to the current rates of use at that time, in existing osteoporosis units in the UK. Assuming a relative cost at that time of £48 per scan, in order to provide such a service would require £25,200 annually for a population of 300,000. The authors[3] do however point out that the availability of adequate facilities and equipment within the UK is patchy, with 90 instruments installed at the time of writing. It was further suggested that provision of adequate access to specialist skill would require a relatively modest allocation of new resources to geographical areas in which they were lacking. In support of this, in their 1994 report on osteoporosis the advisory group to the Department of Health suggested that in those areas lacking in DXA facilities, a bone densitometry service should be established.[20] However in relation to this three important points should be emphasised:

1. Although the additional cost of providing a comprehensive densitometry service may be estimated to be modest, if a policy of referral were to be adopted for all potential candidates seen in a fracture clinic, the demand might be considerably greater than anticipated.

2. It is important to emphasise that the additional cost of treating the numbers in whom it would be appropriate, might make treatment untenable.
3. With more patients receiving treatment, so the demands on DXA would be increased in monitoring such treatment.

Other Roles for DXA in Orthopaedic Practice

The importance of DXA in the diagnosis and treatment of osteoporosis has been well established. More recently other useful applications of DXA have been investigated although this has been mainly within the realms of orthopaedic research. Ingle et al.[35] have used it to demonstrate the patterns of immobilisation osteopenia following wrist and ankle fracture, the hand showing a 9% loss of BMD by 6 weeks after a wrist fracture, which did not recover to normal even up to one year later. In addition it has been used to assess the quantity and rate of formation of regenerate bone during callus distraction procedures.[36] By using software to exclude the effect of metalwork, DXA has been used to assess bone density changes around the components of cemented and uncemented hip arthroplasty, as a measure of ingrowth and osteolysis. Latterly it has also been used to measure BMD within a fracture site and to correlate this with fracture stiffness tests, as an index of fracture healing.

Ultrasound In Bone: an Index of Density and Architecture?

When sound is transmitted through tissue, two of the properties of the wave form are altered: the speed or velocity of the sound wave (speed of sound = SOS) and the amplitude of the sound wave (referred to as attentuation). Recently, considerable attention has been focused on these two parameters to evaluate whether either or both could be used clinically to assess bone structure, bone density and fracture risk. It would appear that the velocity of sound traversing through bone reflects both qualitative and quantitative aspects of its structure, including both density and elasticity. The attentuation of sound in bone (bone ultrasound attenuation = BUA) occurs due to scattering and absorption and in vitro studies suggest that it is highly correlated with both (a) the strength of bone and (b) the trabecular connectivity.[37]

The techniques which are currently available to measure bone density each carry some radiation risk. Therefore the ability to use ultrasound for this purpose particularly considering the portability of the equipment involved, makes this potentially a very attractive option. However, more research work is needed to establish which aspects of the propagating sound wave best reflect the density and the architectural properties of bone, before it can be universally adapted to the clinical setting.

The Future

Osteoporosis has generated enormous clinical and research interest in the past decade which has helped to develop our understanding of the pathological process involved, our capability to diagnosis it and our capacity to treat it. It is a potentially treatable condition and using the popular regimens currently available, the earlier that diagnosis is made, the better the chance of preserving bone mass and subsequently lowering the risk of future fracture.

General screening of the populus is not currently advocated, but the patient who presents to the orthopaedic surgeon with a fragility fracture represents a target group who would and should benefit from investigation and treatment. In particular, those with wrist fractures are a good target group because of the relatively young age at which they present. Indeed, in the future it may be possible to screen patients' bone density levels within the fracture clinic, by the use of peripheral scanners and ultrasound machines. If proven clinically reliable these might reduce the burden on scanning departments, hasten investigation and significantly reduce costs.

Orthopaedic surgeons tend to focus on the orthopaedic management of fragility fractures by which their practice is often swamped. Lamentably their training does not dwell on either the subject of osteoporosis or indeed the pivotal role they might have in liaison with a densitometry and osteoporosis service. The surgeon needs the opportunity to develop the concept of bone as a living, ageing tissue and not just a vehicle for perambulation. Clearly, if the general management of these patients is to improve then the various components of an osteoporosis service need to be available to a fracture clinic and the pair should run smoothly, in concert together. Through education, the orthopaedic surgeon should be motivated towards the importance of early referral where appropriate and should also appreciate the potential for future improvement in their own practice, by encouraging healthier bones within the general populus. This will not only reduce the risk of fracture, but also reduce the risk of future complications and the complexity of the surgery which accompanies such complications (Fig. 8.12). Inevitably there is a substantial financial cost in establishing such a service which includes the acquisition of premises, hardware, softwear, drug treatment, support personnel and a clinician with a personal interest to oversee the general running of and the development of the service.

In addition, through education, both hospital management and the general practitioner should understand the importance of providing this service and in particular the potential health benefits conferred to their local community.

Acknowledgements

I wish to acknowledge the helpful advice given to me by Professor Richard Eastell of the Department of Human Metabolism and Clinical Biochemistry, University of Sheffield, UK and by Dr Mike Davies, Consultant Physician at the Robert Jones and Agnes Hunt Orthopaedic Hospital, Oswestry, UK. I would also like to thank Mr Andrew Biggs, Mr Alun Jones and Mrs Susan Hughes of the Medical Illustration Department and Mrs Marie Carter (Librarian), also of the Robert Jones and Agnes Hunt Orthopaedic Hospital, for their help in preparing the manuscript.

References

1. Consensus Development Conference (1991) Prophylaxis and treatment of osteoporosis. Am J Med 90:107–110.
2. Kanis JA, Melton J, Christiansen C et al. (1994) The Diagnosis of osteoporosis. J Bone Miner Res; 9:1137–1141.

3. Compston JE, Cooper C, Kanis JA (1995) Bone densitometry in clinical practice. BMJ 310:1507–10.
4. Cooper C (1993) Epidemiology and public health impact of osteoporosis. Baillieres Clin Rheumatol 7:459–77.
5. Cooper C, Melton LJ. (1992) Epidemiology of osteoporosis. Trends Endocrinol Metab 3:224–229.
6. Donaldson LJ, Cook RG, Thompson RG (1990) Incidence of fractures in a Geographically defined population. J. Epidemiol Community Health 44:241–245.
7. Seeley DG, Browner WS, Nevitt MC et al. (1991) Which fractures are associated with low appendicular bone mass in elderly women. An Intern Med 115:837–842.
8. Davie MWJ (1996) Fractures at specific sites indicate low bone mineral density at lumbar spine and femoral neck in women. J Orthop Rheumatol 9:41–45.
9. Kanis JA and the WHO study group (1994) Assessment of fracture risk and its application to screening for postmenopausal osteoporosis: a synopsis of the WHO report. Osteoporosis Int 4:368–81.
10. Keene GS, Parker MJ, Pryor GA (1993) Mortality and morbidity after hip fractures. BMJ 307:1248–50.
11. Bonjour J-P, Schurch M-A, Rizzoli R (1996) Nutritional aspects of hip fractures. Bone 18:139S–144S.
12. Arden NK, Spencer TD (eds) (1997) Osteoporosis Illustrated. Current Medical Literature, London.
13. Kanis JA, Pitt FA (1992) Epidemiology of osteoporosis Bone 13:S7–S15.
14. Hollingworth W, Todd C, Parker M et al. (1993) Cost analysis of early discharge after hip fracture. BMJ 306:903–6.
15. Royal College of Physicians (1989) Fractured neck of femur – prevention and management. a Report. Royal College of Physicians, London.
16. Audit Commission (1995) United they stand: co-ordinating care for elderly patients with hip fractures. HMSO, London.
17. Hollingworth W, Todd CJ, Parker MJ (1995) The cost of treating hip fractures in the twenty-first century. J Public Health Med 17:269–276.
18. Wasnich RD, Davis JW, Ross PD (1994). Spine fracture risk is predicted by non-spine fractures. Osteoporosis Int 4:1–5.
19. Eastell R (1996) Forearm fracture. Bone 18:203S–207S.
20. National Osteoporosis Society (1994) Priorities for prevention. osteoporosis a decision-making document for diagnosis and treatment. Policy document. National Osteoporosis Society, Bath.
21. Atkins RM, Duckworth T, Kanis JA (1990) The features of algodystrophy following Colles fracture. J Bone Joint Surg. 72B: 105–110.
22. Eastell R, Riggs BL, Wahner HW et al. Colles' fracture and bone density of the ultradistal radiius. J. Bone Miner Res 4: 607–613.
23. Peel NFA, Barrington NA, Smith TWD et al. (1994) Distal forearm fracture as a risk for vertebral osteoporosis. BMJ 308:1542–1544.
24. Owen RA, Melton LJ,III, Ilsrup DM et al. (1982) Colles fracture and susequent hip fracture risk. Clin Orthop 171:37–43.
25. World Health Organisation (1994) Assessment of fracture risk and its application to screening for post menopausal osteoporosis. World Health Organisation Tech Rep Ser no 843. WHO, Geneva.
26. Ray NF, Chan JK, Thamer M et al. (1997) Medical expenditures for the treatment of osteoporotic fractures in the united states in 1995: report from the National Osteoporosis Foundation. J Bone Miner Res 12:24–35.
27. Cooney LM, Marottoli RA (1993) Functional decline following hip fracture. In: Christiansen C, Riis B (eds) Osteoporosis 1993, Proceedings of IV International Symposium on Osteoporosis and consensus Development Conference. Rodovre, Denmark 480–481.
28. Department fo Health (1994) Osteoporosis. Advisory Group on Osteoporosis. Department of Health Report booklet.
29. Cummings SR, Black DM, Nevitt MC et al. (1993) Bone density at various sites for prediction of hip fractures. *Lancet* 341:72–75.
30. Weiss NS, Ure CL, Ballard JH et al. (1980) Decreased risk of fractures of the hip and lower forearm with postmenopausal use of oestrogen. N Engl J Med 303:1195–8.
31. Cooper C, Eastell R (1993) Bone gain and loss in premenopausal women. Physical activity, calcium nutrition and sex hormone status are important. BMJ 306:1357–1358.
32. Lauritzen JB, Petersen MM, Lund B. (1993) Effect of external hip protectors on hip fractures. Lancet 341:11–13.

33. Pal B, Morris J, Muddu B (1998) The management of osteoporosis-related fractures: a survey of orthopaedic surgeon's practice. Clin Exp Rheumatol 16:61–62.
34. Francis R, Baillie S, Chuck A et al. (1998) New guidelines for hip fracture Newsletter of North East Osteoporosis Regional Advisory Board p. 1–4.
35. Ingle BM, Bottjer HM, Hay SM et al. (1997) Changes in bone mass and bone turnover following wrist and ankle fracture. J Bone Miner Res 12:Suppl 1.
36. Eyres KS, Bell MJ, Kanis J (1993) Methods of assessing new bone formation during limb lengthening. J Bone Joint Surg 75-B:358–364.
37. Van Daele PLA, Burger H, De Laet CEDH et al. (1996) Ultrasound measurement of bone. Clin Endocrinol 44:363–369.

9 Use of Bone Mineral Density Measurement in Primary Care

P. Brown

Introduction

The use of bone mineral density (BMD) measurement in primary care needs to be discussed in the context of the care pathways for management of osteoporosis in the primary care setting. Any such discussion needs to take account of the "new" NHS structure, including the role of primary care groups (PCGs), local health groups (LHGs) and local health care co-operatives (LHCCs) in eventually managing budgets and commissioning services.

To use BMD measurement cost-effectively, primary care teams need to understand the methods available, their strengths and limitations, and how measurement can help them more accurately identify those at high risk of developing osteoporosis, and those who already have the disease. This is turn will allow targeting of treatment to those where it is likely to make most impact on future fracture rates.

With the reorganisation of the NHS, PCGs and LHGs will eventually manage unified budgets for primary, secondary and community care. With this increase in commissioning power, for the first time the cost of diagnosing and managing osteoporosis, and both the acute and long-term costs of fractures, will all be funded from the same budget. In theory this should make it easier to identify the very real financial savings which are possible with early diagnosis and aggressive treatment. However, in the short term, additional funds will need to be provided for diagnostic services, including bone density measurement, and therapy for those with the disease, as there will be a time lag before improved management translates into reduced fracture rates.

Only a few practices are currently proactively identifying patients who are at risk of osteoporosis, and in most practices many of those who have been diagnosed with the disease are not on appropriate therapy. Yet the minimum standards proposed later in this chapter should be achievable by most practices within the next few years, and could make a huge long-term impact on the osteoporosis problem.

Osteoporosis and the New NHS

"Our Healthier Nation"[1] stresses the role that osteoporosis plays in fractures in the elderly and osteoporosis prevention was therefore included as one of the measures recommended to achieve the reduction of accidents by 20% by 2010.

Fractures feature in two of the new clinical performance indicators:

1. Mortality rates in hospital within 30 days of admission with a fractured neck of femur in those aged 65+;
2. Rate of discharge home within 28 days of admission with a fractured neck of femur for patients aged 65+.

The National Osteoporosis Society (NOS) has recently produced "A Primary Care Service Framework for Osteoporosis"[2] which offers practical advice for those commissioning and providing osteoporosis care at a PCG/LHG/LHCC level. This will help them to benchmark their current levels of care and to maximise health gain by providing appropriate services in the future. This activity can be incorporated into programmes of care for the elderly or accident prevention under local Health Improvement Programmes (HImPs)

The key recommendations of "A Primary Care Service Framework for Osteoporosis" are as follows.

1. Include prevention of osteoporotic fractures in the accidents target of each local HImP.
2. Each PCG/LHG/LHCC should identify lead clinicians in primary and secondary care to develop a local osteoporosis programme based on this framework. Each group should have a lead GP for osteoporosis, responsible for monitoring the implementation of the programme.
3. Set up a multidisciplinary local osteoporosis interest group to discuss implementation of the framework.
4. Use a selective case-finding approach to identify those at risk.
5. Provide access to adequate levels of diagnostic and specialist services.
6. Promote the use of care pathways and audit to improve standards of care.
7. Monitor performance to assess health impact.

It is important that there are clear lines of communication between the hospital services, PCGs/LHGs/LHCCs and practices, including clear management guidelines, good referral letters and accurate and timely discharge summaries.

Osteoporosis and Primary Care

Osteoporosis is defined as a "progressive systemic skeletal disease characterised by low bone mass and microarchitectural deterioration of bone tissue, with a consequent increase in bone fragility and susceptibility to fracture."[3] Osteoporosis has been a neglected disease in the past, and indeed not many years ago it was frequently described as a normal consequence of growing old.

Like other primary care diseases such as coronary heart disease and diabetes, osteoporosis is common, it has a high mortality and morbidity rate and we now know it is both preventable and treatable. Those people at greatest risk can often be diagnosed either in the early stages of the disease, or at least at a stage where intervention is worthwhile in terms of preventing future pain, suffering and loss of life. And finally, the drugs used for managing most of these patients are suitable and safe for use in a primary care setting.

Therefore, despite any reluctance on the part of primary care teams to take on the responsibility for osteoporosis in the current climate of restricted drug budgets and limited time and resources, osteoporosis is clearly a primary care disease. The diagnosis and management of osteoporosis will need to be achieved in as cost-effective a way as possible, both in terms of time and people resources, and in terms of financial budgets. Accurate identification of those at risk or those with established osteoporosis by the use of bone mineral density measurement is crucial to allow time and treatment to be targeted to those who need them most.

Primary care goals must be to reduce the number of first and subsequent fractures due to osteoporosis by (a) identifying and treating all those who already have established disease (secondary prevention) and (b) identifying and treating all those who are at high risk of developing the disease (primary prevention).

The Size of the Problem

Osteoporosis and osteoporotic fractures are common. In any five-year period 10% of the population of over 70-year-old women will suffer a hip fracture; 10–20% will die as a result and 50% of the survivors will never return to living independently in their own home.[4]

In 1990 there were 52,000 hip fractures, 40, 500 wrist fractures, 25,000 clinically diagnosed vertebral fractures and 50,000 other osteoporotic fractures in the UK. If we assume that these fractures are distributed evenly among the 500 PCGs, this translates into 104 hip fractures, 81 wrist fractures, 50 clinically diagnosed vertebral fractures and 100 other osteoporotic fractures each year per PCG.[2] That is an average of 335 potentially preventable fractures each year per PCG. Together these are likely to cost the PCG £681 340 for acute costs and £1.5 million when long-term care costs and drug bills are included. These costs take no account of the suffering and loss of independence, to say nothing of loss of life, due to osteoporosis each year.

The numbers of people with osteoporosis who suffer a fracture each year are, however, only the tip of the iceberg. Thousands more in each PCG area will already have undiagnosed osteoporosis. Often the first sign that they are suffering from osteoporosis will be when they suffer their first fracture. Thousands more will be at high risk of developing the disease, and most of them, too, are undiagnosed and untreated.

Yet GPs and their primary care teams are in an ideal position to identify those at risk and those with the disease. About 70% of patients consult their GP in one year and 90% consult over a 5-year period; people in the high risk groups may be seen much more frequently.

Osteoporosis Guidelines

General practitioners are expected to have knowledge of, and a management plan for dealing with, every disease which their patients develop. Guidelines have been criticised and some GPs state that they receive so many sets of guidelines that they do not use any of them. However, many guidelines do provide a simple care pathway and standards for which primary care teams can aim. Many primary care teams find them useful.

There are a variety of recent osteoporosis guidelines available. The Department of Health launched the "Quick Reference Primary Care Guide on the Prevention

Table 9.1. GP use of guidelines[9]

Guideline	% seen unprompted	% seen prompted	% used	% actively adopted
NOS Corticosteroid	10	35	22	14
DoH Guide	3	31	11	6
RCP Guidelines	1	13	3	2
Local guidelines	30	43	33	29
Others	17	16	–	–
None	68	37	15	21

and Treatment of Osteoporosis"[5] in June 1998, and this was posted on the Department of Health's website at www.open.gov.uk/doh/osteop.htm. Unfortunately copies of the Quick Reference Guide and the A4 summary card were only sent out to practices on request. Only GPs motivated enough to request a copy will have seen these guidelines.

The Primary Care Rheumatology Society published "Minimum Standard Guidelines in Osteoporosis"[6] designed specifically for use in the primary care setting. This useful reference card, like the summary card of the DOH guideline document, provides a clear, concise summary of which patient groups need to be identified and the treatment options.

The Royal College of Physicians (RCP) published "Osteoporosis – Clinical guidelines for prevention and treatment"[7] in March 1999. This reference guide includes a database of randomised controlled trials of therapies for prevention and treatment. This document is unlikely to be used by the average general practitioner, although the key recommendations from it can easily be incorporated into "good practice" in the primary care setting.

The National Osteoporosis Society produced "Guidance on the prevention and management of corticosteroid induced osteoporosis"[8] in 1998. This was endorsed by the British Geriatric Society, British League Against Rheumatism, British Society for Rheumatology, National Asthma Campaign, Northamptonshire Health Authority, Primary Care Rheumatology Society, Royal College of Nursing and the Royal Society of Medicine. This provides straightforward guidance on how to manage patients who are taking corticosteroids, and should influence primary care management, including the appropriate use of bone density measurement in this group of patients.

A recent survey of 200 GPs carried out by the National Osteoporosis Society[9] asked GPs whether they had seen, used or actively adopted each of these guidelines. The results are shown in Table 9.1. Initially, 68% of GPs questioned said that they had not seen any guidelines for osteoporosis, although with prompting this dropped to 37%. Almost a third had actively adopted local guidelines, but it is of concern that 21% still have not actively adopted any guidelines. Only 35% of those surveyed had seen the NOS corticosteroid guidelines and surprisingly only 14% had adopted them.

Strategies for Tackling Osteoporosis

Primary care teams need guidance on how they can achieve the greatest reduction in osteoporosis incidence and fracture risk in the most cost effective way. As with the management of other common diseases, two strategies are possible:

1. Population strategies

   Improving the bone mass of the whole population

   Screening the whole population then targeting interventions at those at highest risk

2. Case-finding strategies

   Identifying those at highest risk and targeting interventions to them.

Improving the bone health of all our patients may at first seem an attractive strategy. A 10% increase in the average bone density of all females would result in a halving of the risk of fractures.[10] Lifestyle interventions to attempt to increase bone mass across the whole population would include encouraging smoking cessation, regular weight-bearing exercise, reducing excessive alcohol consumption and ensuring adequate calcium and vitamin D intake.

However, these measures would need to be implemented throughout life to make a major impact on bone mass, and acceptance of such advice and implementation by the general public is likely to be limited. The value of lifestyle advice in improving bone density and ultimately reducing fractures later in life has not been documented. Therefore, although education about the advantages of these lifestyle modifications should begin in school and continue throughout life when recommended as part of a healthy lifestyle to help prevent heart disease and cancer, they should not be relied on at this time to reduce the fracture incidence. Most primary care teams will continue to spend a small amount of time and other resources providing health education and trying to improve the lifestyles of all patients.

Population screening for osteoporosis has been explored in several studies but is currently not cost effective and is not recommended.[7] Practices often undertake population screening for other diseases, such as hypertension and diabetes. However, unlike osteoporosis, these diseases have quick and easy screening tests – blood pressure measurement for hypertension and urinalysis for diabetes – and effective treatments with which most patients will comply. Screening for osteoporosis among groups of patients such as menopausal women may be possible in the future, if a simple and accurate test becomes available and newer drugs result in much higher rates of compliance in those diagnosed with the disease.

Therefore, the most useful approach for primary care teams is to adopt a case-finding strategy, where clinical risk factors, history of fragility fractures and clinical symptoms are used to help identify those who appear to be at greatest risk of osteoporosis or who may have established disease. These patients can then either be treated or, if the need for treatment is unclear on clinical grounds and dual-energy X-ray absorptiometry (DXA) scanning is available, can be scanned and their future management based on the result of the DXA scan. This is the approach recommended by all the guidelines discussed in this chapter.

Management of Osteoporosis in Primary Care

Having established that primary care is the most practical place to manage osteoporosis, and that a case-finding strategy is most appropriate, there are five main tasks which the team need to carry out. These are shown in diagrammatic form in Fig. 9.1, and outlined in more detail in Table 9.2.

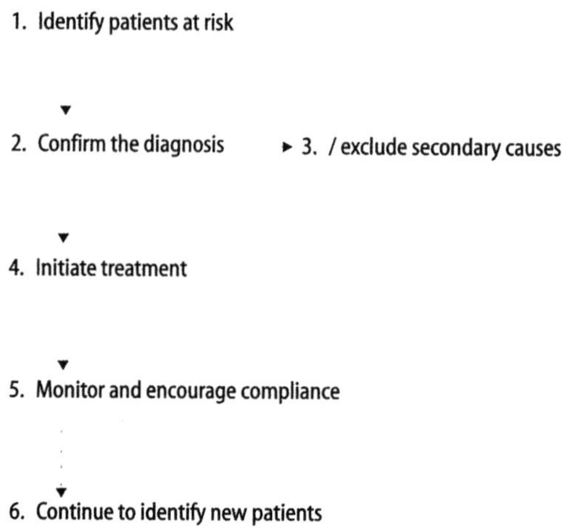

1. Identify patients at risk

▼

2. Confirm the diagnosis   ► 3. / exclude secondary causes

▼

4. Initiate treatment

▼

5. Monitor and encourage compliance

▼

6. Continue to identify new patients

Figure 9.1 Process of management of osteoporosis in primary care.

Table 9.2. Key tasks in the management of osteoporosis in primary care

Identify those who may be at risk
  Those with previous fragility fracture, early menopause or on high-dose oral steroids
  Those with other clinical risk factors
  Those with risk factors specific to increased hip fracture risk
  Those with low measurement on ultrasound or peripheral DXA
  Record all these people in an osteoporosis "high risk" register

Confirm which patients have osteoporosis, or are at high risk of developing it
  Use X-rays to confirm fractures
  Use DXA in those where it will change management
  Use DXA to get baseline measurement in those where treatment options will need bone
  density monitoring

Exclude secondary causes of osteoporosis or other bone disease
  Use blood tests

Provide appropriate treatment
  Lifestyle advice
  Drugs for prevention
  Drugs for treatment

Monitor treatment and encourage compliance
  Use DXA to identify non-responders
  Use "high risk" register to follow up those on treatment

Continue to identify new patients
  Put systems in place to monitor new registrations, hospital letters, new repeat prescriptions
  for steroids
  Feed these patients through the steps identified above.

Each of these tasks will be discussed in more detail in the ensuing sections of
this chapter, including the role of bone density measurement in the appropriate
tasks.

Step 1: Identify Those At Risk

GPs use risk factors, past medical history and current symptoms to identify patients who may be at risk of coronary artery disease. Then more sensitive diagnostic tests, such as exercise ECG testing or angiography, are used in a small number of patients, to confirm who has the disease. In exactly the same way, clinical risk factors, history of fragility fractures and current symptoms and signs (back pain, kyphosis, loss of height) can be used to identify a group of patients who may be at risk of osteoporosis. Then X-rays and bone density measurement are used to more accurately identify those who have low bone mass and are at high risk of developing osteoporosis, and those who already have the disease.

No matter how actively we pursue a case-finding strategy, we will fail to prevent fractures in two groups of patients. Firstly, we will miss those with the disease who do not have any obvious risk factors, symptoms or signs. Their disease will remain silent and undiagnosed until they suffer their first fracture. Secondly, some of the people we identify will not comply with recommendations for lifestyle modification or therapy and their bones will continue to deteriorate. For both these groups, all we can do is implement secondary prevention measures when the first or subsequent fracture occurs.

At present, case-finding and treating those identified as being at highest risk will provide most impact for our effort and funds. It is important that once these patients are identified their details are recorded in some kind of "at risk" osteoporosis register on the practice computer system, so that they can be easily identified in the future. Practices with more sophisticated systems may be able to implement a review programme whereby these patients are brought to a GP or practice nurse's attention at regular intervals so that their compliance with therapy can be assessed.

Previous Fragility Fractures

Patients who have had one fragility fracture are significantly more at risk of further fractures.[10] Usually women lose bone most rapidly at the wrist, sustaining a Colles fracture in their 50s or early 60s. A few years later they develop vertebral osteoporosis and suffer one or more wedge fractures of the vertebrae. However, these may go undiagnosed (around one third are asymptomatic, one third present as back pain which is never accurately diagnosed, and only one third have the fracture diagnosed on plain radiography). Finally, usually in the 70s or 80s, hip fracture occurs. If we could consistently diagnose and treat the osteoporosis even after the first fragility fracture, then this would make a very large impact on the suffering and costs of the disease. This is an important opportunity to target therapy to those at highest risk of future fractures.

Corticosteroid Induced Osteoporosis (CSIO)

Every practice is likely to have a significant number of patients taking long-term, oral corticosteroids. These patients should be easy to identify from the repeat prescribing system in the practice. Most will also be under review for their underlying condition either in the practice or in a hospital clinic.

A practical management plan for identifying and treating these patients according to the 1998 NOS guidelines[8] is shown in Table 9.3 and the summary diagram from the Guidance document is reproduced in full in Fig. 9.2.

Table 9.3. Identification and management of patients at risk of corticosteroid-induced osteoporosis[8]

1. Identify all patients taking long-term corticosteroids
     Repeat prescribing system
     Opportunistically when seen in surgery
     From hospital letters

2. Review notes and identify those taking >7.5 mg daily who are likely to require this for 6 months or more (if in doubt, include rather than exclude the patient)
3. Review notes for evidence of previous osteoporotic fractures, age > 65, or steroid dose > 15 mg. These patients need therapy (see Fig. 9.2)
4. Consider DXA scan for all other patients identified in step 2 above.
5. Follow the guidelines in Figure 9.2 for patients who should have a DXA scan
6. Review the need for continuing treatment and further BMD monitoring in those identified at risk
7. Set up a system for capturing details of new patients at risk

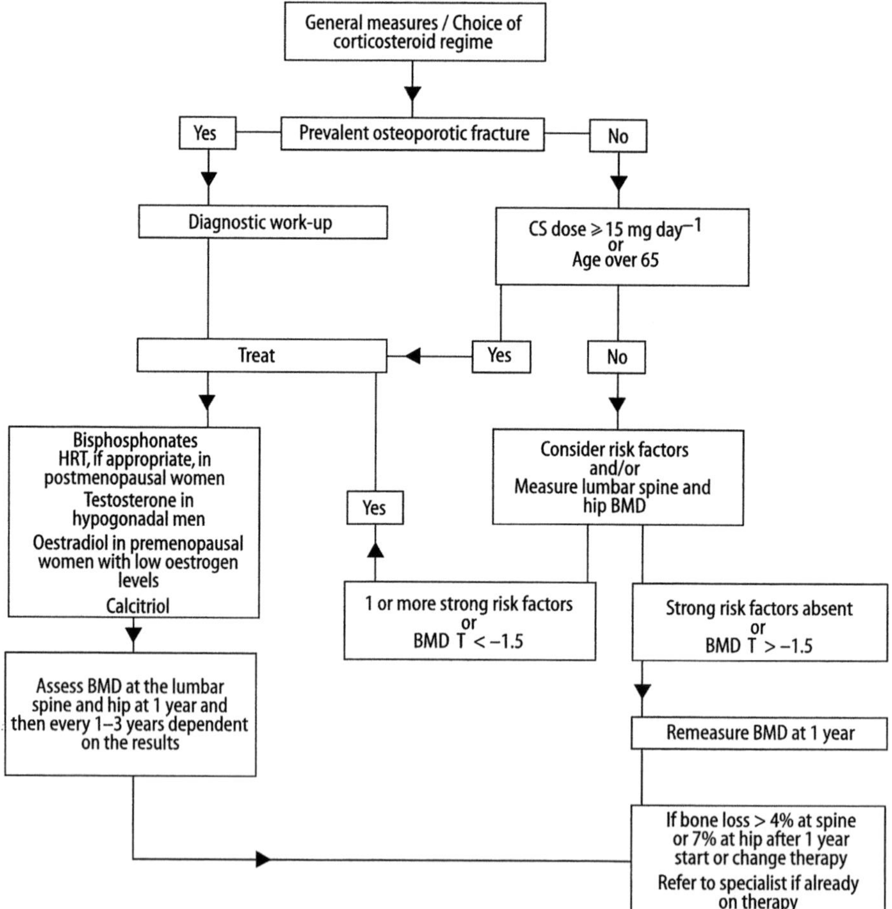

Figure 9.2 Prevention and management of corticosteroid-induced osteoporosis.[8]

BMD measurement may be appropriate for those likely to need high doses for prolonged periods but it should be reserved for those patients where it will alter management. Note that patients who have already suffered an osteoporotic fracture, those taking corticosteroids at a dose of more than 15 mg per day or those who are over 65 years of age, do not need a DXA scan, but should be considered for treatment to prevent or treat osteoporosis. Those taking lower doses need risk factor assessment and/or measurement of BMD at the lumbar spine and hip to guide further management.

Intervention is recommended at a T score of < –1.5, not < –2.5 as is used as the diagnostic level for osteoporosis in the WHO recommendations. This is consistent with the proposed European Regulatory Guidelines[11], and is similar to the baseline mean T-score of placebo treated patients in the study by Adachi[12] where 15% suffered a new vertebral fracture over a 12-month period.

If DXA is not available, then other methods of measurement, such as single X-ray absorptiometry of the forearm (peripheral DXA), may be considered as alternative methods for risk assessment in patients taking long-term corticosteroids. GPs will need to discuss this with their local specialist as there is no treatment threshold identified for this measurement method at present.

Nursing and Residential Homes

Residents in homes are usually elderly and often frail and in poor health. Many will already have established osteoporosis and the remainder are likely to be at high risk of developing the disease. Therefore, many would argue that this group should be identified and managed as actively as those patients taking high-dose corticosteroid therapy. Since the risk of hip fracture in the near future is higher, interventions are likely to be more cost effective.

By the age of 80 years, 80% of women will already have osteoporosis[3] but since they are never seen in surgery they are often forgotten. In some practices, nursing home staff are asked to assess osteoporosis risk of new residents and discuss this with their GP. Very few of this group of patients will need DXA scans to confirm the diagnosis but many will be at risk of other bone diseases such as hyperparathyroidism or osteomalacia therefore some baseline investigations such as alkaline phosphatase and calcium levels may be useful before starting therapy.

Clinical Risk Factors

The RCP Guidelines[7] identify the most important clinical risk factors for the development of osteoporosis. These are shown in Table 9.4. The presence of one or more of these clinical risk factors should make one consider the need for a DXA scan.

Although these clinical risk factors are good predictors of osteoporosis risk for populations, they may not be accurate for individual patients. Therefore, a small number of patients with no risk factors but low bone density will already have osteoporosis and others will be at high risk of developing it. At present the only way to identify these people is to wait until they suffer their first fragility fracture, and ensure that they are identified and treated at that stage.

A recent survey of 200 UK GPs carried out by the NOS[9] showed that 64% of GPs questioned were aware that women who have an early menopause are at increased risk of osteoporosis and are likely to require treatment to prevent bone loss. However, awareness of family history of osteoporosis and being frail and housebound as risk factors was still low at 24% and 13%, respectively.

The use of clinical risk factors to identify elderly patients who are most at risk of hip fracture has also been explored[13]. Sixteen specific risk factors for hip fracture were identified that, when combined, provided a better indication of hip fracture risk than BMD alone (Table 9.5). Patients with five or more of these risk factors are up to 25 times more likely to sustain a hip fracture than those with two or fewer risk factors. Of the 9516 patients over age 65 screened in this study 15% had five or more risk factors.

A questionnaire exploring 14 of the 16 hip fracture risk factors in the Cummings study (the visual perception assessments were excluded) was adminis-

Table 9.4. Risk factors providing indications for the diagnostic use of bone densitometry[7]

1. Presence of strong risk factors

    Oestrogen deficiency:
      Premature menopause (< 45 years)
      Prolonged secondary amenorrhoea (> 1 year)
      Primary hypogonadism

    Corticosteroid therapy
      Prednisolone > 7.5 mg/day for 1 year or more

    Maternal family history of hip fracture

    Low body mass index ($<19 \, kg \, m^{-2}$)

    Other disorders associated with osteoporosis:
      Anorexia nervosa
      Malabsorption syndromes
      Primary hyperparathyroidism
      Post-transplantation
      Chronic renal failure
      Hyperthyroidism
      Prolonged immobilisation
      Cushing's syndrome

2. Radiographic evidence of osteopenia and/or vertebral deformity
3. Previous fragility fracture, particularly of the hip, spine or wrist
4. Loss of height, thoracic kyphosis (after radiographic confirmation of vertebral deformities)

Table 9.5. Risk factors for hip fracture in white women[14]

- Age
- History of maternal hip fracture
- Any fracture since age 50 years
- Poor or very poor health
- Previous hyperparathyroidism
- Anticonvulsant therapy
- Current long-acting benzodiazepine therapy
- Current weight < at age 25 years
- Height at age 25 > 168 cm
- Caffeine intake more than two cups coffee per day
- On feet < 4 hours per day
- No walking for exercise
- Inability to rise from chair without using arms
- Pulse rate > 80 bpm
- Lowest quartile depth perception
- Lowest quartile contrast sensitivity

tered to 100 patients aged over 80 in an inner city general practice in Glasgow (personal communication). The questionnaire was administered by the practice health visitor during over 75 health checks. Of the study patients in this very elderly group 44% were found to have five or more risk factors and therefore to be at greatly increased risk of hip fracture.

Other Methods for Identifying Those At Risk

Radiography

Plain radiography is the best method of diagnosing vertebral and other fractures. Therefore this is the investigation of choice in any postmenopausal or other woman who is at high risk of osteoporosis and who develops sudden onset back pain. However, plain radiographs are very poor at detecting reduction in bone mass – around 30% of the bone mass needs to be lost for osteopenia to be diagnosed on radiography.

Ultrasound

Quantitative ultrasound (QUS) has provoked considerable interest in recent years. It provides a portable, simple, quick and inexpensive method of fracture risk assessment which makes it particularly appealing for use in general practice. It does not use ionising radiation and minimal operator training is needed for effective and accurate use. Detailed information about QUS measurement is provided in Chapter 2. This section concentrates on its potential use in a primary care setting.

There is mounting research evidence that low ultrasound readings at the calcaneum are associated with increased fracture risk, not only in elderly women[16-18] but also in younger age groups.[17,18]

One recently completed study (Hodson, personal communication) explored the use of QUS in an osteoporosis risk assessment clinic in a general practice setting. A total of 500 women aged between 50 and 70 years were invited to attend the risk assessment clinic run by the practice nurse. In a 15 min appointment women were assessed for clinical risk factors, had a QUS measurement at the calcaneum and received "bone friendly" lifestyle advice. Women with low heel ultrasound readings and/or major risk factors were referred for DXA (174 women). Data analysis showed that age, BMI, years since menopause, hormone replacement therapy (HRT) use, hysterectomy, corticosteroid use, previous fracture and radiography changes were predictive of quantitative ultrasound index (QUI). DXA scanning identified 62 women with osteoporosis (36%) and 81 (47%) with osteopenia. There was a highly significant association between QUI and DXA results, but the degree of variability made individual prediction unreliable. Preliminary data analysis suggests that the combination of ultrasound and clinical risk factor assessment to select patients for DXA improved sensitivity and selectivity when compared with either used alone.

The National Osteoporosis Society published a position statement[19] on the use of (QUS) in primary and secondary care in June 1998. This states that although QUS has current and future roles in the clinical assessment of patients at risk of osteoporosis, it does not measure bone mineral content or density directly and therefore cannot be used to diagnose osteoporosis. The statement recommends that women who have a low QUS score are referred for DXA to accurately measure BMD.

This statement provides the following guidance for primary and secondary care teams.

1. Although low QUS of the heel appears to be an independent risk factor for osteoporotic fractures in postmenopausal women, further research is needed to assess its value in predicting osteoporotic fractures in patients taking steroids or in men.

2. QUS appears to be more accurate in predicting low bone mass and future fracture risk than currently recognised clinical risk factors. QUS can, therefore, be used together with risk factors to improve the accuracy of risk assessment.

3. There is only moderate correlation between measurements undertaken with different ultrasound machines.

4. It is currently recommended that those found to have a low QUS measurement are referred for a full assessment of osteoporosis risk, which will usually include a DXA scan.

5. At present there is no evidence that either QUS or DXA would be cost effective for population screening although a few population-based studies have assessed their use.

Step 2: Confirm the Diagnosis Using DXA

DXA uses X-rays to measure bone mineral density at the hip and spine. The technique is described in detail in other chapters. DXA is currently the "gold standard" for BMD measurement and prediction of future fracture risk. In primary care services, DXA can be used to:

1. *Diagnose osteoporosis*: current WHO diagnostic criteria for osteoporosis[3] are based upon bone mass measurement with DXA. The hip is the best site for diagnosis particularly in the elderly;

2. *Predict future osteoporosis risk*: the risk of fracture approximately doubles for each standard deviation reduction in BMD,[20] with variations in the size of the risk depending on the site. The predictive value of BMD for fracture is at least as good as that of blood pressure for stroke;[7]

3. *Monitor continuing bone loss and the effects of treatment*: the lumbar spine is the best site for monitoring and an interval of 1–2 years is required to reliably assess BMD changes;

4. *Save inappropriate therapy use*: by confirming or refuting the diagnosis of osteoporosis, DXA use can help target the use of expensive treatments to the patients who will benefit most.

Diagnose Osteoporosis

WHO criteria for osteopenia and osteoporosis in women using BMD measurement with DXA are shown in Table 9.6. Cut-off levels for diagnosis using DXA are

Table 9.6. Interpretation of DXA results[5]

T-score	Fracture risk
Normal T >−1.0	Low
Low bone mass (osteopenia) T−1.0 to −2.5	Above average
Osteoporosis T<−2.5	High
Established osteoporosis T<−2.5 plus one or more fractures	Very high

Table 9.7. Relative risk (95% confidence interval) of fracture for 1 SD decrease in BMD (measured by absorptiometry) below the age-adjusted mean[7]

Site of measurement	Forearm fracture	Hip fracture	Vertebral fracture	All fractures
Distal radius	1.7 (1.4–2.0)	1.8 (1.4–2.2)	1.7 (1.4–2.1)	1.4 (1.3–1.6)
Hip	1.4 (1.4–1.6)	2.6 (2.0–3.5)	1.8 (1.1–2.7)	1.6 (1.4–1.8)
Lumbar spine	1.5 (1.3–1.8)	1.6 (1.2–2.2)	2.3 (1.9–2.8)	1.5 (1.4–1.7)

less well defined for men but diagnosis at a T-score of −2.5 would seem appropriate as the risk of hip and vertebral fracture is the same in men and women for the same BMD.[21]

Predict Future Fracture Risk

An approximate doubling of the fracture risk occurs with each standard deviation reduction in the T-score as shown in Table 9.7. Higher gradients are found at the hip and lower gradients at appendicular sites. Measurement at the spine is a relatively poor predictor of spinal and other fracture risk, mainly because of calcification of the aorta, arthritis and other artefacts.

Monitoring

About 10–15% of patients will fail to respond to therapy and therefore repeat DXA scan of the lumbar spine after 2 years may encourage change of treatment. This use of DXA is described in more detail in step 6 below.

Save Inappropriate Therapy Use

The appropriate use of DXA to confirm or refute the diagnosis of osteoporosis can save unnecessary use of expensive treatments such as bisphosphonates, allowing these to be targeted to the patients who will benefit most from their use. The average price of a scan is £45, which equates to less than 6 months treatment with the cheapest bisphosphonate.[2]

Access to DXA

Access to bone density measurement has been slow to develop in the UK. A national survey carried out by the NOS in 1995 identified only 13 health authorities (HAs) who were providing services which met DoH recommendations, and many were providing no funding for bone densitometry. In 1997–98 25 units had a contract to provide bone densitometry services to 30 HAs, and this had increased to 41 units supplying services to 49 HAs in 1998–99.

A recent postal survey (prior to April 1999) of 161 centres in the UK believed to have access to bone densitometry[22] showed that of 124 units (77%) who responded, 54 were not providing an NHS service and 31 only provided private scans. Nine only carried out research work, nine had no access to bone densitometry and four had not yet begun to provide their service. Of those providing an NHS service, 52 units (74%) provided open access for GP referrals, 10 provided direct access only for fundholding practices and the remainder provided access only via consultant referral.

The Royal College of Physicians Guidelines stress that all health authorities and other commissioners of health care should implement the recommendations of the Advisory Group on Osteoporosis report[23] and the instructions contained in the NHS Executive Letter EL(96)110[24] which previously recommended that "health authorities should purchase bone density measurement by means of dual X-ray absorptiometry for particular clinical indications". These clinical indications for DXA are as set out in Table 9.4 and discussed below.

Which Patients Should Be Referred for DXA?

The most important point to remember when referring patients for DXA, is that a DXA scan is not necessary unless the result of the scan will alter management. For example, in very elderly patients who have already had one or more fragility fractures confirmed on X-ray, it is reasonable to assume that they have osteoporosis, since 80% of those over 80 will have the disease. As in other age groups, it is important to check that they do not have osteomalacia or secondary osteoporosis, and then to treat the disease appropriately to prevent further fractures. Referral for a DXA scan would not alter management. Likewise in a perimenopausal woman who has already made the decision to take HRT, referral for DXA is inappropriate, as she is already taking the most effective preventive agent. However, at a later stage if she is considering discontinuing HRT then a DXA scan may be useful to assess her BMD, so that a decision to continue HRT or to initiate therapy with another agent can be made.

DXA has a high specificity but a low sensitivity. This means that around 50% of future fractures will occur in people whose DXA scan did not show they were at risk of osteoporosis. DXA scanning and other methods of bone density measurement are not currently recommended for population screening.[7] However, the appropriate use of DXA to confirm or refute the diagnosis of osteoporosis can save unnecessary use of expensive treatments such as bisphosphonates, allowing these to be targeted to the patients who can therefore benefit most from their use. In this context, the use of DXA becomes more cost effective as the cost of the treatment used increases[2] as shown in Table 9.8.

Table 9.8. Estimates of the cost-effectiveness of a treatment strategy with and without assessment of bone mineral density (BMD); effects are assumed to cease when treatment is stopped[7]

Annual cost of treatment (£)	Cost of treatment[a] (£/averted fracture)			Marginal cost per averted fracture (£)
	BMD not assessed	BMD assessed	Ratio	
50	–[b]	–[c]	0.83	–
100	1,207	366	3.3	2,047
150	2,656	870	2.9	4,442
200	4,105	1,374	3.0	6,836
350	8,453	2,887	2.9	14,014
1000	27,294	9,444	2.9	45,143

[a]Both costs and effects are discounted at 6%.
[b]Saves £4,187 per 1,000 women treated.
[c] Saves £5,023 per 1,000 women treated.

The RCP guidelines provide clear guidance on which patients should be considered for DXA as shown in Table 9.4. The Quick Reference Primary Care Guide[5] differs in recommending that DXA be considered for those on high dose corticosteroids for more than 3 months, rather than the 12 months in the RCP guidelines.[7]

Most DXA units which provide open access for GP referrals will have local referral criteria. These are enforced to various degrees, but are usually based on the guidelines discussed above.

A variety of clinical conditions can interfere with the accuracy of DXA scans, for example previous vertebral fractures, aortic calcification and osteoarthritis. These changes are most likely in the elderly and have most impact on the AP lumbar spine scan. Thus in elderly patients a DXA scan of the hip is most likely to reflect the true BMD.

Commissioning DXA for a PCG

It is important for individual practices, and for PCGs/LHGs/LHCCs to be able to estimate the numbers of DXA scans they are likely to need each year, and to budget for their purchase. An estimate of the number of scans required for a typical PCG of 100,000 are shown in Table 9.9. These do not include scans for monitoring therapy. Realistically monitoring will require at least an additional 10%, bringing the total number required to 1000 scans per 100,000 population per year. These requirements may reduce in the future.

It is important to differentiate between the actual unit cost of supplying DXA scans, and the price which is charged by the HA or whoever is providing the service. A recent survey by the National Osteoporosis Society[9] showed that the average charge for scans was £38 for non-fundholders (range £23–£125), £44 for fundholders (£25–£130) and £84 for private scans (£25–£130). The two tier fundholder versus non-fundholder charging system has now disappeared, but it is vital that the new groups budget to continue to purchase appropriate numbers of DXA scans for their population.

Table 9.9. DXA scans required annually for a typical PCG osteoporosis service[2]

Target group	Reason for referral	Number of scans per 100 000 population
Men and women with:		
Previous low trauma fracture	Confirm/assess bone loss if uncertain about management	147
X-ray evidence of osteopenia	As above	194
Corticosteroid use (>7.5 mg daily for 3 months or more)	Identify fast losers/monitor therapy	215
Family history of osteoporosis (especially maternal hip fracture)	Confirm/assess bone loss if uncertain about management	107
Other clinical risk factor: height loss, kyphosis, low BMI (<19 kg/m^{-2})	As above	107
Possible secondary osteoporosis, primary hyperparathyroidism, poorly controlled thyrotoxicosis, malabsorption, rheumatoid, arthritis, liver disease, alcoholism	As above	54
Women with:		
Oestrogen deficiency (menopause or hysterectomy < 45 years, secondary amenorrhoea > 6 months not due to pregnancy, primary hypogonadism)	If HRT contraindicated and in those who are uncertain about or do not wish to take HRT	78
Total scans		902

Based on national survey of DXA provision.[22]

DXA Results and Reports

In order for the DXA assessment to assist in the clinical management of the patient, the result must be presented in a format which the referring GP can understand. The printed report direct from the scanner is highly technical and may contain information which the GP cannot interpret.

DXA results are reported as T-scores (the current measurements compared with the young adult mean scores for the particular machine) and Z-scores, (which provide comparison with reference values for people of the same age as the patient). Table 9.10 summarises the guidance in the NOS National Service

Table 9.10. Actions to consider in patients following DXA scanning[2]

T-score[a]	Action
Normal T>−1.0	Lifestyle advice
Low bone mass (osteopenia) T−1.0 to −2.5	Lifestyle advice HRT/SERMs Calcium and vitamin D supplementation if required
Osteoporosis T<−2.5	Lifestyle advice Treat:HRT/bisphosphonates/ SERMs/calcitonin/calcitriol Calcium and vitamin D supplementation if required
Established osteoporosis T<−2.5 plus one or more fractures	Lifestyle advice Pain control Exclude secondary causes Treat:HRT/bisphosphonates/ SERMs/calcitonin/calcitriol Calcium and vitamin D supplementation if required

SERMs, selective oestrogen receptor modulators.

Framework document outlining the WHO diagnostic criteria and the implications for treatment decisions.

It is important that the results of DXA scans are not considered in isolation. They should be used with the patient's clinical history and risk factor assessment to make a decision regarding the need for therapy to prevent or treat osteoporosis. Ideally this information will have been supplied on the referral form and the specialist clinician assessing the scan will be able to provide advice not only on the diagnosis but on the implications for treatment in the individual patient.

Current GP Use of Bone Density Measurement

A recent survey of 200 GPs carried out by the National Osteoporosis Society[9] showed that 45% of respondents had diagnosed more than six new cases of osteoporosis during the preceding 6 months. The methods of presentation of these new osteoporosis patients are shown in Table 9.11 with 21% being diagnosed following a DXA scan. The findings of a previous survey carried out by the NOS in 1994 among GP readers of a geriatric medicine journal is shown for comparison, although the study populations are different.

When asked about the availability of DXA scans in their area, only 39% said that they were either completely or very satisfied with availability, whereas 36% were either not very or not at all satisfied with access to this investigation; 43% only had access to DXA through consultant referral, 16% only had private access and 3% did not have access to DXA at all. These results show an increased percentage of GPs with direct access to DXA compared with the GPs surveyed in 1994. However, it is of some concern that 31% of the GPs surveyed in 1999 believed that they had access to DXA as a screening tool rather than as a diagnostic investigation.

Table 9.11. Methods of presentation of osteoporosis in general practice: survey results[9]

Method of presentation	1994 survey frequency presented (%)	1999 survey frequency presented (%)
Chance radiograph	32	20
Fracture	32	22
DXA scan	4	21
Other symptoms: back pain, height loss	26	22
Corticosteroid use	N/a	9
Other	6	5

Table 9.12. Which patients should be referred for a DXA scan? Survey results[9]

Patient group	1994 survey frequency referred (%)	1999 survey frequency referred (%)
All menopausal women	36	24
All women 50+	34	13
All men and women 50+	11	5
Anyone with a minimal trauma fracture	75	82
Patient prescribed corticosteroids	67	76
Early menopause	83	80
Family history	N/a	81

When asked specifically which patients they would refer for DXA scan 24% felt it was appropriate to refer all menopausal women, 13% would refer all women over aged 50, and 3% would refer all men and women over 50. The full results are shown in Table 9.12. These show an increase in use for diagnosis in high risk groups compared with the 1994 survey. However, when asked what other technologies they would use to diagnose osteoporosis, 27% claimed to be using bone markers. This demonstrates that despite guidelines and education of GPs, there continues to be confusion about how to diagnose osteoporosis in primary care and specifically, who to refer for DXA.

Peripheral DXA

If lumbar spine and proximal femur bone density measurement with DXA are not available, a measurement of forearm bone density can be used to predict future fracture risk. However, its predictive capacity appears to be slightly less than that of conventional DXA. The details of the technique are described in Chapter 2.

The National Osteoporosis Society has prepared guidance on the current use of peripheral DXA.[25] This recommends that:

Table 9.13. Choice of method for assessing bones in primary care[31]

Clinical need	Use
Identifying those at risk of osteoporosis	Clinical risk factors, biochemical markers of bone turnover, quantitative ultrasound, peripheral DXA
Diagnosing osteoporosis	DXA (especially hip)
Diagnosing fractures	X-rays
Monitoring continued bone loss and effects of osteoporosis treatment	DXA lumbar spine

1. If the T-score is less than –2 SD, treatment is recommended, particularly if there are other risk factors. If monitoring will be required during treatment, referral for a baseline DXA scan is required before initiating therapy;
2. If the T score is between 1 and –2 then a conventional DXA scan of hip and lumbar spine is needed;
3. If the T score is greater than 1, the risk of osteoporosis is low and the patient can be reassured;
4. As with ultrasound, forearm DXA cannot be used for monitoring the effects of treatment as changes in BMD at peripheral sites are small with HRT and bisphosphonates.

A summary of the appropriate uses of DXA, QUS, peripheral DXA and clinical risk factors are shown in Table 9.13.

Step 3: Exclude Secondary Osteoporosis or Other Bone Disease

About 20% of females and 40–50% of males with osteoporosis will have secondary osteoporosis. Therefore, in an ideal world, all patients who have osteoporosis should be investigated to identify the causes of secondary osteoporosis and to exclude other diseases which may mimic osteoporosis, e.g. osteomalacia or malignancy. However, in a world with finite resources, GPs must be selective both in whom they investigate and in which investigations they perform in individual patients. Investigations which should be considered in this situation are shown in Table 9.14 (overleaf).

If all the investigations are normal, but the patient has no obvious reason to suffer from osteoporosis, e.g. they are premenopausal or male, you should consider referral to your local bone clinic, or general physician, for further investigation. One may also want to screen for coeliac disease by carrying out an anti-endomysial antibody blood test. If this is positive, then the patient should be referred to a gastroenterologist for an ileal mucosal biopsy to confirm the diagnosis.

Most men will require referral to a bone specialist for more extensive investigation and specialist management. Although the bisphosphonates can be used in men, they are not yet licensed for this indication.

Table 9.14. Investigations to exclude secondary osteoporosis and other bone diseases

Condition	Investigation(s)
Primary hyperparathyroidism	Serum calcium, vitamin D
Thyrotoxicosis	TSH level
Multiple myeloma	Erythrocyte sedimentation rate, protein electrophoresis
Osteomalacia	Serum calcium, phosphate, alkaline phosphatase, 24 hour urinary calcium
Malabsorption	FBC (anti-endomysial antibodies)
Hypogonadism in men	Free androgen index

TSH, thyroid stimulating hormone; FBC, full blood count.

Step 4: Provide Appropriate Treatment

Managing Osteoporosis in Primary Care

A simplified plan for the management of osteoporosis is shown in Fig. 9.3, but detailed discussion of treatment options is outside the remit of this manual. All patients need to receive education about osteoporosis (ideally both verbal and in written format), advice about lifestyle modification and review of calcium and vitamin D status. Appropriate therapy can then be initiated to prevent or treat the disease. Therapies suitable for use in a primary care setting are described in the "'Quick Reference Primary Care Guide"[5] and in the RCP guidelines document.[7]

Patients in Nursing and Residential Home

Those who are found to have established osteoporosis or to be at high risk can be treated with a bisphosphonate. Other residents who are housebound or eat a poor diet will benefit from supplements of calcium and vitamin D. The vitamin D can be provided orally, for example in a twice daily supplement providing 500 mg and 200 iu of calcium and vitamin D, respectively, in each tablet, or the vitamin D can be provided in a once yearly injection at the time of the influenza immunisation, with a twice daily oral calcium supplement. Calcium and vitamin D therapy in this group has been shown to reduce hip fractures by up to one-third.[26]

The majority of fragility fractures apart from vertebral fractures occur as a result of a fall and residents of homes are particularly at risk of falls. There is no clear evidence that interventions can reduce falls.[7] However, there is good evidence that hip fractures can be reduced in this population by wearing external hip protectors.[27] These are not cosmetically attractive therefore compliance with their use is likely to be poor, even in homes. However, they are relatively inexpensive, a one-off cost, and are easily available, therefore they should be actively considered.

Surgery or Osteoporosis Clinics

Previously GPs were encouraged to provide a variety of special clinics within their practice. A fee was payable for each clinic of 10 patients provided. However, clinic

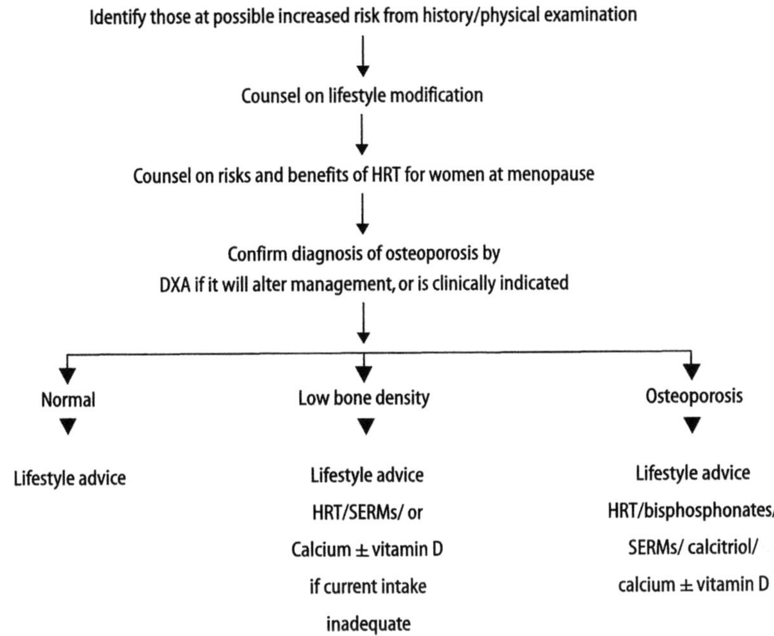

Figure 9.3 Management of osteoporosis in primary care.[5]

fees are no longer paid and as a result most practices now only provide well woman, menopause, antenatal, baby, diabetes and asthma clinics. Diabetes and asthma chronic disease management care continues to attract a fee whether this is provided in a special clinic or during ordinary surgeries.

In the author's own practice, much of the osteoporosis care is provided in the well woman clinics. This are the following advantages.

1. Appointments of 15 minutes allow time for education and examination
2. Patients spend time with the practice nurse as well as the doctor
3. Patients taking HRT for prevention or treatment of osteoporosis would be attending this clinic for review anyway.

The disadvantages are as follows.

1. Men cannot attend this clinic.
2. Other partners who are not involved in the well woman clinics may become less experienced at managing osteoporosis.
3. In some practices the partner with interest and expertise in osteoporosis may not run the well woman clinics.

Step 5: Monitor Treatment and Encourage Compliance

Ideally all patients who have been commenced on treatment following an initial DXA scan should have a repeat DXA scan at least once to check for response.

However, with restricted budgets this may not be possible. About 10–15% of patients fail to respond to treatment[28]. Some patients do not take their medication or take it incorrectly so that it is not absorbed. Others will fail to respond even though they comply with medication. This may be related to malabsorption or an ongoing medical problem causing continued bone loss.

Monitoring may also help compliance. Since treatments for osteoporosis can be expected to reduce fracture risk by 50%, many patients will have a further fracture while on treatment and may perceive this as a treatment failure. Improved BMD on DXA scan can demonstrate that the treatment is working and may improve compliance.

Lumbar spine DXA is most sensitive for monitoring as it contains a high proportion of active trabecular bone which responds fairly rapidly to oestrogen or bisphosphonates and can be scanned with reasonable accuracy (precision around 1%)[28]. Changes in BMD with treatment are smaller at the hip and usually even less at peripheral sites such as the forearm or heel. In addition the precision error is likely to be greater at the hip (1.5–3%).[28]

It is sometimes assumed that any positive change in DXA measurements indicates a response to therapy and any negative change represents continued bone loss. However, to identify statistically significant changes in BMD, the change between scans must be approximately three times the precision of the scanner at this site (1–2% for most DXA scanners).[28] With oestrogen or bisphosphonates, 5–10% increase in BMD can be achieved over the first two years of therapy so this is an appropriate interval between scans.

Since commonly used treatments such as HRT and bisphosphonates only cause very small changes in QUS and peripheral DXA at the heel or forearm over 1–3 years, the National Osteoporosis Society and the RCP do not recommend that QUS or peripheral DXA are used for monitoring treatment

Biochemical Markers of Bone Turnover

The biochemical markers of bone resorption and formation which are specific to bone (eg osteocalcin and deoxypyridinolone) may be particularly useful as monitoring tools and are under active investigation. In the future, these could be used to predict individuals who are fast bone losers and are therefore at risk of osteoporosis, or for monitoring of treatment. The biochemical markers of bone resorption are maximally suppressed in those who respond, by 3 months treatment with HRT or bisphosphonates, and may therefore be more useful for assessing response to treatment than DXA, where changes are not usually measurable for 1–2 years. However, these are still research tools at present.

Ensure Compliance with Treatment

Only a very small proportion of women taking HRT continue with treatment long term. Good patient education (both verbal and written) on the benefits of long-term use of HRT and other osteoporosis therapies may increase compliance. Telephone access to advice from practice nurses, and regular follow-up by an interested primary care team would also be expected to encourage continued use of therapies.

In the author's experience, the first 3–12 months of treatment with HRT or a bisphosphonate are the times when patients are most likely to default. Once patients have stuck with therapy for this length of time, they are much more likely to continue long term.

Motivating patients to implement lifestyle changes is often significantly more difficult than encouraging them to comply with therapy. Brief intervention at each consultation may be the most effective method.

Step 6: Continue to Identify New Patients

All practices need to have in place systems for identifying "new" or previously undiagnosed patients who may be at risk of osteoporosis or already have the disease. This can be achieved by reviewing all new patient questionnaires, hospital letters and new repeat prescription requests for any indication that the patient is at risk of osteoporosis. The key information which should be sought is shown in Table 9.15.

If a patient may be at risk, their notes can be reviewed by a GP or practice nurse, who can decide if further investigation or management is required. If the diagnosis of osteoporosis or osteopenia is confirmed, this should be entered in the patient's electronic and paper-based clinical notes and arrangements made for treatment and review.

The numbers of patients identified in this way each week after the first few months are likely to be small, but without these systems in place, over time many patients at high risk or with established disease will slip through the net. Ideally one member of the team should take responsibility for ensuring that these systems are maintained and updated as appropriate.

Since many of these patients will present in the secondary care setting, it is important that primary and secondary care teams work together on selective case-finding. Some examples of how this could work are shown in Table 9.16.

Table 9.15. Data which may help identify new patients at risk of osteoporosis

New patient questionnaires

    Past medical history of:

        Osteoporosis

        Hysterectomy and/or oophorectomy before age 45 years

        Fractures especially Colles, vertebral or hip

        Back pain in a postmenopausal woman

        Corticosteroids > 7.5 mg daily currently or previously

        Hypogonadism in men

Hospital letters

    Initiation of oral corticosteroid therapy

    Fractures

    Hysterectomy and/or oophorectomy before age 45 years

    DXA scan reports

New repeat prescriptions

    Corticosteroids > 7.5 mg daily

Table 9.16. Examples of opportunities for selective case-finding[2]

High risk group	Setting	Action
Patients with history minimal trauma fracture	Hospital fracture clinic: Advise fracture patients of possible osteoporosis risk and inform GPs of need for follow-up	Warn of possible osteoporosis risk
	Encourage patient to visit GP for follow-up	Offer general lifestyle advice and NOS details
	Offer advice to patients during rehabilitation after hip fracture	Consider referral for diagnostic confirmation and/or treatment
Patients on oral corticosteroids	On initiation of corticosteroid treatment	Warn of possible osteoporosis risk
	In asthma and rheumatology clinic	Review dose of steroid
	On prescription review for patients already prescribed corticosteroids	Offer general lifestyle advice and NOS details
		Refer for densitometry and treat according to NOS CIO Guidelines
Early menopause	At follow-up after hysterectomy	Warn of possible osteoporosis risk
	Review records of women excluded from cervical smear target lists or those	Offer general lifestyle advice and NOS details
	recorded as having a hysterectomy to confirm advice offered	Prescribe HRT unless contraindications. Refer for densitometry if it will change clinical management

Future Trends in Osteoporosis Management in Primary Care

Minimum Standards

In the future, it is hoped that all practices will manage osteoporosis in a proactive way and all will meet the minimum standards of care recommended by the Primary Care Rheumatology Society,[6] Table 9.17. To achieve these standards, primary and secondary care teams will need to work together to provide the "seamless service" that we all aspire to in osteoporosis services.

Genetics

Improved understanding of the genetics of osteoporosis, will allow those at risk to be identified earlier and preventive measures implemented before the disease causes major bone loss.

Ultrasound and Peripheral DXA

In the future there is likely to be continuing interest in, and increased use of quantitative ultrasound, together with clinical risk factors, to screen for those at risk of osteoporosis. Those with low measurements may continue to need a DXA scan to allow a definitive diagnosis of osteoporosis, but as now, only if this will alter management. However, increased use of QUS together with clinical risk factors may improve accuracy of prediction of risk, resulting in more targeted use of DXA scans.

Table 9.17. Minimum standards for osteoporosis in primary care[6]

All patients with previous fragility fractures identified
    Vertebral fractures confirmed on X-ray
    DXA to confirm osteoporosis if it will change the management
    All patients with fragility fractures on treatment and complying
    All patients with new fragility fractures identified and assessed

All patients on oral corticosteroids identified
    All being managed as directed in the NOS Corticosteroid Induced Osteoporosis Guidelines
    All new patients starting oral corticosteroids are identified and assessed

All women with natural or surgical menopause < age 45 years identified
    All encouraged to use HRT
    DXA only if it will alter the management

All housebound nursing and residential home patients identified
    All on calcium and vitamin D or other osteoporosis therapy

All those diagnosed as having osteoporosis investigated for secondary osteoporosis and other bone disease

All men with osteoporosis fully investigated or referred and are on appropriate therapy

Once the main at risk groups have been identified and treated, risk factors can be used to identify other high risk patients. Some of these will also need DXA scanning if available to confirm the diagnosis before treatment starts. **DXA is only required if the result will alter management.**

Peripheral instantaneous X-ray image scanner (PIXI) technology provides DXA scanning at the calcaneum. This is described in detail elsewhere, but is likely to improve accessibility and cost effectiveness of DXA technology. It provides a low cost, very portable method with high precision and reasonable correlation with future fracture risk.

Clinical Risk Factors

Currently clinical risk factors are not very accurate in identifying men and women who later turn out to have osteoporosis on DXA scan. Many high risk people are not identified. In the future, it is hoped that research will identify more and better clinical risk factors, and that we will learn to use them along with information provided by QUS and peripheral DXA assessment, to improve identification of patients with osteoporosis prior to their first fracture.

DXA

Ideally all GPs should have direct access to DXA scans. GPs who do not have access either directly or via a consultant should lobby for access. They can provide their PCG/LHG/LHCC with a copy of "A primary care framework for osteoporosis" produced by the NOS, and the RCG document "Osteoporosis: guidelines for prevention and treatment" which both strongly recommend purchase of these services.

The demand for DXA scans to monitor patients on therapy is likely to increase rapidly over the next few years. GPs need to understand the time interval needed between DXA scans in this situation, and that other methods of bone measurement such as QUS and peripheral DXA are not suitable for monitoring at this time.

Lateral spinal DXA is more accurate than anteroposterior DXA of the lumbar spine in elderly patients who have calcification of the aorta or spinal degenerative disease because it allows the vertebral bodies to be scanned independently of the posterior elements, measuring mainly trabecular bone, free of the degenerative artefacts. Newer machines which offer this facility without repositioning the patient will be faster and more accurate. Lateral spine DXA will also allow accurate diagnosis in elderly patients with bilateral hip replacements.

Biochemical Markers of Bone Turnover

It is likely that biochemical markers of bone turnover will play an increasingly important role as a clinical risk factor in osteoporosis diagnosis and in monitoring in the primary care setting. However, for this to be cost effective, these will need to be available at a much reduced cost.

Therapies

It is anticipated that better and safer therapies for prevention and treatment will become available, and that these will improve compliance rates. This should eventually result in a decrease in fracture rates, which currently continue to rise.

There is little doubt that primary care teams will retain responsibility for osteoporosis in the future. With limited people resources and tight budgets, bone density measurement will have an important role, both at an individual practice level and at a PCG/LHG/LHCC level, in helping teams identify and manage those at risk of osteoporosis.

Acknowledgements

The author would like to acknowledge important contributions from Rosemary Rowe and Dr Jean Hodson during the writing of this chapter, and would like to thank the National Osteoporosis Society for permission to include material from "A primary care service framework for osteoporosis" and various position statements.

References

1. Department of Health (1998) Our healthier nation. Department of Health, London.
2. National Osteoporosis Society (1999) A primary care service framework for osteoporosis. National Osteoporosis Society, Bath.
3. World Health Organisation (1994) Assessment of fracture risk and its application to screening for postmenopausal osteoporosis. WHO Technical Report Series. WHO, Geneva
4. Freemantle N (1992) Screening for osteoporosis to prevent fracture. In: Effective health care no. 1. School of Public Health, Leeds.
5. Department of Health (1998) Quick Reference Primary Care Guide on the Prevention and Treatment of Osteoporosis. Department of Health, London.
6. Primary Care Rheumatology Society (1999) Minimum standard guidelines.
7. Royal College of Physicians (1999) Osteoporosis: clinical guidelines for prevention and treatment.
8. National Osteoporosis Society, London (1998) Guidance on the prevention and management of corticosteroid induced osteoporosis. National Osteoporosis Society, Bath.
9. National Osteoporosis Society (1999) Survey: GP understanding and action regarding osteoporosis. National Osteoporosis Society, Bath.
10. Cooper C, Melton LJ (1992) Vertebral fractures: how large is the silent epidemic? BMJ 304:793–794
11. Compston JE, Audran M, Avouac D et al. (1996) Recommendations for the registration of agents used in the prevention and treatment of glucocorticoid-induced osteoporosis; an update. Calcif Tissue Int 59:323–327.
12. Adachi JD, Bensen WA, Brown J et al. (1997) Intermittent cyclical etidronate therapy in the prevention of corticosteroid-induced osteoporosis N Engl J Med 337:382–387.
13. Cummings SR, Nevitt MC, Browner WS et al. (1995) Risk factors for hip fracture in white women N Engl J Med 332:767–773.
14. Porter RW, Miller CG, Grainger D (1990) Prediction of hip fracture in elderly women: a prospective study BMJ 301:638–41.
15. Hans D, Dargent-Molina P, Schott AM et al. (1996) Ultrasonographic heel measurements to predict hip fracture in elderly women: the EPIDOS prospective study. Lancet 348:511–514.
16. Bauer DC, Gluer CC, Caulay JA et al. (1997) Broadband ultrasound attenuation predicts fractures strongly and independently of densitometry in older women. A prospective study. Study of Osteoporotic Fractures Research Group Arch Int Med 157:629–34.
17. Stewart A, Torgerson DJ, Reid DM (1996) Prediction of fractures in perimenopausal women: a comparison of dual energy X-ray absorptiometry and broadband ultrasound attenuation. Ann Rheum Dis 55:140–142.
18. Thomson P, Taylor J, Oliver R et al. (1998) Quantitative ultrasound (QUS) of the heel predicts wrist and osteoporosis-related fractures in women age 45–75 years. J Clin Dens 1:219–225.
19. National Osteoporosis Society (1998) The use of quantitative ultrasound in the management of osteoporosis in primary and secondary care. National Osteoporosis Society, Bath.
20. Marshall D, Johnell O, Wedel H (1996) Meta-analysis of how well measures of bone density predict occurrence of osteoporotic fractures. BMJ 312:1254–1259.

21. Wasnich RD, Ross PD, Davis JN et al. (1985) Prediction of post-menopausal fracture risk with use of bone mineral measurements. Am J Obstet. Gynecol 153:745–751.
22. Rowe R, Cooper C (2000). Provision of osteoporosis services in secondary care: a UK survey J R Soc Med 93:22–24.
23. Department of Health (1994) Advisory Group on Osteoporosis Report. Department of Health, London.
24. Winyard G, Moores Y (1996) EL (96)110 Improving the effectiveness of clinical services. NHS Executive 1996: Annex B.
25. National Osteoporosis Society (1998) The use of forearm X-ray absorptiometry – a position statement. National Osteoporosis Society, Bath.
26. Chapuy MC, Arlot ME, DuBoef F et al. (1992) Vitamin D_3 and calcium to prevent hip fractures in elderly women. N Engl J Med 327:1637–1642.
27. Lauritzen JB, Petersen MM, Lund B (1993) Effect of external hip protectors on hip fractures. Lancet 341:11–13.
28. National Osteoporosis Society (1998) Fundamentals of Bone Densitometry – Report of a working party. National Osteoporosis Society, Bath.

10 Bone Densitometry in the Elderly

T. Masud and P.D. Miller

Introduction

Osteoporosis is the most prevalent metabolic bone disease in the elderly and causes much morbidity, mortality and cost in terms of health and social services expenditure. It has been estimated that its prevalence will double by year 2044 and that the prevalence of hip fracture, which is one of the most important consequences of the condition, will increase fourfold by year 2050. Although the menopause in women is an important turning point in the development of osteoporosis, the majority of osteoporosis related fractures occur after the age of 65 years and increase exponentially thereafter (Fig. 10.1).

Low bone mass is considered to be the most important predictor of future fracture risk and is as valuable as a predictor of fractures as raised cholesterol and high blood pressure are as predictors of myocardial infarction and stroke

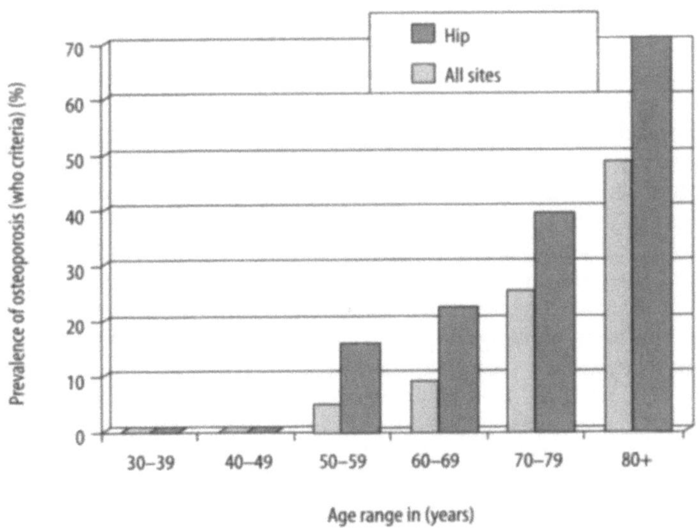

Figure 10.1 Prevalence of osteoporosis in Western women.[53]

respectively.[1] Although bone mass is a surrogate marker for bone strength, accounting for 70–80% of its variability, it has limitations in fracture prediction. Bone density measurements are valuable in assessing an individuals fracture risk but are not good at identifying those specific individual's who will sustain a fracture. Risk factors for low bone density may differ from risk factors for fractures and therefore there is a large overlap in bone mass between fracture and non-fracture subjects.

Age is another important risk factor for fractures, independent of bone mass. A ten year increase in age is associated with a 94% increase in fracture risk whereas a 0.1 g cm^{-2} drop in bone meneral density (BMD) (Ξ to bone loss over 10 years) is associated with a 44% increased risk.[2] Thus for a given BMD fracture risk is greater in the elderly. The predictive value of BMD measurements is likely to be less in the very elderly as extraskeletal factors such as fall propensity assume greater importance with age. If these factors are not considered the importance of BMD measurements alone is overestimated in older subjects. This chapter discusses problems in measuring bone mass in the elderly, the role of bone density and non-skeletal factors in predicting fractures and the relevance of bone mass measurements in clinical practice.

Problems with Measurement of Bone Density in the Elderly

Conventional Radiography: Uses and Limitations

The radiographic features of osteoporosis include "radiological" or "apparent" osteopenia (not to be confused with the WHO term osteopenia which is based on a BMD measurement of between T–1 and T–2.5), abnormalities in trabecular architecture, a decrease in cortical width and the resulting fractures. Traditionally it has been thought that at least 30% of skeletal tissue must be lost before osteopenia is apparent on conventional radiographs and assessing bone density by using radiographs alone is insensitive when compared to bone densitometry techniques.[3,4] Pharmacological treatment for osteoporosis should not be started purely on the basis of a radiological report of apparent osteopenia alone (without prevalent fractures) as a significant proportion of these subjects will have normal BMD on bone densitometry, although in the presence of prevalent fragility fractures, detection of apparent osteopenia on conventional radiography usually implies a low BMD and a case can be made to consider osteoporosis therapy in older subjects if bone densitometry is unavailable.[5]

Changes in trabecular pattern can be associated with low BMD. In the spine, preferential loss of horizontal trabeculae and hypertrophy of vertebral bars gives rise to a striated appearance on radiograph.[6] At the femoral neck site the trabecular pattern, arranged along the lines of compression and tension stresses, has been used (Singh Index) as a measure of low BMD and fracture risk.[7] The risk of hip fracture increases with decreasing score, particularly in the elderly.[8] However, although this method is a simple and reproducible epidemiological tool for estimating bone mass which may detect differences between populations or subgroups within populations, caution should be used in classifying individual patients because of the wide overlap of BMD between grades.[9]

The detection of peripheral fragility fractures by conventional radiography is usually straightforward. The diagnosis of vertebral fractures, however, can be more problematic since the cut-off point between a normal variation and a fracture is not absolute. The term vertebral deformity is therefore often used but it is important to realise that conditions other than osteoporosis such as Scheuermann's disease and longstanding degenerative disc disease can also cause vertebral deformities.[10] In clinical practice spinal radiography and bone densitometry should be regarded as complementary rather than alternative procedures as the principles of the two are essentially different. Whereas the latter provides information on bone mineral content which is independently associated with fracture risk, the former assesses structural changes, including trabeculation and vertebral deformities, which provide information on conditions which may alter BMD measurements such as osteophytosis (see below) and can also diagnose other conditions which may also present with back pain such as myeloma, neoplastic disease, osteomalacia, Paget's disease, disc and bone infections and degenerative disease of the spine.

Factors Affecting BMD Measurements in the Elderly

The prevalence of degenerative disease of the spine increases with age, reaching over 70% in the over 65 year age group.[11] Posterio-anterior (PA) measurements of lumbar spine BMD (via dual-energy X-ray absorptiometry (DXA)) may be artificially raised by the presence of osteophytosis by as much as 32%.[12] Intervertebral disc space narrowing, posterior elements such as facet joint hypertrophy, vertebral collapse and aortic calcification can also spuriously raise BMD readings in elderly subjects. The apparent spinal BMD uniformity is therefore often lost with ageing and differences in BMD exceeding 25% between neighbouring vertebrae are not infrequent. These factors must be taken into account when interpreting PA DXA scans in older subjects to avoid underdiagnosing osteoporosis. The BMD, T- and Z-scores of the individual vertebrae should be considered as well as the average of L1–L4 or L2–L4.

Some of these problems can be overcome by the use of lateral DXA scanning, which excludes the posterior processes. This method potentially has a superior diagnostic sensitivity because age related trabecular bone loss is more pronounced and more strongly associated with prevalent vertebral fractures than with PA measurements. Furthermore, by improving spatial resolution, lateral scanning may identify the presence of vertebral collapse. However, the lateral view is more demanding in acquisition and processing, and reproducibility is poorer due to the greater thickness and non-uniformity of the overlying soft tissue. Furthermore the L2 and L4 vertebrae can be overlapped by the ribs and iliac crests, respectively.

For the above reasons, measurement of hip BMD is thought to be more relevant than spinal BMD in the older age group. Measurements can be made at critical points where fractures occur. The femoral neck region of interest (ROI) is the site of subcapital, midcervical and basicervical fractures which together constitute 63% of all hip fractures, and the trochanter ROI is the site of the remaining 37% of proximal femur fractures. Position of the ROIs with DXA is based on anatomical markers in the proximal femur and is sensitive to errors in positioning of the femur when the scan is performed, especially in older subjects.[13]

This may be particularly important when patients are repositioned for follow-up measurements.

Interprating BMD in Older People: Fracture Thresholds, T- and Z-scores

The concept of the "fracture threshold" is derived from epidemiological data showing that the rate of prevalent fractures increases substantially below a certain BMD value. The threshold value can be set arbitrarily, for example 2 SD below the mean value of young normals. From a clinical perspective this concept provides a simple means for defining the disease similar to the use of arterial pressure for the diagnosis of hypertension. However, the risk of future fractures rises continuously with decreasing BMD and there is a substantial overlap between fracture and nonfracture patients making the term "fracture threshold" misleading and currently out of favour. The proportion of people who have a BMD below such a threshold rises with age and is therefore less useful in an older population where the majority of subjects will be classified as being below the threshold.

BMD can also be expressed as percentage of the mean value of a normal population (either a young adult mean or age adjusted mean). The main drawback to this approach is that it ignores the magnitude of the normal age, although it is a concept which patients find relatively easy to understand. Presenting data as quartiles or quintiles is useful when BMD in a population is asymmetrically distributed. Centiles and percentiles can also be used and the number stated expresses the percentage of the normal population which falls below the measured result.

The WHO definition of osteoporosis using T–2.5 as the cut-off is being increasingly recognised world-wide, although there is still extensive debate about its usefulness in the elderly, as after the age of around 75 years, osteoporosis (defined as $T < -2.5$) becomes increasingly universal. From the health economic point of view, therefore, such a definition for osteoporosis cannot by itself be used as an "intervention threshold". The significance of the WHO term "osteopenia" (T-score between –1 and –2.5) is also quite different at the age of menopause than at an older age (> 75 years). In the former situation a case can be made for prevention therapy as the lifetime fracture risk is high, whereas in the latter situation the remaining lifetime fracture risk is low. Some experts advocate the use of the Z-scores in older subjects at least in terms of "intervention thresholds". A Z-score of worse than –1 either at the spine or hip site is often used arbitrarily in older subjects, as this approach captures approximately the lowest quartile of BMD. The advantages and disadvantages of using T- and Z-scores are summarised in Table 10.1.

Relative Risk, Absolute Risk and Lifetime Risk of Fracture

Although BMD is an important determinant of fracture risk, numerous other factors appear to predict fracture risk independent of BMD (see below). T-scores, Z-scores and fracture thresholds fail to provide a mechanism which incorporates these other important risk factors. One way of expressing the probability of fracture is to use the "absolute risk" which can be calculated from the relative risks of

Table 10.1. Advantages and disadvantages of T- and Z-scores

	Advantages	Disadvantages
T-score	Identifies a high proportion of the elderly population as being at risk of fractures. Recognises the true magnitude of osteoporosis. Concept is supported by fracture data which shows proximal femur fracture rates double every 5–6 years in older females	Does not have the same implications for fracture risk for measurement at all sites in the skeleton or for different methodologies such as ultrasound. Conceptually it is difficult to classify virtually all older women as having a disease and being candidates for treatment
Z-score	Provides a direct comparison of an individual's bone density with other individuals of the same age and provides an accurate assessment of that individuals fracture risk Compensates for variance differences in reference distributions Z-score of –1 at either spine or proximal femur implies approximately the lowest quartile of BMD which can be viewed as an appropriate percentage of the population to consider at risk. It is often stated that a Z-score of –2 or worse implies suspicion of a secondary cause for osteoporosis (although this has not been tested)	The age-related increase in fracture risk is not recognised by the Z-score. If used as an intervention threshold, this method selects the same percentage of women in any age group for treatment, despite the fact that a 50-year-old woman with a particular Z-score has a much lower absolute risk of fracture than an 80-year-old woman with the same Z-score

the relevant factors. Although each individual risk factor has a relatively narrow SD around the estimate of its effect on fracture risk, the cumulative effect of estimation errors using multiple risk factors can be large.

Absolute risks are relatively small over a short time period, but cumulative risk over a person's remaining lifespan can be considerable. The concepts of "lifetime fracture risk" and "remaining lifetime fracture risk" (RLFR) can also be used to quantify the likelihood of future fractures. Few studies of sufficient duration exist to explore how BMD and other risk factors affect lifetime fracture risk and many assumptions are required to extrapolate from short-term risk to lifetime risk. Models for estimating lifetime fracture risk have been explored but applying multiple risk factor data to these models is problematic.[14] Assumptions such as remaining years of life and long-term effect of risk factors which may change (such as BMD) have to be made. The challenge with this concept is to devise a user-friendly model of estimating RLFR, incorporating several risk factors, which can be longitudinally explored. If such a model could be validated it may be possible to use cut-off values for RLFR as intervention thresholds in older as well as younger patients. It is important to appreciate that the RLFR for a younger woman is greater than it is for an older woman with comparable degrees of reduced bone mass because the younger woman has many more years of exposure to low bone mass in the future. In this regard, a young untreated woman with a femoral neck BMD 3 SD below the mean young normal value has a higher lifetime probability of hip fracture than does an 80 year old woman with the same femoral neck BMD. However the short-term (current) fracture risk is higher in the older woman because of the independent effects of age and propensity to fall on fracture risk.

Non-Uniform Reference Databases

An important issue in bone densitometry has been the non-uniform reference databases. A basic principle of statistics is that each sample derived from any given population will yield different mean and SD values. The T-score is calculated from the mean peak adult bone mass (PABM) and the SD from that mean, and therefore an individual may be classified differently if separate populations are used to create the reference databases, as occurs with different manufacturers' machines. This problem has created a potential credibility issue for bone densitometry. One possible solution is the creation of a standardised reference database for each skeletal site and technique that could be adopted by all the major manufacturers. For the total hip and femoral neck sites, the NHANES III (National Health and Examination Survey) common reference data have been incorporated into the databases of the three major central DXA machines which has eliminated the potential for machine specific diagnosis of osteoporosis at the hip.[15] For sites other than the hip, however, a common reference database does not currently exist and as a consequence different devices may yield different T-scores and individual patients may be classified differently by using different machines to measure the same skeletal sites. Further work to develop a uniform database for all existing technologies is currently being developed and has been endorsed in its necessity by the United States FDA regulatory device division.[16]

Risk Factors for Fractures Other Than BMD and Age

Previous Fractures

The existence of a previous fragility fracture confers a significant increase in risk, independent of BMD, of further fractures. Patients with existing vertebral deformities have an increased risk of other vertebral and non-vertebral fractures.[17] Data from the study of osteoporotic fractures (SOF) have shown that a similar increase in hip fracture risk is associated with having experienced a fracture since the age of 50 years. The risk of fractures is also increased in relation to the number of previous fractures. One reason for this independent effect of a previous fracture is that it may indicate structural defects such as changes in microarchitecture which are not measured by BMD. A combination of low BMD and previous fractures further increases the relative risks of subsequent fractures, as shown in Table 10.2.[18] In terms of clinical management these data imply that a patient with a positive fragility fracture history should be considered for intervention earlier with a higher BMD than a patient without.

Propensity to Fall

In later life, BMD becomes increasingly less important in the pathogenesis of non-vertebral fractures at the expense of fall-related factors. Over a third of elderly women aged 65 years and over fall at least once per year, rising to around a half of women aged 85 years and above.[19] Only 5–6% of falls give rise to fractures and 1% to hip fractures in the elderly.[19,20] The frequency of falls is greater in elderly women than in men. A fall in the previous year is a risk factor for further falls and recurrent fallers are particularly likely to be at risk of hip fractures. Of the falls that result in hip fractures, about one half are due to tripping or slipping, one fifth to syncope, one-fifth to one-third to balance problems and the remainder to other miscellaneous factors.[21,22] Direction of the fall (sideways directly over the hip) and reduced soft tissue over the hip (which dissipates forces) are associated with an increased the risk of hip fracture.[23] An increase in body sway, a measure of neuromuscular uncoordination and postural instability, is associated with a doubled increase risk of hip fracture.[24] Although body sway is an epidemiological and physiological tool which may detect differences between and within

Table 10.2. Relative risk of fractures in women according to bone mass, prevalent vertebral and non-vertebral fractures[18]

	Relative risk of further fracture
Low bone mass without previous fragility fracture	2.5
Vertebral fracture without low bone mass	4.3
Non-vertebral fracture without low bone mass	1.8
Vertebral fracture and low bone mass	12.6
Non-vertebral fracture and low bone mass	7.4
Vertebral fracture and non-vertebral fracture and low bone mass	16.6

Table 10.3. Risk factors for falls

Dizziness on standing/postural hypotension (including caused by drugs)
One or more fall in the previous 6 months/12 months
Incontinence
Cognitive impairment
Impaired mobility/balance/low gait speed
Previous stroke/lower limb dysfunction
Chronic diseases (e.g. neurological, musculoskeletal, cardiovascular)
Low physical activity
Inability to walk tandem
Inability to rise from chair without using arms
Reduced vision
Drugs causing reduced alertness (including hypnotics, sedatives and antidepressants)
Environmental (e.g. loose rugs, slippery surfaces, inadequate aids)

populations, it is unlikely to be useful in individual subjects to predict falls because of poor reproducibility of the test.

Easily ascertainable risk factors for falling are shown in Table 10.3. Some of these factors have been used in a risk profile to identify persons aged 70 years and over at high risk of falling. The presence of two or more of the following risk factors in patients aged 70 years or more can identify those at risk of falls: dizziness on standing, postural hypotension, one or more fall in the previous 6 months, incontinence, cognitive impairment, impaired mobility, previous stroke and reduced physical activity.[25]

At a population level there are few data suggesting that the rates of falls can be reduced to a worthwhile extent. One multifactorial intervention in community-dwelling people aged 70 years and over showed that the rates of falling in the intervention group was reduced by 31% compared to controls.[26] However, the cost-effectiveness of such a strategy is not established. Nevertheless, in individual patients causes of falls can be identified and in some cases intervention may reduce the risk of future falls. In a study of elderly people presenting to an accident and emergency department with a fall, a detailed medical and occupational therapy assessment and appropriate intervention significantly reduced the risk of falling in the study group compared to the controls (odds ratio 0.39 (95%CI = 0.23–0.66)).[27] External padded propylene hip protectors have shown promise in preventing hip fractures in elderly institutionalised patients who fall.[28] However, compliance is often poor with these devices, although this may be improved with advances in design.

In an older age group, therefore, assessment of likelihood of falling should therefore be considered in conjunction with other risk factors for fractures such as low BMD and previous fractures in order to target intervention to those most at risk of fractures.

Geometry

The measurement of hip axis length (HAL) (defined as the length along the extended femoral neck axis from below the lateral aspect of the greater trochanter to the inner pelvic brim) has been shown to be associated with an increased risk of hip fracture in women. In a study by Faulkener et al.[29] each standard deviation increase in HAL (0.5 cm) doubled fracture risk in the femoral neck and trochanter areas, independently of age, height, weight and BMD. Automated computer programs are available for modern DXA instruments which allow calculation of the HAL. Another study using conventional hip radiographs showed that after adjusting for age, a combination of the trabecular pattern index (Singh index), femoral neck and shaft cortex thickness and trochanteric width can predict hip fractures at least as strongly as femoral neck BMD.[30] Before any of these measurements are routinely incorporated into skeletal assessments, however, further biomechanical verification will be required.

Clinical Risk Factors

It is important to distinguish between risk factors for low bone density or osteoporosis from risk factors for fractures. Multiple historical risk factors for osteoporosis (such as family history, low body weight, previous hyperthyroidism, corticosteroid therapy) cannot identify the individual patient with low bone mass or predict those who will develop a fracture with adequate certainty.[31] Nevertheless, in the absence of adequate screening strategies, they can be useful in case finding to identify those in whom further assessment is required. As the prevalence of these risk factors is higher in an elderly population, such a strategy may be useful in this age group.

Bone Turnover

Biochemical markers of bone turnover have the potential to be used to identify patients who lose bone rapidly and predict more severe osteoporosis. Algorithms using a single bone mass measurement at the menopause and several biochemical markers of bone remodelling suggest this approach may be useful.[32,33] There is sufficient individual biological variation in the ability of these markers to define the rate of bone loss in individual patients not to warrant the use of these bone markers instead of BMD measurements in individual subjects. Some investigators have also suggested that rapid bone losers may not remain rapid losers and vice versa. In the elderly in particular, however, bone markers may provide a diagnostic role in the future. At the menopause any reduction in BMD is related to low peak bone mass whereas in older subjects the bone loss contributes progressively to resulting bone mass. After the age of 70 years, turnover correlates with bone density more than at the menopause. Further work is required, however, to prove that markers can be used to direct treatments in those patients at risk of future hip fractures. Promising data have come from the EPIDOS study which shows that in women above the age of 75 years, some markers of bone resorption (urinary C-telopeptide and free-deoxypyridinoline) predict the subsequent risk of hip fracture independently of hip BMD, and that combining the measurement of BMD and bone resorption may be useful to improve the assessment of the risk of hip fracture.[34]

Clinical Aspects of Bone Densitometry in the Elderly

Which Site to Measure?

There are three main reasons for measuring BMD. First, confirmation of osteoporosis as defined by the WHO criteria is possible. Secondly, BMD can be used in the assessment of fracture risk. Thirdly, monitoring change in BMD due to ageing, disease process or in response to therapy can be performed. Determining which skeletal site to measure is dependent partly on which of the above issues is prominent.

For diagnosing osteoporosis it is important to realise that BMD is not the same throughout the skeleton. This "discordance" is caused by at least four potential reasons:

1. Differences in development of PABM at various sites;
2. Differences in rates of bone loss between cancellous bone and cortical bone after the menopause (Fig. 10.2];
3. Differences in the accuracy of measuring bone mineral content by various technologies;
4. Differences in manufacturers' young normal reference databases.

Discordance is greater in the early postmenopausal population than in women aged 65 years and over and therefore in the former age group there is a potential problem of misclassification between sites. Greenspan et al.[35] showed that in 129 women, the prevalence of WHO defined osteoporosis varied greatly depend-

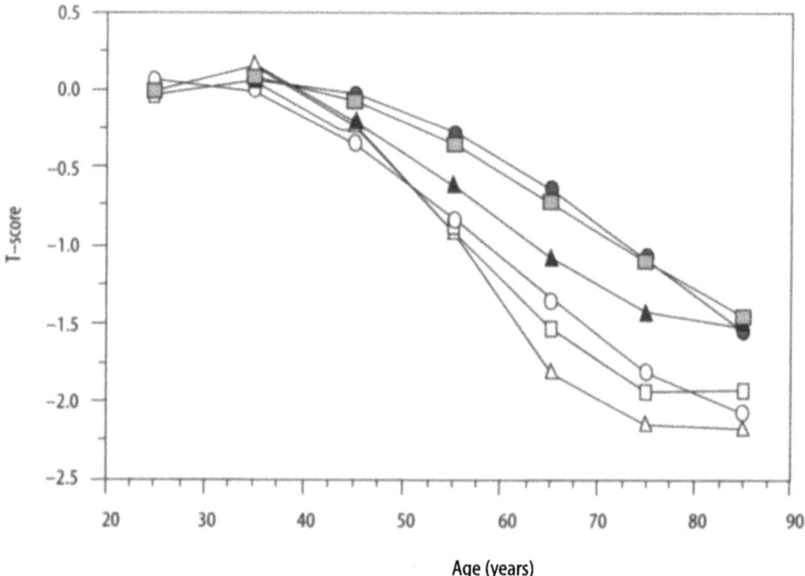

Figure 10.2 T-score age changes for os calcis and axial measurement sites. •, Os calcis BMD; ■, trochanter BMD; ▲, os calcis BUA; ○, femoral neck BMD; □, os calcis stiffness; △, spine BMD.

ing on the skeletal site measured. At the lateral spine 65% of women were classified as osteoporotic compared to < 30% at the PA spine, 55% were osteoporotic at the femoral neck but < 20% were classified as osteoporotic at the greater trochanter.[35] One implication of this difference is, therefore, that it may be appropriate to measure more than one site to reduce the chances of missing a diagnosis of osteoporosis.[36] In general, the concordance in BMD at various skeletal sites in older people is better, which reduces the likelihood of missing a diagnosis of osteoporosis when measuring only one skeletal site such as the wrist, heel, finger or hip. The exception in the elderly is a single measurement of the PA spine by DXA where artefacts may increase BMD values (see above). In individuals 65 years of age and older, therefore, with the exception of PA spine, central measurements and peripheral measurements have similar value for diagnosing osteoporosis.

Most of the data relating BMD to fracture risk relate to elderly, mainly Caucasian, female populations and suggest that fracture prediction is comparable regardless of the skeletal site measured or the technique (central or peripheral) used.[37,38] Thus, low bone mass measured at one site is more likely to represent a global reduction in BMD in an elderly population. The one exception is in predicting hip fracture risk where the predictive value per SD reduction in BMD appears to be greater at the proximal femur sites than at other sites (Fig. 10.3).[37,38] This latter observation does not, however, diminish the strong predictive value that peripheral bone mass measurements have for hip fractures. Although spine and forearm measurements appear to be less sensitive than hip or heel for assessing hip fracture risk, they still have utility, particularly in the elderly. Data on more than 8000 women from the Study of Osteoporotic Fractures show that the relative risks for hip fracture as a function of BMD measured at the hip, heel, spine and forearm were 2.7, 2.0, 1.6 and 1.5, respectively.[37] For vertebral fractures, the Hawaii Osteoporosis Study (mean age 74 years) showed that the relative risks as a function of BMD measured at the spine, heel, forearm and hand sites were 1.6, 1.9, 1.5 and 1.7, respectively.[39] In general therefore, to assess overall fracture

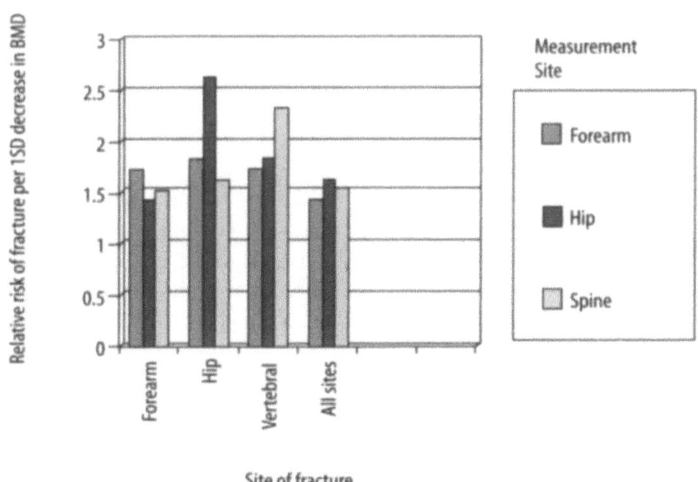

Figure 10.3 Relative risks of fracture for 1 SD decrease in BMD for age-adjusted mean.[38]

risk in the elderly, measurement of any skeletal site is acceptable, although measuring hip BMD provides the best estimate for hip fracture.

In terms of monitoring change in BMD, either to assess the natural progression in time or the response to intervention, the central skeletal sites (spine and hip) currently have an advantage. The metabolically active bone of the spine is the most responsive site particularly around the early postmenopausal period. After the age of 65 years, however, degenerative disease can mask any age-related changes.[35] With pharmacological intervention, the spine shows larger changes than the regions of interest in the proximal femur, whereas little change is seen at the wrist, finger or heel. The reason why the peripheral sites show limited response is unclear. It is unlikely to be related to precision error which is usually low at these sites. Possible explanations are: the difference in bone marrow environment, differences in surface area of bone, and differences in blood flow between the peripheral and central skeleton. The spine may not be the most metabolically active site for all situations. Conditions which influence cortical bone preferentially, such as hyperparathyroidism and calcium malabsorption states, may show little effect at the spine. Thus the forearm appears to be the best site to monitor the effects of excess parathyroid hormone activity and may be useful in deciding timing of parathyroid surgery.[40]

Peripheral Techniques Including Quantitative Ultrasound in the Elderly

Growing realisation of the impact of osteoporosis has led to rapid growth in demand for bone densitometry in the last decade of the twentieth century. Central DXA (hip and spine) has fulfilled this role well because of its high precision. However, in many countries enough central DXA scans are not available to meet potential demand and as central DXA is usually hospital based it is perceived as costly. For this reason peripheral bone mass measurements including single-energy X-ray absorptiometry (SXA) of the forearm, peripheral DXA (pDXA) of the wrist or calcaneus, DXA of the fingers, peripheral quantitative computed tomography (pQCT) of the wrist and quantitative ultrasound (QUS) of the calcaneus, tibia and phalanges have become available for clinical use. These technologies are portable, comparatively inexpensive, associated with little or no radiation exposure, easy and quick to perform and can be easily used in any healthcare provider including primary care. Most experience so far has been with SXA (forearm), pDXA (forearm and calcaneus) and QUS (calcaneus), although the roles for all of the techniques are still being evaluated.

One of the difficulties for the WHO definition based on T-scores is the disparity among T-score results obtained at different skeletal sites and technologies. The causes of this disparity are the differing rates of bone loss (expressed in terms of T-scores) when assessed at different skeletal sites or with different technologies (see Fig. 10.2] and the problem of the T-scores being derived from inconsistent young databases. Thus, dramatically different percentages of patients can be identified as candidates for therapeutic intervention, depending on the site and device utilised. This issue is potentially damaging to the field of osteoporosis and it is important that a solution is found soon as peripheral devices are rapidly being bought and utilised in many countries. One possible solution to this problem currently being discussed among manufacturers and opinion leaders is to define "equivalent T-score thresholds" for any site/device, which would identify the lowest quintile of the 60–69-year-old population. This approach is similar to that used by the WHO in the original definition of the T–2.5 criteria for osteoporosis and by setting equal "prevalence" of osteoporosis by any device/site, the current confusion can be minimised. One proposal is that the femoral neck T–2.5 criteria should be the benchmark against which equivalent T-scores can be calculated. The WHO T–2.5 criteria was based on identifying the lowest quintile and device/site specific equivalent T-score thresholds can be obtained by setting equivalent prevalence (20%) based on 65-year-old Caucasian females. Thus, for example, the equivalent T-score thresholds ($\equiv$ femoral neck T–2.5) for the CUBA heel ultrasound (BUA), SAHARA heel ultrasound (stiffness), ACHILLES heel ultrasound (stiffness) and the PIXI heel DXA (BMD) devices may be –2.0, –1.8, –2.5 and –1.6, respectively, based on current data.

Quantitative ultrasound (QUS) has a potentially valuable role in the assessment of fracture risk, especially in elderly women. The attraction of QUS devices are that they are portable, relatively cheap, easy to perform and do not use ionising radiation. The calcaneus is the site usually chosen because it is easily accessible, has a high percentage of trabecular bone, and is weight bearing with a pattern of loss in osteoporosis similar to the spine. In 1990 Porter et al.[41] reported that heel QUS could predict hip fracture risk in elderly women (mean age 83 years). More recently the French EPIDOS study in 5662 women (mean age 80 years) and the North American SOF study in 6189 women (mean age 76 years) have confirmed these findings.[42,43] These data suggest a twofold increase in hip fracture risk per every SD decline in QUS results. QUS of the heel has recently also shown to predict forearm and other osteoporosis related fractures in middle age to "younger elderly" women (age 45–75 years.[44] Both the BUA and SOS components of QUS have been identified as independent risk factors for hip fracture even after correction for BMD.[42,43] It is possible that this independent association is related to some "structural" or "quality" aspects of the skeleton. This additional information by QUS offers the prospect that combining QUS parameters and BMD may enhance the capacity for predicting hip fracture although this still has to be proven.

Up till now QUS has been used for fracture risk assessment rather than diagnosis of osteoporosis as the WHO criteria is based on BMD related T-scores. If QUS is going to be used in the future as a "diagnostic" or "intervention" threshold, then each QUS device needs to define what T-scores these thresholds should be for their relevant parameters (BUA, SOS or stiffness), as the WHO BMD T-score threshold of –2.5 may not apply. It remains to be shown whether this technique can be used in screening to reduce fracture rates in older people. However, the incorporation of quantitative ultrasound as a pre-screen for all women in the seventh decade provides a better referral procedure than is currently achieved by clinical referral criteria (both in sensitivity and specificity) for identifying osteoporotic subjects. It was also estimated to reduce the cost per osteoporotic subject correctly identified.[45]

One common problem encountered in older people using the direct system ("dry") QUS machines is the presence of peripheral oedema which can influence measurements of QUS parameters. The presence of oedema may reduce both BUA and SOS by amounts equivalent to a quarter of one standard deviation of the reference range. As the severity of oedema varies throughout the day, and from day to day, measurement protocols for bone ultrasound should pay attention to the confounding effects of oedema.[46]

Using Bone Density in Treatment Decisions

In clinical decision-making the ability to assess fracture risk is of greater importance than just determination of bone density, particularly in the elderly. The task of the clinician is to be aware of the limitations of BMD (or QUS parameters), to interpret the results alongside the clinical risk and fall-related factors and to decide on the best treatment for the individual patient. The precise application of bone mass measurements in conjunction with these other factors will benefit from further research, but this should not delay the use of the data already gained on the additional risk factors for fractures.

Intervention thresholds are not necessarily the same as diagnostic thresholds. Factors other than BMD which influence treatment decisions include patient perceptions and preferences, presence of other risk factors for falls and fractures, relevant medical co-morbidity and the risk/benefit and cost of the candidate treatments. Intervention thresholds may vary according to the type of treatment being considered. A drug which is cheap, free of side effects and effective will have a less stringent threshold than one which is costly and not well tolerated. Indeed BMD measurements may not be always necessary prior to considering treatments, particularly in areas where densitometry is not freely available. In patients with past or prevalent non-traumatic fractures, the diagnosis of osteoporosis can be presumed in the absence of bone densitometry, and a case can be made for treatment without prior BMD measurements. The drawback to this approach is that monitoring cannot be performed. In the elderly, low bone mass is almost universal and thus densitometry (particularly using T-scores) is rarely helpful in making decisions. If the aim is to target treatment to only those most at risk, then using the Z-score may be more appropriate (see above) and using non-BMD risk factors for fractures assume more importance. The desirability of monitoring BMD depends partly on availability of densitometry, type of densitometry available (central DXA but not peripheral techniques) and partly on what treatment is proposed. The growing evidence that vitamin D and calcium reduce fracture risk, especially in the frailer elderly population, argues for routine supplementation, an approach that is likely to be more cost-effective in this population than selection by bone densitometry for treatment. In some situations bone densitometry may be useful in choosing treatments. For example if hip BMD is particularly low bisphosphonates may be chosen rather than say a selective oestrogen receptor modulator as the former therapy has a better evidence base for the prevention of hip fractures. It is important, however to consider the age group in which the pivotal trials have been performed. Thus there is no prospective evidence published yet that beyond the age of 81 years bisphosphonates can reduce hip fracture risk although current studies may answer this question.

Monitoring of Therapy

The rationale for monitoring bone mass during treatment in both younger and older patients is that it provides reassurance both to the clinician and the patient that medication with potential side-effects is actually providing beneficial effects and that it may increase compliance with treatment.[47] The common practice of performing annual central DXA scans is controversial on cost-effectiveness grounds, it lacks in credible evidence and needs to be re-examined. Detection of treatment effect or failure reliably takes 2–3 years (spine and hip respectively), and the extent to which a further scan (or scans) improves compliance or patient management is not fully established. Most therapies used in the treatment of osteoporosis generally have low non-responder rates at least in clinical trials. If availability of bone densitometry is already limited, a certain maximum number of scans can be performed in a year, and if everyone is rescanned in the following year, then it would not be possible to scan any new patients during the new year. In this situation one approach is to rescan at the end of a defined period (such as 5 years) to ascertain if further therapy is indicated or whether treatment can be stopped. In some situations, however, it may be important to monitor changes in bone mass more often, for example those patients taking high dose long-term corticosteroids or in groups where response rates are not known as in men and transplant patients.

Peripheral techniques have the potential to become more widely available, but as discussed before, these are currently less useful in monitoring change. With respect to QUS, precision between the different types of machines varies widely although with the newer imaging adaptations utilising various region of interests, this may improve. Recent data showing the ability to discriminate between different groups treated with various treatments indicate that in the future QUS may have the ability to monitor treatment in individuals, although at present not enough evidence is available.[48]

An alternative approach is to use biochemical markers of bone turnover in monitoring treatment. The development of newer more specific bone turnover markers (such as the pyridinoline crosslinks) may allow prediction of changes in BMD. Responses to bone resorption inhibition is often complete by three months and thus an assessment of response can be made much earlier than the two years required for DXA. Although this approach has potential, further data on its use for monitoring various treatments are required before it is widely utilised in clinical practice.

Differential Diagnosis of Low Bone Mass

It is important to realise that a patient with low bone mass does not necessarily have osteoporosis. Some patients may have concomitant osteomalacia or other metabolic bone diseases. The presence of osteomalacia in patients who appear to have osteoporosis is unknown. The incidence of osteomalacia in the elderly population with hip fractures is not insignificant.[49] This may be related to the high prevalence of occult vitamin D deficiency (vitamin D "insufficiency") which leads to secondary hyperparathyroidism and increased bone turnover but without the clinical features of osteomalacia. A low serum calcium or phosphate, a high alkaline phosphatase may point to vitamin D deficiency or insufficiency and a raised parathyroid hormone level and, if available, a low 25-hydroxy vitamin D_3 may be helpful in confirming the diagnosis, although in difficult cases a quantitative histomorphological evaluation of a non-decalcified bone biopsy may be required.

In the geriatric population, it is important to consider several secondary causes of osteoporosis. The diagnosis of coeliac disease has been made easier by the development of anti-gliadin and endomysial antibody tests. In primary hyperparathyroidism hypercalcaemia may occur as well as low bone mass, and the latter finding may be one factor on which to make a decision regarding parathyroidectomy. Multiple myeloma may present with low bone mass with or without fractures and in older people an erythrocyte sedimentation rate (ESR) and serum and urine electrophoresis should be considered especially in the presence of vertebral fractures. Hyperthyroidism and possibly overtreatment with thyroid replacement therapy may lead to accelerated bone loss.

Evaluation in Men

The epidemiology, diagnosis and treatment of osteoporosis in men have not been studied to the same extent as in women. Up until the fifth decade the incidence of all fractures is higher in men than women, mainly related to trauma. After this age there is a reversal in trend with the incidence of non-traumatic fractures becoming much more common in women. These fractures are less common in elderly men in comparison to women because firstly, accumulation of skeletal mass during growth is greater in men resulting in larger bone size which is independently associated with better mechanical strength. Secondly, women lose more bone with ageing than do men and thirdly older men fall less often than women do. In addition, lifespan in men is several years shorter than in women, and so they are exposed to a low BMD for a shorter period. Nevertheless, the incidence of these fractures in men also increases rapidly with age reflecting increasing skeletal fragility and therefore osteoporosis in men is also becoming a major healthcare problem. Furthermore, age-adjusted mortality rates for hip fracture in males is higher than it is for females.

The WHO definition for osteoporosis applies to women only and suitable diagnostic BMD threshold values for men are not well defined. However, observational data show that the risk of spine and proximal femur fractures is similar in both sexes for a given BMD and therefore appropriate diagnostic BMD threshold values for men may be the same as in women, namely 2.5 SD below the mean for women.[50] Currently available data suggest that HAL does not independently predict hip fracture in elderly men, unlike in women[51] and the role of biochemical markers in men is not yet adequately established.

An important aspect in clinical management of male osteoporosis is the higher proportion of conditions which cause secondary osteoporosis (approximately 50%) in comparison to women. The commonest causes are corticosteroid therapy, alcohol abuse, hypogonadism and previous gastric surgery although it is important not to miss other rarer causes such as neoplasia (particularly myeloma) and endocrine disorders (including thyrotoxicosis and hyperparathyroidism). Clinical evaluation should therefore include tests to investigate for these conditions as management of osteoporosis will be directed to the treatment of the specific cause. The exact role of bone densitometry, including peripheral techniques such as QUS, in elderly men will benefit from more research, as will the development of treatment strategies.

Managing Osteoporosis in Patients with Fractures

The occurrence of a non-traumatic fracture makes future fractures including hip fracture more likely. It is important, therefore, to consider the diagnosis and further management of osteoporosis in all cases of a non-traumatic fracture. The peak incidence of Colles' fractures occurs between the ages of 60 and 70 years. In many cases, however, once the fracture is fixed, the general lack of guidelines on further management means that an ideal opportunity is missed to try and reduce the risk of further fractures. Similarly the opportunity for secondary prevention is often missed following other osteoporotic fractures including those at the spine, pelvis, upper arm and the hip. Local guidelines on management of osteoporosis in patients with fractures are therefore necessary. These guidelines may vary from area to area depending on local availability of bone densitometry. One such guideline for patients with hip fractures has been developed by The North East (UK) Osteoporosis Regional Advisory Board (Fig. 10.4), although many of its recommendations also apply to other fractures. These guidelines stress the importance of "falls assessment" as well as "osteoporosis assessment" on all patients.

Medical assessment and investigations including where necessary cardiological tests such as 24 hour Holter monitoring, echocardiography and tilt testing should seek underlying causes of falls. Secondary causes of osteoporosis should also be sought. Routine biochemical profile is worthwhile as hypocalcaemia and hypophosphataemia may indicate osteomalacia, although these measurements lack sensitivity and specificity in diagnosing osteomalacia in the elderly. Serum 25-hydroxyvitamin D and intact parathyroid hormone estimations are potentially useful in excluding vitamin D deficiency in patients with limited sunlight

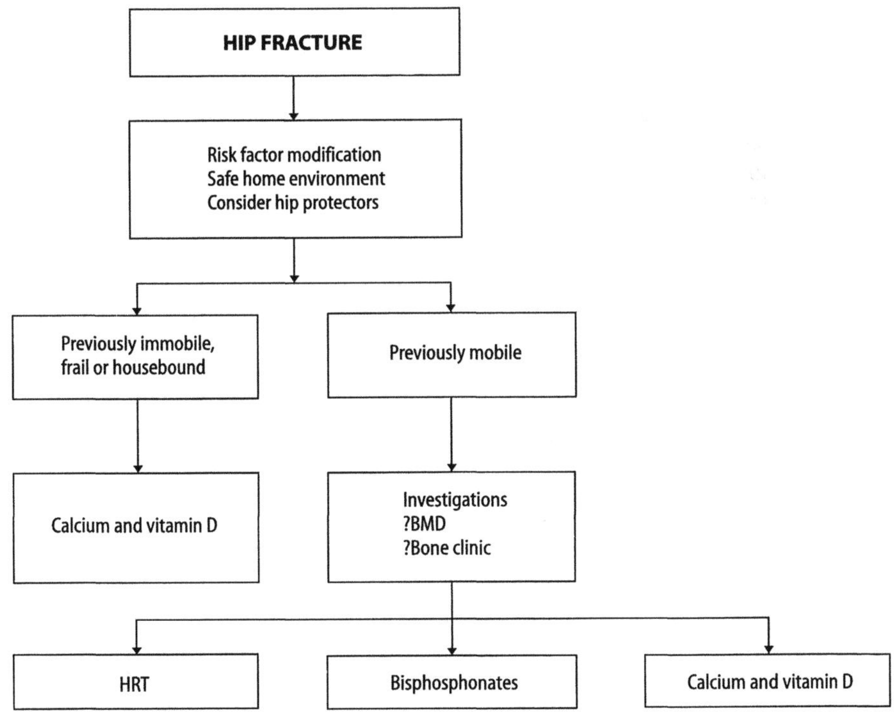

Figure 10.4 Management of osteoporosis in patients with hip fractures. From: New guidelines for hip fracture, North East Osteoporosis Regional Advisory Board, UK.

exposure, but are probably unnecessary if treatment with calcium and vitamin D is the planned intervention. Thyroid function tests are of value in the non-acute situation as the classical signs and symptoms of osteoporosis are not always present in the elderly.

Bone density measurements are of limited value in the diagnosis of osteoporosis in elderly patients with hip fractures, as the vast majority will have reduced BMD and results are unlikely to influence management. Nevertheless in some situations, serial BMD measurements may be used to assess the efficacy of therapeutic intervention. A reasonably pragmatic approach is to divide patients with hip fractures into two broad groups. The first group comprises mainly older frailer patients, many of whom were immobile, housebound or institutionalised before fracture whereas the second group is generally younger (< 75–80 years) and previously mobile and independent. Patients in the first group have limited life expectancy and so it is probably inappropriate to perform extensive investigations to exclude secondary causes of osteoporosis or to request BMD measurements. These patients are more likely to benefit from calcium and vitamin D supplements than other therapeutic interventions. Patients in the second group would benefit from more active management as life expectancy and quality of life could be improved by decreasing the risk of further fractures, and therefore investigations to exclude secondary cause of osteoporosis should be performed and BMD measurements considered prior to deciding on intervention.

Screening and Health Economics Issues in the Elderly

The Health Economic case for universal screening for osteoporosis at the time of menopause is not proven. The beneficial effects of hormone replacement therapy given at the menopause for a few years wears off with ageing so that the effect on hip fractures will be minimal.[52] As therapy is not usually taken for life and since hip fractures occur in the later stages of life, starting treatment at an older age has theoretical advantages. Treating 70-year-old women compared to immediately menopausal women would save more hip fractures, and therefore screening, as well as case finding, at a later age may be more appropriate. The cost benefit of later intervention is thought to be greater.[53] From the standpoint of an individual, a treatment which reduces the risk of a fracture by 50% may seem trivial if the fracture risk is low. From a public health perspective the most efficient use of therapy is in the treatment of the highest risk subjects. Those with established osteoporosis (who have already had a non-traumatic fracture) would fall into the latter category and should be treated. In women with osteoporosis but without a fracture, the assessment of risk based on BMD alone is currently unlikely to be accepted as a general strategy on economic grounds and therefore other estimates of fracture risk should be included in the case-finding approach.

Conclusion

Low bone density is an important predictor of fracture risk, even in older subjects. It has limitations, however, if used by itself because of the wide overlap in bone density between fracture and non-fracture subjects. Measurements of spine BMD in the elderly can be affected by many confounders including degenerative spine disease, vertebral collapse and vascular calcification. For this reason hip BMD in the elderly is more useful compared to the spine in diagnosing osteoporosis, although positioning difficulties in frail older patients affects hip BMD precision. Spine BMD remains the best option for monitoring purposes in the elderly. On health economic grounds the use of fracture thresholds and the WHO definition of osteoporosis (T = −2.5) are problematic in older subjects if used as intervention thresholds as a high proportion of older people will be classified as osteoporotic. The Z-score allows comparison with normals of the same age and is one way of identifying those subjects at higher risk of fracture. An alternative approach using the remaining lifetime fracture risk may prove to be useful in older people.

The best prediction of fractures require combining BMD with other risk factors for fracture. The most important of these risk factors in the elderly are the presence of previous fractures and fall related factors, although in the future, geometrical factors (such as hip axis length), bone turnover markers and quality of bone measures (such as quantitative ultrasound) may play a role. Historical clinical risk factors perform poorly in identifying those subjects who will fracture, but in the absence of validated screening strategies they can be useful in a case finding approach.

The greater concordance in BMD at various sites in older subjects means that in general measuring any site has value in predicting fractures. The rapid growth of peripheral bone density techniques including peripheral DXA and QUS means that there is potential for many more older subjects to have access to some form of bone mass measurement. However, disparity among T-score occurs at different skeletal sites and with different technologies can lead to different classification of the same subjects according to which site and technology is used. This issue in particular has to be resolved if the peripheral techniques are to have a major impact in the future. Another disadvantage of the peripheral techniques is that at present they have not been fully validated for the purposes of monitoring treatment, although further technological advances should resolve this issue.

The decision regarding when and how often to perform bone densitometry in the elderly depends on many factors, including availability of the scans, personal preference of patients and clinicians, presence of other non-BMD risk factors for fractures and the type of treatments being considered. In the frailer, very elderly patients, life expectancy may be low and bone densitometry is unlikely to influence management which often consists of calcium and vitamin D supplementation combined with reducing fall risk. In the fitter mobile older subject life expectancy and quality of life may be improved by reducing fracture risk and a more aggressive approach which may involve the use of bone densitometry and treatment with newer agents such as bisphosphonates is warranted.

References

1. Cooper C, Aihie-Sayer A (1994) Osteoporosis: recent advances in pathogenesis and treatment. Q J Med 87:203–209.
2. Melton LJ, Kan SH, Frye MA et al. (1989) Epidemiology of vertebral fractures in women. Am J Epidemiol 129:1000–1011.
3. Ardran GM (1951) Bone destruction not demonstrable by radiography. Br J Radiol 24:107–109.
4. Masud T, Mootoosamy I, McCloskey EV et al. (1996) Assessment of osteopenia from spine radiographs using two different methods: the Chingford study. Br J Radiol 69:451–456.

5.   Scane AC, Masud T, Johnson FJ et al. (1994) The reliability of diagnosing osteoporosis from spinal radiographs. Age Ageing 23:283–286.
6.   Steinbach HT (1964) The roentgen appearance of osteoporosis. Radiol Clin North Am 2:191–207.
7.   Singh M, Nagrath AR, Maini PS (1970) Changes in trabecular pattern of the upper end of the femur as an index of osteoporosis. J Bone Joint Surg 52A:457–467.
8.   Wickham CAC, Walsh K, Cooper C et al. (1989) Dietary calcium, physical activity and risk of hip fracture: a prospective study. BMJ 299:889–992.
9.   Masud T, Jawed S, Doyle DV et al. (1995) A population study of the screening potential of assessment of trabecular pattern of the femoral neck (Singh Index): the Chingford Study. Br J Radiol 68:389–393.
10. Dequeker J (1997) Inverse relationship of interface between osteoporosis and osteoarthritis. J Rheumatol 24:795–798.
11. Lawrence JS (1969) Disc degeneration: its frequency and relationship to symptoms. Ann Rheum Dis 28:121–138.
12. Masud T, Langley S, Wiltshire P et al. (1993) Effects of spinal osteophytosis on bone mineral density measurements in vertebral osteoporosis. BMJ 307:172–173.
13. Maggio D, McCloskey EV, Camilli L et al. (1998) Short-term reproducibility of proximal femur bone mineral density in the elderly. Calcif Tissue Int 63:296–299.
14. Melton LJ, Kan SH, Wahner HW et al. (1988) Lifetime fracture risk: an approach to hip fracture risk assessment based on bone mineral density and age. J Clin Epidemiol 41:985–994.
15. Looker AC, Wahner HW, Dunn WL et al. (1995) Proximal femur bone mineral levels of US adults. Osteoporosis Int 5:389–409.
16. Faulkner KG, Von Stetten E, Miller P (1999) Discordance in patient classification using T-scores and their discrepancies. J Clin Densitometry 2:343–350.
17. Ross PD, Davis JW, Epstein RS et al. (1991) Pre-existing fractures and bone mass predict vertebral fracture incidence in women. Ann Intern Med 114:919–923.
18. Wasnich RD, Davis JW, Ross PD (1994) Spine fracture risk is predicted by non-spine fractures. Osteoporosis Int: 1–5.
19. Winner SJ, Morgan CA, Evans JG (1989) Perimenopausal risk of falling and incidence of distal forearm fracture. BMJ 298:1486–1488.
20. Gibson MJ (1987) The prevention of falls in later life. Danish Med Bull 34 (suppl 4):1–24.
21. Clark ANG (1968) Factors in fracture of the female femur: a clinical study of the environment, physical, medical and preventative aspects of this injury. Gerontol Clin 10:257–270.
22. Dias JJ (1987) An analysis of the nature of injury of fractures in the neck of femur. Age ageing 16:373–377.
23. Greenspan SL, Myers ER, Kiel DP et al. (1998) Fall direction, bone mineral density, and function: risk factors for hip fracture in frail nursing home elderly. Am J Med 104:539–545.
24. Nguyen T, Sambrook SP, Kelly P, Jones G et al. (1993) Prediction of osteoporotic fractures by postural instability and bone density. BMJ 307:1111–1115.
25. Van schoor, Lips P, Bouter L (1999) Can the number of hip fractures be reduced by external hip protectors. Calcif Tissue Int 64 Suppl 1):S69.
26. Tinnetti ME, Baker DI, McAvay G et al. (1994) A multifactorial intervention to reduce the risk of falling among elderly people living in the community. N Engl J Med 331:821–827.
27. Close J, Ellis M, Hooper R et al. (1999) Prevention of falls in the elderly trial (PROFET): a randomised controlled trial. Lancet 353:93–97.
28. Lauritzen JB, Peterson MM, Lund B (1993) Effect of external hip protectors on hip fractures. Lancet 341:11–13.
29. Faulkener KG, Cummings SR, Black D (1993) Simple measurements of femoral geometry predicts hip fractures: the study of osteoporotic fractures. J Bone Miner Res 8:1211–1217.
30. Gluer CC, Cummings SR, Pressman A et al. (1994) Prediction of hip fractures from pelvic radiographs: the study of osteoporoti c fractures. J Bone Miner Res 9:671–677.
31. Pouilles JM, Ribot C, Tremollieres F et al. (1991) Risk factors of vertebral osteoporosis: results of a study of 2279 women referred to a menopause clinic. Rev Rheum Mal Osteoarticulaire 58:169–177.
32. Delmas PD. (1990) Biochemical markers of bone turnover for the clinical assessment of metabolic bone disease. Endocrin Metab Clin North Am 19:1–18.
33. Miller PD, Baran D, Bilezikian JP et al. (1999) Practical Clinical application of biochemical markers of bone turnover consensus of an expert panel. J Clin Densitometry 2:323–342.
34. Garnero P, Hausherr E, Chapuy MC et al. (1996) Markers of bone resorption predict hip fracture in elderly women: the EPIDOS Prospective Study. J Bone Miner Res 11:1531–1538.
35. Greenspan SL, Maitland-Ramsey L, Myers E (1996) Classification of osteoporosis in the elderly is dependent on site-specific analysis. Calcif Tissue Int 58:409–414.

36. Miller PD, Bonnick SL, Johnston CC et al. (1998) The challenges of peripheral bone density testing. Which patients need additional central density skeletal measurements? J Clin Densitometry 1:211–217.

37. Cummings SR, Black DM,Nevitt MC et al. (1993) Bone density at various sites for prediction of hip fracture. Lancet 341:72–75.

38. Marshall D, Johnell O, Wedel H (1996) Meta-analysis of how well measures of bone mineral density predict occurrence of osteoporotic fractures. BMJ 312:1254–1259

39. Ross P, Huang C, Davis J et al. (1995) Predicting vertebral deformity using bone densitometry at various skeletal sites and calcaneus ultrasound. Bone 16:325–332.

40. Silverberg SJ, Shane E, de la Cruz L et al. (1989) Skeletal disease in primary hyperparathyroidism. J Bone Miner Res 4:283–291.

41. Porter RW, Miller C, Grainger D et al. (1990) Prediction of hip fracture in elderly women: a prospective study. BMJ 301:638–641.

42. Hans D, Dargent-Molina, Schott AM et al. (1996) Ultrasonographic heel measurements to predict hip fracture in elderly women: the EPIDOS study. Lancet 348:511–514.

43. Bauer DC, Glue CC, Caley JA et al. (1997) Broadband QUS attenuation predicts fractures strongly and independently of densitometry in older women. A prospective study. Study of Osteoporotic Fractures Research Group. Arch Intern Med 157:629–634.

44. Thompson PW, Taylor J, Oliver R et al. (1998) Quantittive ultrasound (QUS) of the heel predicts wrist and osteoporosis-related fractures in women 45–75 years. J Clin Densitometry 1:219–225.

45. Langton CM, Ballard PA, Langton DK et al. (1997) Maximising the cost effectiveness of BMD referral for DXA using ultrasound as a selective population prescreen. Technol Health Care 5:235–241.

46. Johansen A, Stone MD (1997) The effect of ankle oedema on bone ultrasound assessment at the heel. Osteoporosis Int 7:44–47.

47. Miller PD, Zapalowski C, Kulak CAM et al. (1999) Bone densitometry: the best way to detect osteoporosis and to monitor therapy. J Clin Endocrinol Metab 84:1867–1871.

48. Gonelli S, Cepollaro, Podrelli C et al. (1996) Ultrasound parameters in osteoporotic patients treated with salmon calcitonin: a longitudinal study. Osteoporosis Int 6:303–307.

49. Aaron JE, Gallagher JC, Anderson J (1974) Frequency of osteomalacia and osteoporosis in fractures of the proximal femur. Lancet i:229–233.

50. Delaet CED, Bjarnason NH, Mitlack BH et al. (1997) Bone density and risk of hip fracture in men and women: a cross-sectional analysis. BMJ 315:221–225.

51. Nelson DA, Jacobsen G, Barondess DA et al. (1995) Ethnic differences in regional bone density, hip axis length and lifestyle variables amomg healthy black and white men. J Bone Miner Res 10:782–787.

52. Kanis JA (1995) Treatment of osteoporosis in elderly women. Am J Med 98 (suppl 2A):60s–66s.

53. WHO (1994) Assessment of fracture risk and its applications to screening for postmenopausal osteoporosis. WHO technical report series 843. World Health Organisation, Geneva.

Index

Absolute risk   202
Accuracy   40–1
Advisory Group on Osteoporosis (AGO)   89, 92, 94, 111, 112
Age effects   200
  bone mass   159
  bone mineral density (BMD)   63
  see also bone densitometry in the elderly
Age groups   5
Age range and reference ranges   43–4
Alcoholism   83–4
Alendronate   59
Amenorrhoea   82–3
Amenorrhoeic athletes   83
American Medical Association   123
Anabolic steroids   79
Ankylosing spondylitis   86
Anorexia nervosa   83
Anticonvulsant therapy   85
Artefacts
  bone density scans illustrating   102–9
  effects on BMD measurements   100–1
Audit   109–11
  CPGs   136–7
  criteria   7, 9
  referral patterns for BMD measurement   137
Audit Commission   155
Autoimmune deficiency syndrome (AIDS)   34

Biochemical markers   15, 57, 60, 192, 196, 207, 213
Bisphosphonates   60, 72, 79, 98, 109, 183, 192, 212
BMC
  compared with BMC   42
  measurement   5
  quantitative values   20–1
BMD   42, 67
  absolute value   60
  age effects   63
  and fracture risk   58, 67, 209
  and risk factors   63
  calculation   19
  clinical context   55–66
  clinical practice issues   62–6
  data interpretation   134–5

menopause   49
monitoring   59–60, 210
percentage of expected (%)   60–1
quantitative values   20–1
tabular/graphical approach   50–1
three decimal places   46
treatment decisions   212
BMD measurement   1–16, 67
  checking   101
  criteria   182
  current GP use   187
  current systems   25–6
  current techniques   17–35
  factors affecting   101
  in primary care   171
  interpretation, difficulties in   102–9
  methods   12
  of multiple sites   62
  orthopaedic practice   147–70
  presentation of results   50–2
  principles   11–15
  rationale   90–2
  report forms   64–5
  reporting   61–2, 66
  rescan interval   98–9
  results   60–1
  role in osteoporosis services   89–123
  secondary benefits   92
  sites   24–5
  techniques   18–24
  see also bone densitiometry and specific methods
Bone densitometry
  access to   92–7
  clinical indications   112, 160
  compact systems   29–30
  costs of service provision   113–14
  diagnostic use *see* diagnosis; diagnostic tests
  effect of artefacts on measurements   100–1
  in the elderly   199
    clinical aspects   208–17
    factors affecting   201
  indications and indications with resources constraints   111
  interpretation of results   99–109
  potential service costs   166–7
  reasons for referral   94

Bone densitometry (*continued*)
  referral request 94
  request form 93
  rescanning 97–9
  selection criteria for patients 92
  see also osteoporosis services
Bone density, low 55
Bone formation 57
Bone health questionnaire 94, 96
Bone loss 69, 71, 99, 153, 155, 159
Bone mass 159, 199, 200
  and age 159
  and fracture risk 205
  differential 213
  in the elderly 161
  monitoring during treatment 212–13
Bone mineral content *see* BMC
Bone mineral density *see* BMD
Bone resorption 57, 59, 160
Bone turnover 57, 59, 60, 207
  see also biochemical markers
Bowel disease 84–5
Broadband ultrasonic attenuation (BUA) 12, 22, 23, 56

Calcaneus 210
Calcitonin 79
Calcitriol 78
Calcium 74, 78, 149, 161, 175
Cancellous bone 23, 99
Carbamazepine 85
Case-finding
  opportunities 194
  strategies 175
Chemical markers 59
Clinical effectiveness 5–6
Clinical Practice Guidelines *see* CPGs
Clinical risk assessment 11
Clinical risk factors 179, 196, 207
Coefficient of variation (CV) 40
Coeliac disease 84
Collagen, type I 15
Colles' fractures 3, 153, 215
Committee on the Medical Aspects of Food and Nutrition Policy 90
Compact densitometry systems 29–30
Compliance encouragement 191–3
Computed tomography (CT) 21
Contact systems 31
Continuing education 118
Cortical bone 21, 23, 69, 99
Corticosteroid-induced osteoporosis (CSIO) 177
  bone densitometry 80
  pathogenesis 77–8
Corticosteroid therapy 77–80
Corticosteroid users 15
CPGs 121–45
  acceptance 126–7
  audit 136–7
  availability for consultation 131–2
  baseline information on current practice 136–7
  clinical areas 132–6
  definition 121–2
  development
    and content 127–8
    for BMD measurement and osteoporosis management 131
    general considerations relevant to 131
    pitfalls 122–3
  development committee 137
  dissemination 139–40
  factors to be considered 129–31
  further investigation 135
  general hints on preparation 123–31
  general practice 137
  guide to past experience 141–2
  hospital practice 136–7
  implementation 128–31, 139–40
  need for 123
  points to be considered 123
  principles of 131
  publication considerations 138–9
  quality assurance 140
  risk factors 133–4
  starting the development process 137–8
  treatment strategy 135–6
  validity 127
Cushing's Syndrome 77

Deoxypyridinoline 15, 60
Department of Health 155, 173
Diagnosis 55–6, 216
  confirmation 182
  use of bone densitometry 180
Diagnostic tests 11
  clinical usefulness 13
  properties 13
Differential diagnosis of low bone mass 213
Distal forearm fractures 3
DMS UBIS5000 31
DPX-IQ 27
DPX-MD 26–7
Dual energy X-ray absorptiometry *see* DXA
Dual photon absorptiometry (DPA) 12, 25
Dual photon/X-ray absorptiometry 19–20
DXA 12, 15, 33, 34, 37, 59, 67, 89, 90, 112, 115, 155–7, 162, 182
  access 184, 196
  appropriate use 183
  commissioning for PCG 185
  interpretation of results 135, 144
  orthopaedic practice 167
  patient referral for 184
  pencil beam systems 26–7
  reference data 46
  reports 186–7
  results 187–8
  terminology 39–42
  see also peripheral DXA; reference ranges

Eating disorders   34
Echocardiography   215
Effectiveness test   6
Efficiency test   6
Elderly persons *see* bone densitometry in the
      elderly
Eli Lilly National Clinical Audit Centre   7, 9
EPIDOS Study   114, 207, 211
Epilepsy   85
Ethnic groupings and reference ranges   42–3
Etidronate   74, 75
European Commission   7–11
European Community   90
European Foundation for Osteoporosis (EFFO)
      132
Evidence-based medicine   5–6
EXCELL densitometer   27
Exercise   9–10, 85
EXPERT XL fan beam densitometry system
      28–9

Falls   205
causes   215
prevention of, and protection against   9–10
risk factors   206
Fan beam DXA systems   27–9
FDA   114
Femoral neck   71, 75, 95, 97, 99, 101, 115, 117,
      118, 150, 151, 158, 201, 204
Femoral shaft fracture   162
Femur   33
Fingers   210
Fluoride salts   73–4, 80
Forearm   81, 115, 188, 210
Forearm fractures   3–4, 152–9
Fracture patient management   163
Fracture risk   90, 91, 200
   and BMD   58, 67, 209
   and bone mass   205
   factors increasing   143
   prediction   56–8, 183
Fracture threshold   202
Fractures, miscellaneous sites   4
Fragility fractures   201
   previous   177, 205

Galactosyl hydroxylysine   60
Gastric surgery   84
Gender (sex) and reference ranges   43
General practice, CPGs   137
Genetics   195
Guidelines for primary care groups   173

Haemochromatosis   81
Hawaii Osteoporosis Study   209
Health economics, elderly persons   216
Health Improvement Programme   6
Heel   56, 95, 115

Hip   99, 158, 201, 204, 217
Hip axis length (HAL)   206
Hip fractures   2, 97, 149, 205
   average length of hospital stay   151
   disability following   154
   management   155, 215
   prevalence   199
   risk factors   180
Hip replacement   162
Hologic   26–8, 31, 34
Holter monitoring   215
Hormone replacement therapy *see* HRT
Hospital practice, CPGs   136–7
HRT   15, 59, 60, 78, 79, 86, 91, 94, 98, 109, 115,
      129, 159, 184, 192
Hydroxylysine glycosides   15
Hydroxyproline   15, 60
Hyperparathyroidism, primary   82
Hyperprolactinaemia   81, 83
Hyperthyroidism   82
Hypogonadism   81–2

Identifying new patients at risk   193
Idiopathic hypogonadotrophic hypogonadism
      81
IGEA DBM sonic 1200   31
Immobilisation   85
Intervention   6–7
   efficacy   216
   indications for   179
   non-pharmacological   9
   response to   92
   thresholds   212
Intracapsular fracture   150
Inverse care law   14

Joint disease   85–6

Klinefelter's syndrome   81

Least significant difference (LSD)   39, 42, 46
Lifetime risk of fracture   202
Local health care co-operatives (LHCCs)   171
Local health groups (LHGs)   171
Low bone density   55
Lumbar spine   33, 43, 45, 59, 60, 70, 71, 74, 75,
      81, 95, 97, 99, 100, 110, 115, 117, 118, 158,
      201
Lumbar vertebra, computed tomogram   21
Lunar   26–9, 34
Lunar Achilles+   31

McCue CUBA Clinical   31
Magnetic resonance imaging (MRI)   24
Magneto-optical disk storage system   26
Malabsorption   84–5

Male hypogonadism   81–2
Menopause, BMD   49
Meta-analysis   7
Methodological considerations   37–53
Metra Biosystems QUS2   32
Minimum standards   195
Monitoring   58–60, 183
    BMD   59–60, 210
    bone mass during treatment   212–13
    treatment   191–3
Monofluorophosphate   73–5
Mortality   68
Myocardial infarction   13
Myriad Soundscan Compact   31

National Health and Nutritional Examination
        Surveys (NHANES)   34, 49, 204
National Institute of Clinical Excellence (NICE)
        125
National Osteoporosis Foundation   56, 100, 154
National Osteoporosis Society (NOS)   95, 109,
        126, 132, 162, 172, 174, 181, 184, 187,
        188
Negative predictive value   13
New patients at risk, identifying   193
NHS, new structure   171
Non-pharmacological interventions   9
Non-steroidal anti-inflammatory drugs
        (NSAIDs)   6
Non-uniform reference databases   204
Norland   27, 29–30, 34
Nursing homes   179, 190
Nutrition   9–10

Orthopaedic practice
    BMD measurement   147
    DXA in   167
    osteoporosis management in   136
Orthopaedic surgeon
    guidelines for   161
    role for   155
    selecting patients for investigation   161
Os calcis   115, 117, 118
Osteocalcin   15
Osteomalacia   84
Osteometer DTU-one   31
Osteopenia   14, 159, 182
    definition   90
Osteoporosis   182
    administrative frameworks   6
    classification   147
    definition   67, 90, 147, 157, 172, 202
    diagnosis see diagnosis; diagnostic tests
    drug treatments   159
    epidemiology   1–4
    established   55
    future directions   167–8
    guiding principles   4–6
    in men   68–75, 165

incidence   90
intervention see intervention
investigation in men   70–1
management   1–16
    in men   71–5
    in orthopaedic practice   136–7
    primary care, future trends   195
    primary care groups   175
operational definition   55
pathogenesis in men   69–70
presentation   11
prevalance   199
prevention levels   5
preventive strategies   7
    costs   10–11
primary prevention   5
public health approach   15–16
secondary   71, 75–80, 164
size of the problem   173
strategies for tackling   174–5
treatment   158–61
see also corticosteroid-induced osteoporosis
    (CSIO)
Osteoporosis in the European Community   90
Osteoporosis services
    development   6
    doctors' indications for referrals   110–11
    functional components   95, 97
    future developments   114
    outline   95
    personnel/facilities   97
    planning   5
    population needs   112–14
    Primary Care Groups   186
    provision of   5, 92–9
    role of BMD measurements   89–123
    St Peter's Hospital   142–3
    see also bone densitometry
Osteoporosis specialist   165–6
Osteoporotic fractures   11, 12, 205
    age- and sex-specific incidence   149
    cost   154–5
    in men   69–70
    size of the problem   173

Pamidronate   79
Parathyroidectomy   82
Peak adult bone mass (PABM)   204
Pelvic fractures   4
Pencil beam DXA systems   26–7
Percentiles   51–2, 61
Periarticular osteoporosis   85
Peripheral bone measurements   63
Peripheral DXA   29, 114, 188, 195
Peripheral quantitative computed tomography
        (pQCT)   29, 210
Peripheral scanning, advantages and
        disadvantages   115, 116
Peripheral sites   97
Peripheral techniques   95, 114, 210–11

Phalanges   210
Phenobarbitone   85
Phenytoin   85
Plain radiographs   12, 181
Planning services   5
Population screening   14, 175
Population strategies   175
Positive predictive value   13
Postmenopausal women
    osteoporosis in   80
    risk factors   57
Precision   39–40, 99
Pregnancy   86
Presymptomatic disease, criteria for population
        screening   14
Primary care
    BMD measurement in   171
    osteoporosis management in, future trends
        195
Primary care groups (PCGs)   171, 172
    guidelines for   173
    osteoporosis management   175
    osteoporosis service   187
Primary Care Rheumatology Society (PCRS)
        132, 175, 195
Primary Care Service Framework for
        Osteoporosis   172
primary hyperparathyroidism   82
primary testicular failure   81
Protection of Persons Undergoing Medical
        Examination or Treatment (POPUMET)
        24
Proximal humerus fractures   4
Publication considerations, CPGs   138–9
Pyridinoline   15

QDR 4000   26
QDR 4500 Acclaim   27–8
QDR 4500 SL   28
QDR 4500 W   28
Quality assurance   32
    CPGs   140–1
Quantitative computed tomography (QCT)   12,
        20–2
    see also peripheral quantitative computed
        tomography (pQCT)
Quantitative ultrasound (QUS)   181–2, 192, 211
elderly persons   210–11
Quantitative ultrasound index (QUI)   181

Radiation Protection Service   24
Radiography   12, 181
    uses and limitations   200
Randomised controlled trials (RCT)   7
Receiver operator characteristics (ROC)   117,
        118
Reference data
    DXA system   46
    ideal requirements   49–50

locally collected   47
multiple centres   48
NHANES   49
Reference ranges   38–9, 59
    and age range   43–4
    and densitometry systems   42
    and ethnic groupings   42–3
    and gender (sex)   43
    construction   44–5
    currently available to DXA users   46–9
    development   42–6
    inclusion and exclusion criteria   44
    men   63
    regional, national or international   44
    source of   62–3
Reference value   37, 38
Referral
    criteria   142–3
    doctors' indications for   110–11
    patterns for BMD measurement   137
    procedure   143, 184
    request for bone densitometry   94
Relative risk   202
Remaining lifetime fracture risk (RLFR)   204
Reporting considerations   37–53
Reproducibility   39
Residential homes   179, 190
Response concept   58–9
Rheumatoid arthritis (RA)   85
Risk assessment, clinical   11
Risk factors   5, 56, 133, 159, 160, 177, 202
    and BMD   63
    clinical   179, 196, 207
    CPGs   133–4
    falls   206
    hip fracture   180
    identifying   179
    other than BMD and age   205
    postmenopausal women   57
Royal College of Obstetrics and Gynaecology
        132
Royal College of Physicians (RCP)   7–9, 89, 90,
        92, 109, 132, 151, 155, 175, 184
Royal College of Surgeons   132

St Peter's Hospital, osteoporosis service   142–3
Scanning sites   95, 97
Screening
    elderly persons   216
    population   14, 175
Secondary osteoporosis   71, 75–80, 164
Secondary prevention   5
Selective case finding   15
Sensitivity   13
Sex (gender) and reference ranges   43
Sex hormone binding globulin (SHBG)   69
Singh index   25, 200
Single-energy X-ray absorptiometry (SXA)   12,
        210
Single photon absorptiometry (SPA)   12, 25

Single photon/X-ray absorptiometry   18–19
Sodium valproate   85
Specificity   13
Speed of sound (SOS)   12, 22, 56
Spinal fractures   152
Spine   149, 200, 201, 217
Standard deviation (SD)   67
Steroid-induced osteoporosis   136
Stratec XCT 2000 peripheral QCT system   29
Sunlight Omnisense   31
Systemic lupus erythematosis (SLE)   86

T-scores   34, 39, 41, 51, 55, 56, 61, 63, 66, 67, 70, 81, 115, 118, 136, 159, 179, 202, 203, 210, 211
Telopeptides   15, 60
Tertiary prevention   5
Testosterone   72–5
Testosterone replacement therapy   81
Tibia   210
Tilt testing   215
Total hip   71
Trabecular bone   69, 119
Trabecular content   21
Training requirements   118
Transplantation osteoporosis   80–1
Treatment decisions   212

Trochanteric BMD   71
Type 1 collagen   15

Ultrasound measurements   12, 22–4, 115, 181, 195
    index of density and architecture   171

Vertebral fractures   2–3, 70, 73
Vitamin D (deficiency and supplements)   74, 78, 84, 149, 161, 175, 213

Well Woman clinics   191
Whole body scanning   25
World Health Organisation (WHO)   14, 25, 55, 67, 90, 147–8, 157
Wrist   95, 149, 210
Wrist fracture   153, 160

X-rays   6

Z-scores   39, 41, 45, 51, 58, 61, 62, 66, 136, 202, 203, 212, 217